Mobile Communications
Safety

TELECOMMUNICATIONS TECHNOLOGY AND APPLICATIONS SERIES

Series editor:
Stuart Sharrock, Consultant,
The Barn, Sugworth Lane, Radley, Abingdon,
Oxon, OX14 2HX, UK

This series covers research into and the development and application of a wide range of techniques and methods used in telecommunications. The industry is undergoing fundamental change under the combined impact of new technologies, deregulation and liberalisation, and the shift towards a service oriented philosophy. The field of communications continues to converge, encompassing all of the associated technologies of computing, networking, software, broadcasting and consumer electronics. The series presents this material in a practical and applications-based manner which equips the reader with the knowledge and tools essential for an engineer working in the industry.

Titles available

1. **Coherent Lightwave Communications Technology**
   Edited by Sadakuni Shimada

2. **Network Management**
   Concepts and tools
   Edited by ARPEGE Group

3. **The Informatics Handbook**
   A guide to multimedia communications and broadcasting
   Stewart Fist

4. **Mobile Communications Safety**
   Edited by N. Kuster, Q. Balzano and J.C. Lin

JOIN US ON THE INTERNET VIA WWW, GOPHER, FTP OR EMAIL:

WWW: http://www.thomson.com
GOPHER: gopher.thomson.com
FTP: ftp.thomson.com
EMAIL: findit@kiosk.thomson.com

A service of **I(T)P**®

Mobile Communications Safety

Edited by

Niels Kuster
Swiss Federal Institute of Technology (ETH)
Zurich
Switzerland

Quirino Balzano
Motorola Inc.
Ft. Lauderdale, Florida
USA

and

James C. Lin
University of Illinois at Chicago
Chicago, Illinois
USA

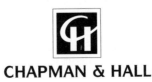

CHAPMAN & HALL

London · Weinheim · New York · Tokyo · Melbourne · Madras

Published by Chapman & Hall, 2–6 Boundary Row, London SE1 8HN, UK

Chapman & Hall, 2–6 Boundary Row, London SE1 8HN, UK

Chapman & Hall GmbH, Pappelallee 3, 69469 Weinheim, Germany

Chapman & Hall USA, 115 Fifth Avenue, New York, NY 10003, USA

Chapman & Hall Japan, ITP-Japan, Kyowa Building, 3F, 2-2-1 Hirakawacho, Chiyoda-ku, Tokyo 102, Japan

Chapman & Hall Australia, 102 Dodds Street, South Melbourne, Victoria 3205, Australia

Chapman & Hall India, R. Seshadri, 32 Second Main Road, CIT East, Madras 600 035, India

First edition 1997

© 1997 Chapman & Hall

Printed in Great Britain at T.J. Press (Padstow) Ltd., Padstow, Cornwall

ISBN   0 412 75000 7

A catalogue record for this book is available from the British Library

∞ Printed on permanent acid-free text paper, manufactured in accordance with ANSI/NISO Z39.48-1992 and ANSI/NISO Z39.48-1984 (Permanence of Paper).

Contents

Preface

The beginning of 1993 saw intense press and television coverage of a lawsuit filed in Tampa, Florida by a husband for the death of his wife. In the lawsuit the husband, David Reynard, alleged that his wife died of a brain tumor which was caused or accelerated by her use of a portable cellular phone, approximately one and a half years before her death. Because of the widespread use of portable cellular phones, there was substantial public concern about a possible connection between the radio frequency energy emitted by the phone and the growth of brain tumors. The media coverage caused a briefing session by the Telecommunications Subcommittee in the House of the United States Congress during February, 1993 and a similar proceeding in the Bundestag of Germany in May, 1993. The use of portable cellular phones had become a matter of public health concern in several industrialized countries.

During the peak of media interest, the Food and Drug Administration of the United States issued a 'talk paper' which gave a summary of the specific available scientific evidence. In the 'talk paper' was stated,

> 'How much evidence is there that handheld cellular phones might be harmful? Briefly, there is not enough evidence to know for sure, either way. Although it is known that high levels of radiofrequency energy that are absorbed by the body can be harmful, the effect of lower levels, such as those emitted by handheld cellular phones, is far less clear. A few studies suggest that these levels can accelerate the development of cancer in laboratory animals, but there is much uncertainty among scientists about whether these results apply to the use of cellular phones.'

Since then, research has been conducted in the United States and Europe on the dosimetry and biological effects of RF at the power levels of the signals from cellular phones, in order to build up the scientific basis for analysis.

The results have been slowly accumulating, as happens when a scientific task of this complexity is tackled by researchers. The present book summarizes the available scientific evidence up to early 1996. This book is a compendium of the knowledge of well recognized and renowned experts in the research of RF energy bioeffects in the frequency band of cellular phone communications.

The book is divided into four parts. In the first part, there is a summary of the present and future technologies of mobile cellular telephony. In the second part, the dosimetry, interference, biological effects and epidemiological studies regarding the RF energy emitted by portable cellular phones are reviewed with sufficient detail to inform an interested reader without advanced knowledge in these areas. Formulas and scientific notations have been kept to a minimum. In the third part, the current efforts of biological research on the RF signals from cellular phones are presented, grouped by region of the world where the research is performed: North America, Europe, and Asia Pacific Rim. In the fourth part, the regulatory and standard activities for human exposure to RF energy are discussed by world region. A discussion of the criteria for the acceptability of the results of future research on the biological effects of RF energy concludes the book.

The authors and the editors put forth their efforts in the hope of clarifying the available scientific evidence and stimulating future scientific research in the area of biological significance, as clearly shown by the content of this book.

The statements contained in this book do not necessarily reflect the views of the editors. The editors gratefully acknowledge the efforts and commitment of Thomas Schwitter, who translated the text, tables and figures into the appropriate formats.

N. Kuster
Q. Balzano
J.C. Lin

September 1996

Contributors

Dr. W. Ross Adey
Pettis Memorial Veterans' Hospital, Dept. of Veterans Affairs, 11201 Benton Street, Loma Linda, CA 92357, USA.

Mr. Howard I. Bassen
Center for Devices and Radiological Health, HFZ-133, Food & Drug Administration.

Dr. Ulf Bergqvist
National Institute for Working Life, Department of Neuromedicine, S-171 84 Solna, Sweden.

Mr. Mark Bogers
Satellite Communication Policy, Wetstraat 200, BU31 2/40, B-1049 Brussels, Belgium

Dr. Craig V. Byus
University of California, Riverside, Biomedical Science Division, Riverside, CA 92521-0121, USA.

Dr. Robert F. Cleveland
Office of Engineering and Technology, Federal Communications Commission, 2000 M Street, NW, Rm. 230, Washington, D.C. 20554, USA.

Dr. Leo Hawel, III
University of California, Riverside, Biomedical Science Division, Riverside, CA 92521-0121, USA.

Mr. Raymond J. Millington
Motorola Cellular, 600 North U.S. Highway 45, A-N283, Libertyville, IL 60048-1286, USA.

Dr. Michael Repacholi
World Health Organization, Avenue Appia 20, 1211 Geneva 27, Switzerland.

Dr. Peter Semm
University of Frankfurt, Department of Zoology, Siesmayerstrasse 70, 60323 Frankfurt, Germany.

Dr. Asher R. Sheppard
Asher Sheppard Consulting, 108 Orange Street, Suite 8, Redlands, CA 92373-4719, USA, and Department of Physiology, Loma Linda University, Loma Linda, CA, USA.

Dr. Masao Taki
Tokyo Metropolitan University, Departement of Electronics & Information Engineering, 1-1, Minami-Osawa, Hachioji-shi, Tokyo 192-03, Japan.

Dr. Bernard Veyret
Laboratoire de Physique des Interactions Ondes-Matière (PIOM), Ecole Nationale Supérieure de Chimie et de Physique de Bordeaux, F-33402 Talence Cedex, France.

PART I

Technology

1

Mobile and personal communications in the 90s

Raymond J. Millington

Today's two major consumer wireless communications services, paging and cellular telephony, both grew out of services which began in the 1950s. At the outset of both services, industrial applications dominated. Paging and Cellular Telephony applications have grown dramatically and are rapidly becoming commonplace in the consumer marketplace. At the end of 1994, paging had grown to a worldwide market serving 50 million users, a 40% growth rate in a market some 'experts' had expected to all but disappear as a result of cellular. Cellular telephone users numbered 52 million worldwide at the end of 1994, representing a 58% growth rate. Both markets have been fueled by increasing functionality, shrinking acquisition cost, enhanced portability and ever improving coverage of service.

The industrial or private mobile radio (traditional two-way radio) is served by 40 million transceivers (radios with a transmitter and a receiver). Private customers, such as utilities and governments, are demanding more sophisticated system capabilities including encryption, data, telephone interconnect and messaging. Also trunked radio (multiple base transceivers networked to provide wide area coverage) customers are evolving their systems to compete in the era of personal communications. At the same time, there seems to be a growing need for people to be in touch at all times. Thus, even at the entry level, consumers are purchasing pairs of low cost radios to keep in touch while hiking, fishing, camping, etc.

Where does this growth in paging, cellular telephony and two-way radio stop? The answer is not at all clear since the applications and the penetration of the customer base is still embryonic. Cellular penetration, for example is only 20% in the more developed countries. In lesser developed countries, cellular is being used to either supplement wired telephony or to provide basic telephony as these countries struggle to develop their communications infrastructure.

Mobile Communications Safety
Edited by N. Kuster, Q. Balzano and J.C. Lin
Published in 1997 by Chapman & Hall, London. ISBN 0 412 75000 7.

In developing countries, ranging from Indonesia to Eastern Europe, cellular telephony is emerging as the wireless technology of choice for basic telephone service. One can set up a working telephone system just by putting up a few antenna towers. Deployment of a modern cellular system is measured in months, as compared to years or even decades required to bring wired telephone service to customers on waiting lists. In Latin America, for example, where cellular service substitutes for wired telephony, the minutes of usage per subscriber are 2 to 3 times higher than in the United States. When you factor in the future of wireless data, satellite systems like Iridium, cordless phones, wireless systems for home and office and enhanced two-way paging messages, you can see that we've just scratched the surface.

A number of key market and technology forces are driving the growth in wireless communications:

1. The push to improve productivity, emergency/safety communications, responsiveness and the quality of life that wireless communications can provide.

2. The changing political and economic scene in international markets as well as a shift to a global economy has opened up new opportunities for all technologies. Over half of the people in the world have never used a phone. The efficiency and cost-effectiveness of new wireless systems will have a profound and positive effect on these emerging markets.

3. Smaller more powerful semiconductor components coupled with improved battery technologies are both lowering the cost and improving the portability of communications equipment.

4. As wireless communications networks mature and more antenna sites are added to handle the traffic load, lower power is required for both the end user equipment as well as the antenna site equipment. This has several positive effects; longer battery life for the end user equipment and a reduction in interference being key benefits derived from shorter antenna site distance.

5. As manufacturers leverage new technologies and bring down their costs, they increasingly attract and serve consumer as well as industrial markets.

Of course, sustained growth is accompanied by constraints. There is only so much capacity available in the radio spectrum; channels are becoming crowded. Two factors are being used to alleviate that constraint. The first is the creative technical effort being applied globally to more efficiently use the spectrum and the second is the allocation of new spectrum. The amount of spectrum per user is being driven down through frequency division, time division, spread spectrum and packet radio. It is beyond the scope of this article to address the cost and size burden of these new radios owing to their increased complexity; a contradiction to the need to provide ever more cost-effective products to the consumer market. Time and market experience will ultimately provide insight into the balance between spectrum utilization and cost.

Table 1.1 lists the existing conventional cellular systems which provide for a

Table 1.1 Constant envelope cellular systems.

System	Where used
NMT	Scandinavia
NTT	Japan
JTACS	Japan
NTACS	Japan
AMPS	North America, South America and Asia
NAMPS	North America, Israel and South America
ETACS	United Kingdom and Asia

Table 1.2 Digital cellular systems.

System	Where used
IRIDIUM	Global[†]
GSM and DCS*	Europe, Asia and Australia
DECT	Europe
CT2	Asia and Europe
NADC*	North America and Hong Kong
ETDMA	North America[†]
CDMA*	North America and Asia
PDC	Japan
PHP*	Japan
ESMR	USA and Japan

* Are candidates for upbanding to US PCN frequency band of
  1850 – 1990 MHz.
[†] Not in commercial service.

single user per radio frequency channel. Table 1.2 lists the digital cellular systems which use compression techniques described above to provide increased utilization of radio frequency channels. Table 1.3 describes some of the key characteristics for conventional cellular portable systems. Table 1.4 further describes key characteristics for digital cellular portable systems.

Whether a system uses conventional cellular technology or digital cellular technology, capacity gains are achieved by shrinking the area served by individual antenna sites. This has several beneficial effects; greater reuse of the radio frequency spectrum, ability to handle dense traffic loads and a lower operating power for both the antenna site and the end user equipment. One of the key attributes in Tables 1.1 to 1.4 is the wide range of power levels noted

Table 1.3 Attributes of constant envelope portable cellular systems.

	NMT	JTACS	AMPS	NAMPS	ETACS
Frequency range					
– uplink (MHz)	890–915	898–925	824–849	824–849	872–905
– downlink (MHz)	935–960	843–870	869–894	869–894	917–950
Modulation	FM	FM	FM	FM	FM
Power levels	1 – 0.1 W in 1 step	0.6 – 0.006 W in 4 dB steps			
Frequency spacing	12.5 kHz interlaced	25 kHz	30 kHz	10 kHz	25 kHz
Duplex type	Frequency division duplex				
Speech coding	None				
Times slots/frames	None				
Frame length	None				
Channel bit rate					
– signaling (kB/s)	1.2	8	10	0.01–0.2	8
– supervisory tone	4 kHz	6 kHz	6 kHz	200 B/s	6 kHz

for each technology. The ability of the cellular systems to dynamically control power levels with a general reduction in required power as a system matures and handles a greater number of users will allow cellular users to enjoy longer battery life and improved coverage. Figure 1.1 shows this effect graphically: as systems mature, portable cellular phones become increasingly popular.

The second factor working to alleviate the capacity of constraint is the increased spectrum being provided to extend the growth of personal communications. Regulators are allocating spectrum and deferring to free market principles to achieve competitive environments. In virtually every country, two to three times today's spectrum is being made available to current and new operators to fuel and satisfy the demand for service. Figure 1.2 shows the spectrum allocations at 800 to 960 MHz and Figure 1.3 shows the more recently allocated spectrum at 1.4 to 2.0 GHz.

This cycle of new spectrum allocation along with technology expansion is a key part of the wireless industry growth process. In the next 15 years, the wireless industry will increase tenfold, reaching more than $ 600 billion by 2010. Over the same time frame, telecommunications will triple to $ 3 trillion. Wireless will increase its share of the telecommunications market from roughly 6% to 20% in 2010.

Another key factor in driving wireless telecommunications is the need to increase productivity. Virtual offices and the need to communicate in 'real time' with people on the go are becoming necessities. The wireless infrastructure will

Table 1.4 Attributes of digital portable cellular systems.

	IRIDIUM	GSM	DCS	NADC
Frequency range	1616–1626.5			
– uplink (MHz)		890–915	1710–1785	824–849
– downlink (MHz)		935–960	1805–1880	869–894
Modulation	DEQPSK	GMSK (0.3)	GMSK	$\pi/4$ QPSK
Power levels		5 – 0.02W	1 – 0.01W	0.6 – 0.006W
		in 2dB steps	in 2dB steps	in 4dB steps
Frequency spacing	41.67 kHz	200 kHz	200 kHz	30 kHz
Duplex type	TDD	TDD/FDD	TDD/FDD	TDD/FDD
Speech coding	2.4/4.8 kB	13 kB	13 kB	8 kB
	VSELP	RELP	RELP	VSELP
Times slots/frames	8+	8	8	3
Frame length	90 ms	4.615 ms	4.615 ms	20 ms
Channel bit rate	50 kB/s	270.83 kB/s	270.83 kB/s	48.6 kB/s

	CDMA	PDC	ESMR
Frequency range			
– uplink (MHz)	824–849	810–830	806–821
– downlink (MHz)	869–894	940–960	851–866
Modulation	QPSK	$\pi/4$ QPSK	16-QAM
Power levels	1W – 0.01μW	0.6 – 0.006W	1 – 0.01W
	in 1dB steps	in 4dB steps	in 5dB steps
Frequency spacing	1.23 MHz	25 kHz	25 kHz
Duplex type	FDD	TDD/FDD	FDD
Speech coding	8 kB	6.8 kB	4.2 kB
	QCELP	VSELP	VSELP
Times slots/frames	None	3	6
Frame length	20 ms	20 ms	90 ms
Channel bit rate	1.288 MB/s	42 kB/s	64 kB/s

have ever increasing demands placed on it for data and message delivery. Some future paging services will require 'ack back' (acknowledge back) paging devices so that lengthy messages can be delivered efficiently by only transmitting to the geographic area that the paging device is located in. There are many examples where wireless communications will have societal benefits. For example, improved health care delivery is made possible with on-site diagnosis. Additionally, wireless communication devices are increasingly being used to improve peoples 'peace of mind' as these devices are used for emergency or safety notification. Although, this chapter has highlighted portable communication

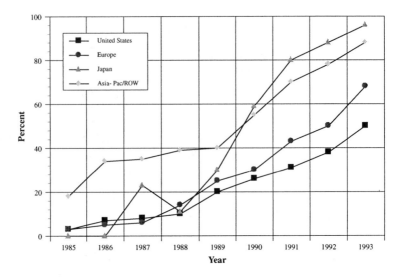

Fig. 1.1 Percent portable mix.

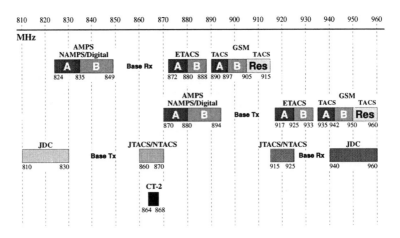

Fig. 1.2 Frequency spectrum 800 to 960 MHz.

devices, industrial applications for mobile or fleet dispatch radios are growing in sophistication as businesses find ways to enhance the productivity of their vehicles.

In summary, wireless communications will continue to grow in consumer and industrial markets. Although the emergence of this market has mushroomed over the last decade, its roots go back to 'walkie-talkies' used during the Second World War. The combination of lower cost, improved performance of

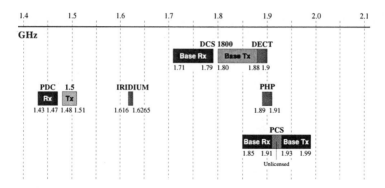

Fig. 1.3 Frequency spectrum 1.4 to 2 GHz

semiconductor and battery components along with a recognition of the life style and productivity enhancements made possible by wireless communications have popularized this industry. Additional uses and growth for this industry is forecast particularly in light of the demands in countries emerging into the global market.

PART II

State of Knowledge

2

Experimental and numerical dosimetry

Niels Kuster and Quirino Balzano

2.1 INTRODUCTION

The objective of this chapter is to document the state of the art of experimental and numerical dosimetry with emphasis on those aspects relevant to mobile communications. This includes the evaluation of the suitability of various tools developed for dosimetry in the frequency range of mobile communications (40 MHz – 6 GHz). Since the suitability of a tool is here determined by the physical requirements defined by the specific applications, the dose rate, the energy absorption mechanism and the two major application areas are discussed first.

2.2 DOSE RATE AND SAFETY STANDARDS

In 1982 the American National Standards Institute (ANSI) became the first organization to introduce the *Dosimetric Concept* for protection from nonionizing radiation (ANSI, 1982) . This represented a marked improvement, since all previous standards, e.g. the ANSI Standard of 1974, were based strictly upon exposure quantities, such as power densities and field strengths. This new approach was subsequently adopted by most national and international standards commissions, e.g. DIN/VDE (1984), NCRP (1986), NRPB (1986), IRPA (1988), TTC/MPT (1990), CENELEC (1995).

The dosimetric concept was initially developed for and successfully applied to protection from ionizing radiation. The ionizing standard is based on an established correlation between the dose and the biological effects, whereby the 'dose' is defined as the energy absorbed per unit mass. Derived values, such as the incident radiation in terms of radiometric quantities, and the definition of dosimetric terms, such as whole body and organ dose, population dose, and relative biological effectiveness, were also defined.

Although this is quite a straightforward approach for protection from ionizing

Mobile Communications Safety
Edited by N. Kuster, Q. Balzano and J.C. Lin
Published in 1997 by Chapman & Hall, London. ISBN 0 412 75000 7.

Table 2.1 Examples of SAR limits proposed in the USA (ANSI, 1992), Europe (CENELEC, 1995) and Japan (TTC/MPT, 1990) for the frequency range of mobile communications (40 MHz – 6 GHz).

	ANSIC95.1-1992	prENV50166-2	TTC/MPT
Group 1:	controlled env.	workers	condition P
whole-body av. SAR	0.4 W/kg	0.4 W/kg	0.4 W/kg
spatial peak SAR	8 W/kg	10 W/kg	8 W/kg
averaging time	6 min.	6 min.	6 min.
averaging mass	1 g	10 g	1 g
shape of volume	cube	cube	cube
Group 2:	uncontrolled env.	general public	condition G
whole-body av. SAR	0.08 W/kg	0.08 W/kg	0.4 W/kg
spatial peak SAR	1.6 W/kg	2 W/kg	8 W/kg
averaging time	30 min.	6 min.	6 min.
averaging mass	1 g	10 g	1 g
shape of volume	cube	cube	cube

radiation, it is much less suitable for nonionizing radiation. The reason is that the interaction path between exposure, dose and biological effects depends on many more parameters than in ionizing radiation. Hence, several further additions were required to make the dosimetric concept applicable to frequencies below 300 GHz. These are discussed in the following for the frequency range of mobile communications, i.e. 40 MHz – 6 GHz.

2.2.1   Dose rate or basic limits

In the mobile communications frequency range all current standards are based on the premise that the underlying mechanism, which correlates well with the biological endpoint, is the temperature increase in the tissue caused by the absorption of nonionizing energy, i.e. thermal effects. At the frequency range of 40 MHz – 6 GHz the electromagnetic field penetrates deeply into tissue, causing an increase in the random molecular motion. Since the body's capability to detect temperature increases at greater tissue depth is lower than at the skin, the exposure cannot directly be compared to that of infrared or light exposure, which is absorbed within the first few millimeters of the skin tissue.

One of the difficulties in developing a safety standard was that a straightforward definition of a dose which correlates well with heating effects is not possible. The reason is that whole-body or local temperature increases not only depend upon the amount of energy absorbed and the effects of passive heat dissipation but also to a very large extent upon complex thermoregulatory processes in the human body. Since those processes depend upon a number of parameters (e.g. specific organs, environment, health status, etc.), it is not the initial temperature increase in the tissue that is used to define the dose but the **power absorbed per unit mass (W/kg)**, called the specific absorption rate (SAR). SAR is defined (ANSI, 1982) as the incremental electromagnetic power (dP) absorbed by an incremental mass (dm) contained in a volume element (dV) of given density (ρ):

$$SAR = \frac{dP}{dm} = \frac{dP}{\rho dV} \qquad (2.1)$$

However, in order to maintain the relation between the absorbed power and the induced heat (i.e. the increase of tissue temperature due to absorption), the SAR must be averaged over a certain period of time (see Table 2.1).

The available experimental data allows the postulation of a correlation between biological effects and whole-body average temperature increases. Very little is known about the possible biological effects induced by local temperature increases, especially when these are small. The only effects that have been thoroughly investigated at the cellular or single organ level are thermal necrosis (in connection with hyperthermia cancer treatment) and ocular effects (cataracts).

However, despite this lack of knowledge, limits for local absorption or spatial peak SAR have had to be defined (see Table 2.1), since near-field exposures can lead to considerable local heating long before the whole body average SAR limit has been exceeded. Aside from the averaging time, a minimum mass of tissue over which the SAR must be averaged was defined, in order to account for the effects of strongly localized heating at the skin, which are annoying but not hazardous (e.g. caused by spark discharges). The choice of these masses has been the subject of much discussion, since the biological basis for defining these averaging masses is at best tenuous. Furthermore, the physical rationale for describing these masses as cubes is also unsettled. The cube was merely chosen because of former experimental and numerical limitations. The evaluation is further complicated by the fact that a variety of tissues of different specific weights can exist within the averaging volume. Many other definitions of the averaging volumes or masses would be physically more plausible. For example, if a hot spot distribution is assumed to be the most general occurrence, a spheroid with the local peak SAR at the center would be much more appropriate. Additional definitions are necessary if the sphere intersects with the surface of the body, as would be necessary for the cube. In this case the sphere must be enlarged so as to contain the appropriate mass of tissue, whereby the maximum would be at the center of the sphere and the intersecting surface would correspond to the surface of the body.

It is obvious that the SAR distribution caused by a given exposure can be assessed only by using human equivalent phantoms and by drawing on considerable technical resources. Hence, as in the field of ionizing radiation, exposure limits had to be derived to achieve a workable standard.

2.2.2   Exposure limits

Exposure limits must have a direct relation to the dose, preferably being proportional. However, in contrast to ionizing radiation, the relationship between the exposure and the induced dose or SAR distribution is significantly dependent on various exposure parameters, such as the frequency and field polarization, as well as on the exposed biological bodies. The human body has complex surfaces and internal geometries and is composed of tissues with spatially varying dielectric properties. Furthermore, the mere presence of the body significantly alters the field distribution. In the case of near field exposures, the coupling between the body and the electromagnetic source can even alter the performance of the source.

Consequently, exposure limits are possible only if they are based on worst case conditions, i.e. when they ensure that the basic limits are satisfied under all conditions. Absorption under various exposure conditions was extensively investigated in numerous studies in the late 70s. From these studies the current exposure limits for electric and magnetic field strengths have been derived. These field quantities can be easily measured using existing equipment (IEEE, 1992). The gist of these studies was that the most efficient absorption occurs under plane wave conditions with an upright human body parallel to the incident E-field. Other, more unusual body postures might also result in enhanced absorption. However, for most body postures other than the upright with parallel field polarization, the derived limits substantially overestimate the actual absorption. This is especially true when the body or body parts are in the close near field of the radiation source and re-radiating structures. For example, in the closest vicinity of low power transmitters, these exposure limits are easily exceeded, although the actual induced absorption might only be a small fraction of the SAR limits.

In other words, the exposure limits are of no use for the safety assessment of handheld telephones. Subsequently, the testing of compliance of handheld mobile communication transceivers with safety limits has lately become the key problem in the area of dosimetry. In view of the importance of this issue, the focus of this chapter will be on the discussion of methods and procedures to assess the basic dose for current standards, i.e. the SAR distribution inside biological tissues. However, one should keep in mind that the importance of time-averaged and volume-averaged SAR values as the only physical quantities of biological relevance is still frequently questioned. The implications of this consideration will be discussed in the following chapters. Even if another measurable quantity proves to be more suitable in future, the following discussions would still be largely applicable.

2.2.3   Exclusions for mobile telecommunications equipment

Right from the onset of the development of the dosimetric concept, it became obvious that handheld mobile telecommunications equipment (MTE) would exceed the derived safety limits. ANSI C95.1-1982 (ANSI, 1982) simply by-passed this problem by an exclusionary clause for low power handheld devices. In this clause all transceivers operating below 1 GHz and radiating less than 7 W were excluded from the requirement to demonstrate compliance with the basic safety limits. This exclusionary clause was adopted worldwide by most standard-setting organizations, although there was no real scientific back-up for this assumption. It was dropped or modified in the beginning of the 90s, when it became well known that transceivers with an input power of 7 W may result in spatial peak SAR values of well above 100 mW/g (Kuster, 1992a; Meier *et al.*, 1996a). However, the 7 W exclusion, together with an extended frequency range of up to 3 GHz, is still valid in some national standards (e.g. Sweden and Japan).

The scientific data available in the early 80s and used to substantiate this exclusion were from experimental studies that had been performed on various transmitters operating at frequencies between 30 and 900 MHz (Balzano *et al.*, 1977; 1978a; 1978b). However, they did not supply any supporting evidence of the soundness of the 7 W exclusion clause.

During the eighties the absorption induced by sources in the close vicinity of biological bodies were studied in several laboratories (Chatterjee *et al.*, 1985; Guy and Chou, 1986; Stuchly *et al.*, 1986a; 1986b; 1987; Kuster and Ballisti, 1989; Cleveland and Athey, 1989; Fujiwara *et al.*, 1990). The results proved to be difficult to interpret and contradictory with respect to the conclusions about the validity of the exclusionary clause. A study in 1992 on the absorption mechanism of biological bodies in the near field of dipole sources clarified the situation and showed conclusively that the exclusionary clause is in clear contradiction of the spatial peak SAR limits (Kuster and Balzano, 1992).

These contradictory findings from distinguished research groups demonstrate the difficulties in performing accurate and reliable dosimetric studies, especially in the close near field of sources. This is just as true for the evaluation and design of optimized exposure setups to be used for *in vitro* and *in vivo* experiments.

It is interesting to note that NCRP (NCRP, 1996), which defined the same basic restrictions in their guidlines as ANSI (ANSI, 1982), did not adopt the 7 W exclusion in 1986. However, it permitted the use of MTE exceeding the limits of the general population as a personal decision by the individual, provided the exposure of the user does not exceed the recommended occupational guidelines and provided that people other than the user are not exposed above the population guidelines. A tighter criterion was added for modulated exposures: 'If the carrier frequency is modulated at a depth of 50 percent or greater at frequencies between 3 and 100 Hz, the exposure criteria for the general population

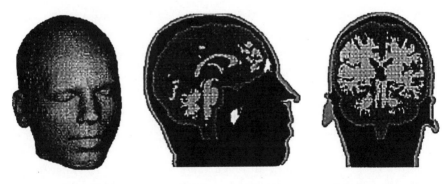

Fig. 2.1 Human head phantom discretized on the basis of MRI images. The voxel size is 1 mm in all three cartesian dimensions, whereby 13 tissue types were distinguished. The brain region was segmented very carefully, but the lower part of the head, which is of minor interest, was assigned only one tissue type. The source is a 900 MHz calibration dipole 0.45λ in length and 15 mm from the head, with an orientation parallel to the body's axis. Reproduced from Hombach *et al.* (1996).

shall also apply to occupational exposure.' Furthermore, the shape of the 1 g mass of tissue had not been defined.

2.3   ENERGY ABSORPTION IN THE NEAR FIELD OF MTE

General electrodynamic problems still are difficult to solve, despite the immense increases of computer power and the various numerical techniques developed during the last twenty to thirty years. The difficulties appear most pronounced if the involved structures or scatterers are in the range of the wavelength, as in the case of mobile communications. So far, no reliable validation procedures are known for assessing the uncertainties of the results. Cursory eye-balling of the field distribution is still the most widespread technique for judging the qualitative accuracy of the results. This technique, even questionable for qualitative control, is certainly not adequate to assess the quantitative uncertainties of the calculated values.

On the other hand, an approximation based on simple assumptions often gives good results, since a single interaction mechanism is dominant in many cases. From the point of view of the engineer, it is useful to distinguish between capacitive coupling (i.e. dominantly E-field induced currents) and inductive coupling (i.e. dominantly H-field induced currents). For resonance phenomena antenna models are often suitable. Although these considerations are less suitable for predicting results beforehand, they are often very useful for validating numerical results or deriving simple approximation formulas. The reason is the

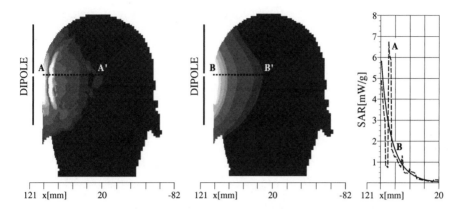

Fig. 2.2 Left: SAR distribution in the xz-plane of head phantom described in the previous figure. Middle: SAR distribution in the same plane but with the parameters of all 13 tissues assigned to those of brain tissue ($\varepsilon_r = 41$, $\sigma = 0.88$ mho/m). Right: Absolute SAR values on the indicated lines A/A' and B/B' respectively for an antenna feedpoint current of 100 mA. The simulations were performed with the FIT code MAFIA. Reproduced from Hombach *et al.* (1996).

difficulty of surveying all possible effects which could render the simplifications invalid.

For example, the most relevant biological tissues have a high water content, i.e. a relatively high permittivity ($\epsilon_r > 30$). The capacitive coupling is therefore poor in most cases, whereby the inductive coupling is often found to be a dominant factor, especially at higher frequencies and in low impedance fields.

2.3.1 Absorption mechanism for homogeneous bodies

For dipole-like transmitters in the vicinity of the body, inductive coupling has proven to be a very efficient model to describe absorption (Kuster and Balzano, 1992). The model is all the more valid for sources generating a dominantly reactive H-field in their vicinity, such as loops, helix antennas or wires. The same study has further concluded that the absorption mechanism is scarcely affected by the shape of the body. Because of the very dominant inductive coupling, a simple but reliable approximation formula has been derived for the SAR induced at the surface (SAR_s) of a flat phantom as a function of only the tissue material (σ, ϵ) and the incident magnetic field ($H_{t_{inc}}$):

$$SAR_s \approx \frac{\sigma}{\rho} \frac{\mu\omega}{\sqrt{\sigma^2 + \epsilon^2\omega^2}} (1 + c_{corr}\gamma_{pw})^2 H_{t_{inc}}^2 \qquad (2.2)$$

in which γ_{pw} is the plane-wave reflection coefficient for the H_t-field

$$\gamma_{pw} = \frac{2|\sqrt{\epsilon'}|}{|\sqrt{\epsilon'} + \sqrt{\epsilon_0}|} - 1 \qquad (2.3)$$

with the complex permittivity $\epsilon' = \epsilon - \sigma/i\omega$. The correction coefficient c_{corr} is introduced to take into account the changed reflection properties from small distances d of the antenna from the scatterer. It was empirically approximated to be:

$$c_{corr} = \begin{cases} 1 & : \quad d \geq 0.08\lambda/\gamma_{pw} \\ \sin(\frac{\pi}{2}\frac{\gamma_{pw}}{0.08}\frac{d}{\lambda}) & : \quad d < 0.08\lambda/\gamma_{pw} \end{cases}$$

Because of the relatively large dimensions of the human head and high conductivity above 800 MHz (dimension with respect to the skin depth δ and wavelength inside the tissue), this approximation is well suited for estimation of the exposure of sources in the vicinity of the head or body. If the H-field can be assessed from the current distribution on the transceiver, the spatial peak SAR averaged over a cube of side length Δx (SAR$_{av}$) can be approximated for a homogeneous representation of the head by

$$SAR_{av} \approx \frac{\delta_{skin}}{2\Delta x} SAR_s (1 - e^{-\frac{2\Delta x}{\delta_{skin}}}) \qquad (2.4)$$

whereby δ_{skin} is the skin depth of the tissue and SAR_s the surface SAR value approximated by (2.2). In many cases it is sufficient to calculate the incident magnetic field $(H_{t_{inc}}^2)$ from the assumed current distribution by simple quasi-static considerations.

An analytically based approach for a layered box (corresponding to the head) has recently been published (King, 1995a). The problem of the evaluation for exposure assessments has been transferred to the assessment of the equivalent dipole moment. This paper does, however, confirm the more easily applicable empirical approximation formula (2.4).

For body cross-sections significantly smaller than the wavelength (e.g. small animals), the SAR distribution is similar to induced eddy currents, with high absorption at the peripheral regions and small values in the center. An example is illustrated in the Figures 2.8 and 2.13. Another example is the absorption in Petri-dishes (Burkhardt *et al.*, 1996), where a good approximation could also be obtained by separately considering capacitive and inductive coupling.

In the frequency range below 200 MHz the body is capacitively coupled to the handheld device, which is often operated with electrically short antennas. In this case the body is an integral part of the antenna system and simple antenna models might be useful for dosimetric estimations.

2.3.2   Considerations for nonhomogeneous bodies

The validity of the above discussed energy absorption mechanism has been widely questioned for strongly nonhomogeneous bodies, such as the human head. This has been addressed recently in two studies about the dependence of electromagnetic energy absorption upon human head modeling for the frequency range below 900 MHz (Hombach *et al.*, 1996) and for 1.8 GHz (Meier *et al.*, 1997). The studies have been conducted using several numerical and experimental phantoms. Phantoms in the context of this chapter are physical or numerical bodies which simulate the electrical properties of living biological bodies. They can be of varied complexity with respect to tissue composition as well as to shape. The most complex phantoms used in this study of the absorption dependence upon modeling were three independently discretized head phantoms based on MRI scans of three different adults, whereby 13 different tissue types were distinguished. One of them is shown in Figure 2.1. The most simple phantom was a homogeneous sphere of 200 mm diameter. The findings of these studies can be summarized as follows:

- The global SAR distribution is similar for homogeneous and nonhomogeneous modeling, i.e. the energy absorption mechanism is not changed (Figure 2.2). In other words, the absorption distribution is strongly related to the expected incident magnetic field, i.e. to the RF current distribution versus the distance. Most of the power is absorbed close to the radiating structure and focusing effects are negligible.

- The local SAR distribution depends significantly on the local distribution of the electrical tissue properties. In humans, however, the local tissue distribution for various individuals varies largely and can even change with time. For example, the outer shape depends on the individual profile and on any movement of the mouth or the eyes. The electric parameters of a human body vary with levels of physical and metabolic activity, health, and age.

- The spatial peak SAR values also depend on the local anatomy. On the other hand, the homogeneous modeling led to results which also overestimated the values of the nonhomogeneous head with the highest absorption. However, the overestimation is surprisingly small for the site above the ear, i.e. <10% for the 10 g averaged values and <25% for the 1 g averaged values .

- Small shifts (<10 mm) of the source parallel to the surface of body can result in variations of the spatial peak SAR of larger 3 dB in the case of nonhomogeneous modeling. For homogeneous bodies such shifts do not lead to any changes in the spatial peak SAR values, which always overestimate the values of the nonhomogeneous case.

- The effects due to the shape of the head are negligible for a given distance of the RF current source from the body.

- The human hand is an anatomically and geometrically complex structure which can cover an MTE in almost an infinite number of configurations.

Studies of a large number of different devices have shown that the largest spatial peak SAR values measured for different ways of holding the devices is well represented by not considering the hand (Meier, 1996).

- The two parameters which determine the SAR distribution most are clearly the actual current distribution on the device and the distance of these currents from the tissue.

In a follow-up study possible enhancement effects of external metallic accessories such as optical glasses or jewelry are investigated. Enhancement of several dBs are possible for nonhomogeneous modeling. The effects become negligible with homogeneous exposure (Meier, 1996).

2.3.3   Influence of the scattered fields on the source

Conductive scatterers in the close vicinity of the antenna generally affect the source. This has been studied for a dipole source at different distances from a head-shaped body (see Figure 2.4). Whether a change in the feedpoint impedance results in a significant increase or decrease of the feedpoint current (i.e. of the absorbed power) depends on the actual design of the final RF amplifier. Although the radiating structures of most devices have rather low Q-values, the actual current distribution on the device could be significantly modified by the vicinity of the body, which may in turn have a large effect on the spatial peak SAR value.

2.4   APPLIED DOSIMETRY IN MOBILE COMMUNICATIONS SAFETY RESEARCH

2.4.1   Introduction

A broad variety of dosimetric tools and different dosimetric strategies have been developed during the last two decades. Before their suitability for dosimetric assessments can be evaluated, the actual dosimetric needs in the area of mobile communications will be discussed. Two major areas with significantly different dosimetric requirements can be distinguished. These are: (1) the dosimetric evaluations and optimizations of exposure setups to be used in biological experiments; (2) the dosimetry for compliance testing of certain products with the basic restrictions of the safety guidlines. Specifically, the dosimetry required for compliance testing of handheld MTE needs careful consideration, since the absorption may vary greatly between individuals and may strongly depend on the position of the MTE with respect to the head and the body of the user. A possible approach is presented and discussed in the following Section 2.5.

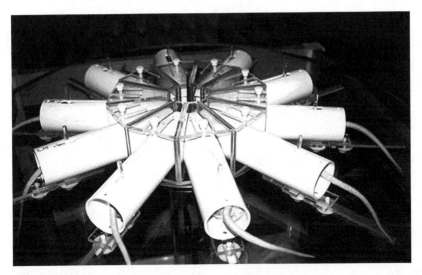

Fig. 2.3 Near field exposure setup used by different laboratories to study possible effects of electromagnetic exposure on the central nervous system (CNS) at the MTE frequency bands 800–900 MHz. Ten adult rats are grouped around a symmetrical dipole. The distance between feedpoint and snout was kept constant to approximately 30 mm by restraining the animals in the shown tubes (Burkhardt *et al.*, 1997).

2.4.2   Dosimetric evaluation of biological experiments

In biological experiments the field strengths induced in the tissues should be defined as well as possible. It is usually desirable that the fields in the target tissue or organ are much larger than those in the rest of the body, in order to prevent the investigated effects from being masked by other factors. For example, when investigating the possible effects of wireless technology on the central nervous system (CNS) using animals, the exposure should simulate real life exposures during the use of MTE as far as possible. This requires: (1) identical signal characteristics; (2) identical SAR distributions and identical field strengths in the brain tissue of the animal; (3) low exposure in the rest of the body; and (4) low stress levels caused by the exposure setup. If the latter two cannot be satisfied, the CNS effects may be masked by other effects, such as whole-body heating or stress caused by restraining the animal movement. However, it is often very difficult, if not impossible, to satisfy all of these requirements, especially since the setup must be practical and of reasonable cost.

Profound knowledge of the absorption mechanism is needed for evaluation of an optimal exposure system. However, any setup should be complemented by numerical or experimental dosimetry, since a thorough dosimetry is a prerequisite for a good biological study. Field strength variations in the target tissues (e.g. due to different anatomies and movement) must be determined with the greatest precision. The exposure of the remaining tissues should be reliably assessed as well. In most cases this can be best achieved using numerical techniques. Since the possible errors in numerical simulations are numerous, solutions must be validated. The correctness of the simplifications must also be validated. This is best achieved by measurements in critical areas or by applying a second independent numerical technique. Figures 2.8, 2.7 and 2.13 illustrate such a dosimetric approach. The details are described in Burkhardt *et al.* (1997). Another dosimetric analysis of an *in vitro* exposure setup is presented in Burkhardt *et al.* (1996).

2.4.3   Compliance testing with safety standards

Compliance of a given exposure situation with safety standards is demonstrated, when it can be shown that both the whole-body, as well as the spatial peak SAR, are not exceeded for any person in any position with respect to the radiation source. It is obvious that the dosimetric requirements largely differ from those of analyzing exposure setups for biological experiments. In the latter very accurate SAR values in specified body parts are required, whereby position and orientation with respect to the incident field is well defined. The test subjects are also largely identical in size and weight.

In compliance tests the highest possible SAR value must be determined given a multitude of various conditions, e.g. anatomical variations (differing sizes, body weights) and a wide range of possible positions and orientations (polarization, different postures). The best dosimetric technique for compliance testing is, therefore, not the one with the best resolution, but the one in which the worst-case exposure conditions can be most efficiently and reliably determined.

Compliance with basic restrictions is most easily assessed by testing compliance with exposure limits, since these values are derived from worst-case studies. Only one field component, i.e. electric or magnetic field strength, needs to be measured, if the exposure approximately corresponds to far field conditions and if the frequency is above 300 MHz. In the near field of active radiators or passive re-radiators, both the incident electric and the incident magnetic field strengths should be independently measured. However, there is no commercial instrument available yet for magnetic field measurements at these frequencies. It is often mistakenly assumed that the most appropriate measure would be the time-average power flux density or Poynting vector. However, the power flux density only badly correlates with the absorption in the near field, because the coupling mechanisms with biological tissues are more correlated to the electric or magnetic components of the exposure than with the Poynting vector (see Section 2.3).

Measurements in the close near field of RF sources are difficult and require great precaution. (1) Only isotropic probes which are electrically small should be used, otherwise the greatest care is necessary to ensure that all three

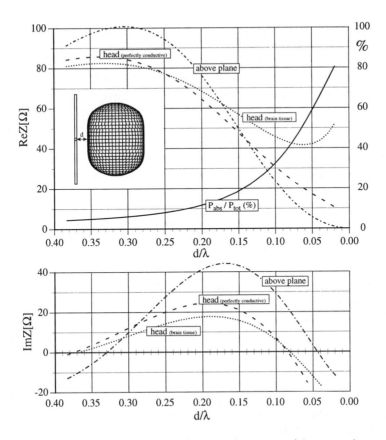

Fig. 2.4 Diagram of the computed feedpoint impedance (above: real component $Re(Z)$, below: imaginary component $Im(Z)$) as a function of the distance d between the antenna axis and the surface of the head. Additionally, the portion of the total power available at the feeding gap which is absorbed in the head is plotted. The two other curves show the corresponding impedance curve of the same dipole, which is 1) in front of a geometrically identical but perfectly conducting head and 2) above a perfectly conducting plane. Dipole: frequency $= 575\,$MHz, diameter $= 6\,$mm, length $= 24.4\,$cm (free space feed point impedance: $Z = 73.5\Omega$); head: $\varepsilon_r = 45$, $\sigma = 0.65\,$mho/m (correspond to brain tissue). Reproduced from Kuster (1992c).

orthogonal components are measured at the same location. (2) If no minimum distance between probe and radiator is specified in the probe manual, (IEEE, 1992) recommends a minimum distance between sensors and metal structures of greater than 5 times the largest dimensions of the sensor. Otherwise the sensor characteristics might change considerably, due to capacitive coupling with metal parts of the RF source.

If exposure limits are exceeded in the near field, compliance with basic restrictions can also be demonstrated by directly determining the SAR distribution in experimental or numerical phantoms representing the human body. Such dosimetric assessments, however, are generally difficult to perform, especially because the body may strongly interact with the radiation source or the reradiating structures nearby. The absorption depends on various parameters, such as the position of the RF source near the body, posture, size and anatomy. In addition, possible error sources in the experimental and numerical dosimetry are numerous. Testing compliance with the basic restrictions is therefore time consuming and expensive and should be considered as a solution of last resort.

The easiest way to enforce safety limits is to implement appropriate measures to prevent access to critical areas where the exposure limits are exceeded. If access is required under certain circumstances (e.g. for maintenance purposes), the operator of the installation can stipulate a procedure (e.g. shutdown of the transmitter or wearing of protective clothing), to avoid exposure exceeding the safety limits.

Some equipment, however, need to be operated in the close vicinity of users for functional reasons (e.g. portable and handheld MTE). Exclusionary clauses can be defined but should satisfy the worst case criteria. This may not be the case for the exclusionary clause for low power devices defined in ANSI C95.1-1992 (ANSI, 1992). A better basis to define a sound exclusionary clause might be the approximation formula (2.4). However, further studies are needed to verify its general validity and its range of uncertainty.

However, many cellular phone systems do not fall under such an exclusion, since their maximum input power is large enough to theoretically exceed the spatial peak SAR limits. This has the consequence that a special procedure must be implemented to demonstrate compliance with basic restrictions. Since this is one of the key problems in the dosimetry of mobile communications, special requirements for compliance testing of handheld MTE are necessary and are discussed in the following Section 2.5.

2.5   SPECIAL REQUIREMENTS FOR COMPLIANCE TESTING OF MTE

2.5.1   Introduction

In recent years handheld mobile telecommunication equipment (MTE) have become a common and widely used consumer product. Their use is shifting from mainly business oriented to personal. With falling operational costs more frequent and more prolonged conversations can be expected (see also Chapter 1). However, the operation of transmitters in very close proximity to the head subjects the exposed parts of the user's body to electromagnetic fields which are several magnitudes above the average background fields. The locally induced field strength is significantly higher than any exposure the broader public has been exposed to before, except during certain common medical treatments (e.g. MRI, diathermy, hyperthermia, etc). Recent studies have even shown that some current cellular phones are close to or even exceed recommended limits under certain operational conditions (Meier *et al.*, 1995).

In view of this, it is reasonable that some health agencies are urgently calling for dosimetric type approval and require compliance with safety limits under all operational conditions (Strahlenschutzkommission, 1992; Bundesamt für Gesundheit, 1993). Such a worst case approach is directly analogous to the commonly applied safety considerations for chemical and physical agents. Some manufacturers and service providers, on the other hand, prefer to test under intended use or normal positions only, a position which is described in their user manuals. This is because of their concern that more strict requirements cannot be satisfied with current technology, especially in view of the consumer's desire to purchase smaller and lighter devices. It is clear that desired growth can only be realized with an attractive high-tech consumer product.

The rationale is often brought up that since large safety factors have been incorporated in the standards, exceeding these limits under certain circumstances is acceptable. However, this argument is contradictory to the basic idea of safety standards, since these factors consider the uncertainty of the extrapolation from animal experiments to the human organism. In addition, they should also incorporate possible variations among humans with respect to their biological responses on physical stimulus. It would therefore not be consistent to apply them for the uncertainty of the exposure as well.

Other arguments are that it is unlikely that a user would hold the device in the same position during the entire averaging period (see Table 2.1) or that the device would be continually radiating at maximum power during the entire averaging period. Power levels of the devices undergo constant adjustment according to radiation conditions. Furthermore, when the discontinuous transmission mode (DTX) is used, the averaging power level is reduced according to the talk-listening ratio. These combined improbabilities might justify less rigid test requirements than those initially requested by some health agencies.

On the other hand, intended or normal positions do not reflect the actual average use. Hence, the exposure assessment under this intended use position would differ from those of many daily life situations, since tests have shown (Meier and Kuster, 1995) that this position results in spatial peak SAR levels which are close to the minimum among the various operational positions.

Considering all these aspects, a certification procedure could only be considered to be sound if it satisfy the following basic requirements.

2.5.2   Basic requirements

- The procedure should ensure that the assessed spatial peak SAR values do not underestimate the actual exposure of any MTE user for the operational conditions.

- The procedure should also allow for testing the effects of manufacturing variations and tolerances on the SAR.
- The tests should be conducted at the highest power of the MTE under operational conditions. It is also important to require that the tests be conducted for each configuration (e.g. with all antennas provided for a particular MTE) and multi-system MTE should be tested using each system.
- A fundamental requirement is a high reproducibility of the tests.

Before a procedure satisfying these basic requirements can be developed, a number of conditions have to be carefully defined, such as the operational conditions, technical requirements and compliance criteria. Because this discussion is ongoing, a possible approach is discussed in the following sections which could satisfy both the interests of the industry as well as the safety requirements of the consumer. They also reflect to some extent the current discussion of some health agencies and regulatory committees.

2.5.3   Operational conditions

The physical embodiment and handling differ significantly among MTE. Hence, the operational conditions for each class of MTE must be well defined for testing. In the following, three different classes of MTE are briefly discussed.

Handheld mobile phones

The first class are handheld mobile phones. These MTE consist of a single unit with integrated microphone, ear piece, transceiver and antenna. Most of these mobile phone systems are open systems and not technically and administratively restricted to workers. In these cases the limits for the general public should also be applied when the MTE is provided by the employer for business use only.

It is usually specified in the user manuals how the MTE shall be used, i.e. in the **intended use position**. Nevertheless, handheld mobile phones are generally used like wireline phones. Various operational conditions (e.g. antenna retracted or partially extended, etc.) can be seen on the street and the phone is held in various positions with respect to the body (e.g. right or left side of the head, at various angles).

There are two aspects to be considered. On one hand, the manufacturers cannot be made responsible if the phone is not handled properly, particularly if the user has been adequately warned in the user manual. On the other hand, usage at slight variance of this intended use position can unavoidably occur.

Since even small variations of the position may considerably alter the spatial

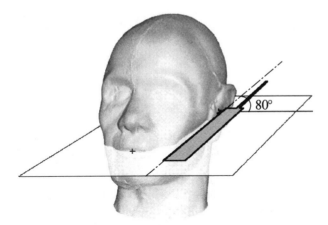

Fig. 2.5 Illustration of the **intended use position** as suggest by a working group of CENELEC drafting a report under EU mandate M/032 (see Chapter 11). The intended use position is generally established by fully extending the antenna of the MTE. Definition: (1) The center of the ear-piece should be placed directly at the entrance of the auditory canal. (2) The reference line of the phone is defined as the line (on the surface of the phone's case facing the phantom) which connects the center of the ear-piece with the center of the bottom of the case (typically near the microphone). (3) The reference line defined above should lie within the reference plane defined by the following three points: auditory canal openings of both ears and the center of the closed mouth. (4) The intended use position is defined by an angle of 80° between the reference line of the phone and the line connecting both auditory canal openings. If this position is not applicable, the manufacturer should specify in detail the intended position of use.

peak absorption, the test should ensure that the MTE complies with the safety standard for the usual variations of the intended use. The suggestion of a limited number of positions which cover well the possible range of SAR values has recently been advanced by a CENELEC working group drafting a report under EU mandate M/032 (see Section 11).

The intended use or normal position is a position which is convenient and provides good acoustic coupling. It is defined and illustrated in Figure 2.5.

Three additional positions have also been suggested which are set to cover the normal variations of the intended use position. They are illustrated in Figure 2.6. These definitions do not cover small shifts parallel to the surface, which is valid if the used phantoms are invariant to such shifts. For phantoms not having this property, additional tests would be necessary for the proof of compliance.

Tests should be performed in all four positions with the antenna fully extended

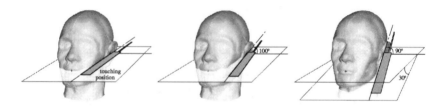

Fig. 2.6 Illustration of the three additional operational test positions: (left) The angle between the reference line of the phone and the line connecting both auditory canal openings is reduced until the device touches the face of the phantom. (center) The angle between the reference line of the phone and the line connecting both auditory canal openings is increased to 100°, provided that the antenna does not touch the head. If the antenna does touch the head before an angle of 100° has been reached, this position should be tested. (right) As an additional position, the reference plane should be tilted by 30° in the direction of the body's axis, whereby the angle between the reference line of the phone and the line connecting both auditory canal openings is 90°.

and fully retracted, if the antenna can be extended. Tests could be limited to just one phantom (righthand or lefthand phantom), depending on the phone, since higher SAR values occur when the antenna is mounted on the side of the upper ear, because of the closer proximity to the upper head area.

Dispatch MTE

Another important category are dispatch radios, which, however, are not as extensively used as mobile phones. They are usually held in front of the face. For dispatch radios which are used like handheld mobile phones, the operational conditions discussed above should apply. The appropriate minimum operational distance between the center of the mouth and the microphone should be clearly indicated in the user manual, or preferably on the device. A minimum distance between mouth and microphone of larger than 5 cm are hard to justify on the basis of performance.

A reasonable test position is defined when the vertical axis of the radio is parallel to the axis of the phantom, whereby the line perpendicular to both axes goes through the center of the closed mouth and the center of the microphone, which in turn faces the phantom.

Portable MTE

Portable MTEs are devices for which the antenna is usually not mounted on the handset but on a separate portable unit. The antenna is nevertheless often in the close vicinity of the body. Most user manuals specify the minimum distance to be kept between the antenna and the human body.

2.5.4 Basic technical requirements

Requirements for modeling of the MTE

Since absorption is strongly dependent on the design details of the handset, it is preferable to perform the tests on the actual unmodified MTE. The highest possible operational output power at which the test must be performed can be established by an air link between the device and a system test set or by programming the device for maximum power output in a test mode.

   If the compliance test procedure cannot be performed with the actual physical MTE (i.e. if a modeling or modification of the handset is required), it is necessary to establish a procedure to ensure that the safety limits are not exceeded by the actual MTE.

Requirements for modeling of the human body

The fundamental requirement for the modeling of the human body is the ability to assess SAR values which are unlikely to be exceeded in any user under the operational conditions defined in Section 2.5.3. Furthermore, the phantoms should ensure current distributions on the MTE similar to those which occur in real situations in close proximity to the head.

   As outlined in Section 2.3.1, this could well be satisfied by homogeneous modeling of the human head. However, the shape of the head is a crucial factor, since the positions are defined in terms of angles and not in terms of distances between device and body. In order to satisfy requirement (1), the shape of the head must be optimized, so that it provides a good representation of the minimum distances between the parts of the MTE and the surface of the head, as found in all potential users under the defined operational positions.

Requirements for the dosimetric simulation software

The basic requirements for a numerical approach include: (1) accurate electromagnetic modeling of the MTE in the defined operational positions and conditions; (2) ability to model a phantom satisfying the above requirements; (3) accurate simulation of the near-field coupling between phantom and device; (4) capability of assessing the solution and modeling uncertainties.

   As will be discussed in Section 2.7, the disadvantage of numerical compliance testing is seen in satisfying requirements 1 and 4. The latter is especially difficult to satisfy, since the uncertainty analysis has to include:

• Uncertainties of each assessed SAR value. Note that every simulation may have its own potential sources of error (e.g. due to the wide variety of different antenna structures operating in the closest vicinity of the lossy scatterer).

- Uncertainties due to modeling of the MTE.
- Uncertainty of the chosen head phantom with respect to the maximum exposure occurring among all users.
- Uncertainty due to the unknown effect on the output circuit from the proximity of the scatterer to the MTE.

Requirements for the dosimetric measurement system

The basic requirements for a dosimetric measurement system can be summarized as follows: (1) As the spatial peak SAR can occur inside the body tissue which is closest to the MTE, the three-dimensional SAR distribution must be determined in this region of the body. (2) If the local SAR at and close to the surface cannot be directly determined, a procedure should be established through which an accurate extrapolation to the surface can be performed.(3) Appropriate measures must be taken to avoid significant errors due to reflections from nearby objects. Special consideration with respect to the test environment is required for frequencies below 400 MHz. (4) The system must ensure accurate time-averaged SAR values for pulsed or amplitude modulated systems. (5) It is important that all ambient sources which may induce SAR values of higher than 10 mW/kg are eliminated.

Since the actual MTE is tested, the overall uncertainty of the entire setup need only be carefully assessed once. The analysis should included:

- Uncertainty of the electrical parameters of the phantom.
- Error due to deviation from isotropy of the probe response.
- Error due to deviation from linearity of the probe response.
- Error induced by unwanted interactions of the measurement equipment with ambient low and high frequency fields.
- Error at or close to a dielectric material discontinuity.
- Uncertainty of the probe calibration (required for each frequency and tissue simulating material for which the system is used).
- Uncertainty due to the limited spatial resolution.
- Uncertainty due to the extrapolation to the surface and interpolation between the measured points.
- Uncertainty due to the implemented averaging procedure (volume, time).
- Uncertainty of the chosen head phantom with respect to the maximum exposure occurring among all users.
- Uncertainty due to errors in positioning the MTE according to the test positions.
- If the actual MTE must be modified for testing purposes, the uncertainties due to these modifications must be assessed as well.

2.5.5 Testing procedure

The applied measurement or simulation procedure and the phantom should satisfy the outlined requirements. The tests should be performed with the highest power available under operational conditions (e.g. fully charged batteries, highest power level specified by the system). The values with which the basic restrictions should be compared are achieved by adding the corresponding uncertainty to the measured or numerically obtained spatial peak SAR value.

The most simple compliance criteria would require that the SAR values of all tested positions be below the basic restrictions. An alternative for handheld mobile phones, which would also be easy to justify, could be the average between the intended use and the maximum value found among the additional operational conditions and positions.

A detailed documentation of the results of any measurement should be part of the requirements, such that possible errors of contradictory results can be traced.

2.5.6 Final remarks

At first sight the compliance test criteria and requirements outlined above might seem to be extensively rigid. However, the authors are of the view that a sound technical approach would have distinct advantages and could be made available at a moderate cost. The possible negative implications of an implausible or controversial testing procedure should not be underestimated. A questionable approach can lead to negative publicity and criticism by government agencies responsible for the safety of the public. This in turn can lead to expensive legal actions against both manufacturers and service providers and to lack of confidence among consumers.

In view of the potentially serious economic implications, a sound procedure is more than justified. The experimental and numerical tools currently available to implement such a certification procedure is the topic of the following sections.

2.6 RECENT ADVANCES IN EXPERIMENTAL DOSIMETRY

2.6.1 Introduction

The most obvious approach towards dosimetric analysis is to experimentally determine the SAR distribution in phantoms simulating animal and human bodies as well as in real cadavers. One way of determining the local or whole-body SAR is by temperature measurements. The SAR is proportional to the temperature increase only when the effects of heat diffusion can be neglected.

Because of thermodynamic processes, this is only the case at the moment the exposure begins $(t \rightarrow +0)$ and when the thermal equilibrium was prevalent at the site of measurement prior to the exposure.

$$SAR = c \left. \frac{\partial T}{\partial t} \right|_{t \rightarrow +0} \tag{2.5}$$

where c is the specific heat of the tissue at the site of measurement. Since the heat transfer mechanisms that lead to thermal equilibrium are relatively slow, SAR can be determined by evaluating $c \Delta T / \Delta t$ if the effects of thermal conduction, convection and radiation are negligible in the time interval Δt. In fluids with relatively low viscosity, convection is the dominant heat transfer mechanism. Since convection is a nonlinear process, assessment of the SAR by taking measurements over a longer period of time and accounting for heat exchange processes is very intricate and should be avoided. The advantages and drawbacks of this approach will be discussed in Section 2.6.3.

Another way of determining the SAR distribution inside tissue-simulating materials is by measuring the electric field (E) inside the exposed tissue.

$$SAR = \frac{1}{2} \frac{\sigma}{\rho} |E|^2 \tag{2.6}$$

where σ is the conductivity, ρ the density of the tissue at the site of measurement, $|E|$ is the Hermitian magnitude of the local electric field vector. The advantages and drawbacks of this method will be discussed in Section 2.6.4.

Both approaches have some common requirements. Any measurable field disturbance caused by the probe must be avoided. A further requirement, which is often but not necessarily concomitant with the previous, is that any signal picked up by any parts of the probe other than the sensor itself should be sufficiently suppressed. For many dosimetric assessments, the sensitivity of the probe is not a key issue, since low sensitivity can be compensated for by applying high power exposures. However, for tests of compliance with safety limits a sensitivity of considerably better than the safety limits is required, since it is preferable to test unmodified equipment (see Section 2.5.4). A sensitivity of at least 0.1 W/kg would certainly satisfy these requirements, which approximately corresponds to 0.03 mK/s or 10 V/m for current liquids or gels simulating tissues rich in water.

The spatial resolution should be better than the smallest spatial dimension of any local field maxima or minima, in order to enable accurate assessment of the SAR distribution. Compliance tests and most dosimetric assessments require the determination of the SAR distribution in the tissue volume of interest. In larger volumes with greatly non-uniform distributions, measurements in several hundred points might be necessary. Since the location of the sensor must be precisely known, stereotactic or robot positioning is a costly but often necessary solution.

2.6.2   Tissue-simulating materials

The dielectric properties of tissue simulating materials at a specific frequency and at room temperature should accurately correspond with the dielectric properties of living tissues at body temperature. Since the SAR is defined as the time rate of energy absorption per unit weight, only the macroscopic simulation of the tissue's permittivity ϵ, permeability μ and conductivity σ are required. For SAR determination through temperature increase measurements, material with low specific heat and high viscosity would be advantageous. The use of E-field probes does not have any prerequisites, except that the material should be liquid. The reason is that E-field probes are relatively large. Holes in solid material would significantly alter the field distribution in the phantom and would also severely limit the number of spatial points of measurements. For practical reasons, the material should be inexpensive, stable, nonpoisonous and easy to handle.

Animal tissues are generally used as the sources for assessing the dielectric properties of the various tissues. The values for living tissue parameters presently found in literature show large variations. This is due to the difficulties encountered when handling living or freshly excised tissues during data collection and due to the natural variations of tissues. The most recent dielectric data from living tissue are provided by MCL Consultants (Microwave Consultants, 1994) and by the University of Maryland (Davis *et al.*, 1996) which, however, differ considerably in both permittivity and conductivity. Additional data can be found in Pethig (1984), Hartsgrove *et al.* (1987) and Foster (1995).

Most biological tissues in the head have high water contents ($\approx 75\%$). These tissues (e.g. skin, muscle, various brain tissues, blood, cerebrospinal fluid) can be easily simulated as simple water-based solutions. Exceptions are bone and fatty tissues. In the frequency spectrum of mobile communications the relative permittivities ϵ_r of those tissues range between 35 and 55, the conductivity levels between 0.5 mho/m and 2.8 mho/m. The magnetic permeability of all tissue is accurately simulated by that of a vacuum, i.e. $\mu_r = 1$. To decrease the high permittivity of the solvent water (deionized), sugar (sucrose) is dissolved in the water. To increase the conductivity, sodium chloride is added. Water, sugar and sodium chloride allow the simulation of a wide variety of tissue types in the frequency range between 200 MHz and 1 GHz (Meier, 1996). However, for frequencies higher than 1 GHz bound sugar-water complexes alone determine the conductivity levels. The smallest values that can be reached at a given relative permittivity of 45 are around 1.6 mho/m (at 2 GHz). To nevertheless simulate low conductivity tissues, such as white brain matter, which has a higher fat content, water can be substituted by an organic solution (e.g. butyldiglycol) (Meier *et al.*, 1996a). A summary of relevant tissue types for the human head, their simulating liquids and corresponding recipes are given in Meier *et al.* (1996b) and Hartsgrove *et al.* (1987).

The dielectric parameters of liquids can either be measured by the slotted line method or by the open coaxial method. The latter method is simple to implement and gives the value of complex dielectric parameters over a broad frequency range. A commercial measurement kit is available from Hewlett Packard (HP 85070A Dielectric Probe Kit). The achievable accuracy is ±5% for the permittivity and ±10% for the conductivity. A better accuracy for the conductivity of about ±6% can be achieved by the slotted line method.

2.6.3 Temperature measurement methods

Introduction

An important advantage of the temperature measurement method is that temperature is a scalar value, which makes it easier to produce probes of very small size and short time constants. One major difficulty is to achieve high SAR sensitivity, i.e. ≪ 1 W/kg. Another important drawback is that the time derivative can only be determined by temperature measurements at two discrete times, whereby the thermodynamic state prior to exposure must be known and preferably be in equilibrium. Since the exposure alters thermal equilibrium, means must be provided to re-establish equilibrium after each measurement cycle, which is usually time consuming.

Implantable electrical temperature probes

The temperature probe based on a high-resistance thermistor connected to high-resistance leads was first described by Bowman (1976). By using the four-lead configuration, a high impedance current source and a voltage amplifier, the temperature can be measured accurately, despite the instability and temperature dependence of the leads. Such probes are commercially available and have been successfully used in dosimetry in the last two decades. They have nonetheless received little attention compared to fiber-optical temperature probes. Superior sensitivity (Table 2.2) has recently been achieved by using specialized electrometer grade amplifiers and sophisticated software for filtering and data evaluation (Burkhardt *et al.*, 1996). One disadvantage is that the leads of these probes are not totally unaffected by electromagnetic fields. However, if the measurements are performed with the necessary precautions and a well designed setup, the effect of RF exposure on the probe compared to the induced temperature increase can be kept below −20 dB.

Implantable optical temperature probes

In the eighties temperature sensors utilizing optical temperature effects were developed and commercialized for applications such as temperature control in high voltage transformers, industrial microwave heating, hyperthermia, dosimetry, etc.

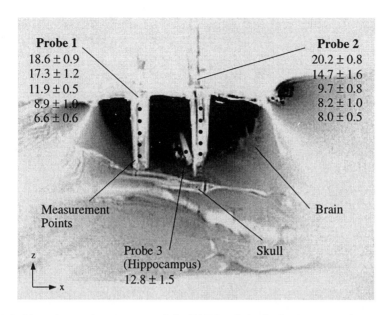

Fig. 2.7 Experimental assessment of the SAR levels in the brain tissue of rats exposed in the setup shown in Figure 2.3. Fiberoptical temperature sensors were positioned by stereotactic means in the brain tissue of a rat cadaver. After assessing the exact position of the probes by a high resolution MRI scan, the rat cadaver was placed at the same location in which the rats were exposed during the experiments. The maximum available antenna input power was 82 W. Shown is the measured temperature rise in mK/s at the different locations. Reproduced from Burkhardt (1997).

One of the effects employed for temperature measurements is the rate of fluorescent decay from a phosphorescent layer on the tip of an optical fiber. An exponentially decaying material with a long half life is preferably used (e.g. magnesium fluorogermanate activated with tetravalent manganese excitable by Xenon flash light) (Wickersheim and Sun, 1987). Currently commercially available devices typically do not have a noise level of better than ±0.1°C (averaging time 1 s). Multichannel devices with a wide operational range from −200°C to 450°C are now available.

Another effect that has been utilized for optical probes is the interferometric microshift of a cavity resonator, which is filled with a material of very high refractive index that is temperature dependent. The short-term drifts and noise is about 10 mK/s for practical applications. This can be reduced by improved data processing. In small animal cadaver a sensitivity of about 2–3 mK/s was achieved, due to the larger thermal constant in the tissue compared to liquids (Burkhardt et al., 1996).

Table 2.2 Comparison of commercially available temperature measurement systems.

Physical principle	Fluorescent decay	Cavity resonator	Thermistor
Noise level/short term drifts (sampling time)	±0.1°C (1 s)	±0.1°C	±0.005°C (0.1 s)
Sensitivity (10 s of exposure)	±15 mK/s	±10 mK/s	±0.15 mK/s
Sensitivity to RF exposure (835 MHz)			
- resistive lines parallel to E-field	<noise	<noise	<0.5 mK/s*
- resistive lines normal to E-field	<noise	<noise	<0.1 mK/s*

* Measured by exposing the first 6 cm of the line from the tip to an incident field of 950 V/m.

Radiation thermometry

Radiation thermometry is an obvious technique to perform measurements without disturbing the field. Since entire surfaces can be efficiently scanned, this was one of the first methods utilized for SAR measurements (Guy, 1971). Thermographic cameras have been used to evaluate the distribution of the SAR on phantom surfaces and on the cut of a bisected cadaver (Figure 2.8), as well as on full size (Guy, 1971) and scaled (Guy, 1984) phantoms comprised of a fiberglass shell filled with a tissue-simulating jelly-like material. In Nojima *et al.* (1991) a full-size dry head phantom composed of various kinds of ceramics, carbon powder and resins is described, which has been used to assess the exposure by mobile communication equipment. To achieve sufficient sensitivity at larger distances (15 cm) of the antenna from the phantom surface, an antenna input power of 200 W had to be used.

The technology for infrared imaging has been continuously improved in the past few years, and sophisticated devices for various applications (e.g. medical diagnosis, infrared sensing, etc.) are today available. For the precise measurement of small temperature changes, as required for SAR assessments, several error sources must be carefully considered: (1) The radiative properties and specific heat of materials under study must be carefully determined. (2) The object must receive only uniform background radiation. (3) Evaporative cooling or air flow convection may cause significant errors and must be well controlled. (4)

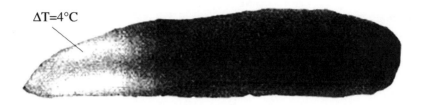

ΔT=4°C

Fig. 2.8 The dosimetric assessment for the exposure setup of Figure 2.3, here shown as performed by radiation thermometry. The rat was frozen and sagitally cut in half, with the cut surfaces covered by a silk tissue. The thawed and reassembled rat was exposed in the exposure setup, whereby the antenna input power was 204 W applied for 60 s. Immediately after the exposure, the cut surfaces were scanned by the IR camera FLIR System IQ 325, from which the SAR distribution can be assessed.

Considerably differing viewing angles will also result in different temperatures being read (Cetas, 1978).

Radiation thermometry entails interesting features for SAR measurements, since the temperature profile on surfaces can be efficiently scanned with high spatial resolution and without disturbing the incident field. It is an especially interesting alternative to other methods if qualitative assessments through certain cross sections are being studied. However, this method is unsuitable for standardized compliance testing of low power handheld devices, not only due to its limited sensitivity (>10 W/kg) and demanding requirements for ambient control, but primarily because of its practical limitation to certain cross sections.

Calorimeters

A variety of calorimeters have been used to measure the total energy delivered to a whole-animal cadaver. Although this method is accurate in the determination of whole-body averaged SAR, it cannot provide information about the SAR distribution within the body.

Conclusions

The required sensitivity of better than 100 mW/kg for compliance tests can only be approximately achieved by thermistor probes, since the measurements must be performed within 20 s to avoid convection problems. On the other hand, the achievable spatial resolution is excellent. Because of the strong limitations on the minimum measurement time per spatial point, temperature measurements are not suitable for the implementation of a certification procedure for MTE. Nevertheless, temperature measurements at high power levels provide the most accurate means of calibrating electric field probes. If point measurements in very small structures (e.g. in a small animal cadaver) are of interest, temperature measurements are often the only possibility, because significantly smaller outlines can be realized compared to E-field probes, i.e. $<1\,\mathrm{mm}^2$. An example is given in Figure 2.7.

2.6.4   Electrical field measurement methods

Introduction

E-field probes have been utilized since the early 70s for experimental measurement of internal microwave fields (Johnson and Guy, 1972). The first prototype of a miniature isotropic diode loaded E-field probe for dosimetric assessments was presented by Bassen *et al.* (1975). The utilization of fiberoptical E-field sensors for dosimetric assessments was suggested as far back as 1978 (Bassen and Ross, 1978), although it has taken present day technology for commercial application.

Since the field polarization is unknown in the close near fields of radiators, only probes with an isotropic response in the tissue simulating material should be used. This is usually accomplished by measuring the field components with three orthogonal sensors. Because of the short wavelength in the tissue and since the induced field may have relatively large spatial gradients, the probe size should be as small as possible. Furthermore, the interaction of the probe with the field should be negligible.

These requirements are difficult to satisfy, because the usually fragile probes must be mounted on a supporting core and covered with an outer shell to strengthen the probe tip and to protect the single probes from contact with the tissue-simulating material. However, any dielectric material around electric probes has an effect on the local signal strength, depending on the surrounding material. A good orthogonal response in a particular material might be greatly impaired in another media. Ways of realizing isotropic probes within tissue-simulating materials have been discussed in Schmid and Kuster (1997). In addition, the sensitivity of these probes in lossy media depends upon the frequency and to a lesser extent on the relative permittivity of the media (Meier *et al.*, 1996a).

Diode-loaded dipole sensors

Isotropic diode-loaded dipole sensors consist of three small orthogonally arranged dipoles which are directly loaded with Schottky diodes. Direct conversion of the high frequency voltage across the gap into a DC voltage and highly resistive lines (RF transparent) are used to transmit the DC signal to the data acquisition unit. This approach is appropriate since the SAR is proportional to the square of the Hermitian magnitude $|\mathbf{E}|$ of the internal electric field vec-

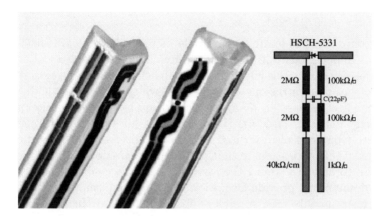

Fig. 2.9 Tips of 'rectangular' (left) and the 'triangular' (center) probes (without shell encasement) and the equivalent circuit representation of the probe (right). The employment of the thick-film technique permits the use of different sheet resistances on the same substrate. Reproduced from Schmid *et al.* (1996).

tor, i.e. SAR $\sim (|E_x|^2 + |E_y|^2 + |E_z|^2)$. Hence, information on the polarization is not needed. The first commercially available sensors used transmission lines of relatively low resistance per unit length $<50\,\mathrm{k\Omega/cm}$, realized either by carbon-impregnated Teflon strips or thin-film technology on a ceramic or quartz substrate. The theory of this type of probe has been discussed in various publications. An excellent review is given in Bassen and Smith (1983). A similar probe is still commercially available (NARDA, 1995).

The limitations of this approach are principally due to the secondary modes of reception, constructional asymetries, etc. These problems have recently been analyzed and an improved design has been presented, showing significantly improved performance compared to the previous approach (Schmid *et al.*, 1996) and (Pokovíc *et al.*, 1996). This was mainly achieved through incorporation of a distributed filter and a precise symmetrical construction. Two different isotropic configurations are shown in Figure 2.9. The 'triangular' design has proven to be very suitable for scanning the SAR distribution in tissue-simulating liquids over a frequency range of 10 MHz to >3 GHz. The 'rectangular' design, which has a slightly larger outline, was developed for use in air or low dielectric materials, for which an excellent isotropic response was achieved (Schmid and Kuster, 1997). Although the improved probe characteristics were obtained at the cost of increased demands on the signal amplifiers (increased source impedance of the probe of 5 to 8 MΩ), a high sensitivity and a broad dynamic range ($1\,\mu\mathrm{W/g}$ to $>100\,\mathrm{mW/g}$) has been realized by specialized data acquisition hardware and software. The probes and hardware are described in (Schmid *et al.*, 1996).

Fiberoptical E-field sensors

Several groups worldwide are currently developing fiberoptical E-field sensors for various applications (e.g. EMC, measurements on ICs, etc.) utilizing the Pockels effect. The Pockels effect describes the change in the optical dielectric permittivity of noncentrosymmetric crystals, which is linear with the electric field. This effect is used in many integrated optics devices to alter the real or imaginary index of refraction (i.e. tuning of a filter, optical switches, modulators, etc.) but can also be used to realize E-field sensors. The promising advantages of this approach are that these sensors are non-metallic, extremely broad band (practically from DC to several GHz) and enable measurements in the time domain, i.e. provide frequency and phase information. Such sensors are already commonly used in high voltage applications. In Kuwabara *et al.* (1992) a small wideband sensor realized on a $LiNbO_3$ substrate is presented, whereby the E-field induced in the crystal is enhanced by attached metallic dipole arms. Another approach has been recently presented, which is based on a CdTe (cadmium telluride) crystal and has relatively low permittivity (Cecelja *et al.*, 1994). The one-dimensional probe has no attached metallic dipole arms but a sensing crystal of about 10 mm length.

Calibration of E-field probes

Reliable and accurate standardized procedures must be available to calibrate E-field probes in different tissue-simulating liquids and to assess the uncertainties in assessing the spatial peak SAR values. Keeping uncertainties small is crucial for compliance tests, since all uncertainties must be added to the measured values. Large uncertainties would therefore unnecessarily enhance the compliance criteria and might imply severe economical consequences.

The calibration is equivalent to quantitatively determining the relationship between the field in the absence of the probe and the sensor signals. This depends on various factors:

- design and construction materials of the probe;
- electrical properties of the surrounding media;
- direction and polarization of the field;
- field gradient at the measurement site;
- higher order modes or different reception modes in the probe; and
- RF characteristics of the sensor, the transmission line and the processing circuit.

In addition to the calibration parameter, it is important to know the absolute uncertainty and the validity range of the calibration.

In view of the significance of, and the difficulties involved in, accurate calibration, surprisingly little has been published about broadband calibration of isotropic E-field probes in dielectric materials. In Hill (1982) a calibration procedure in an S-band waveguide at a single frequency of 2.45 GHz is described. However, the calibration uncertainties due to the dependence of the probe sensitivity on polarization, frequency, dielectric parameters of the surrounding media and spatial resolution have only been marginally addressed. In a recent study (Meier *et al.*, 1996a) these issues have been analyzed in detail and an experimental procedure has been developed which allows an absolute calibration of the probes for dosimetric assessments with an uncertainty of less than ±10%.

In addition, the possibility of determining the conversion factor (i.e. the ratio of the sensitivities in the tissue simulating liquid and in air) by numerical simulations has been investigated. For symmetrical probes, such as the 'triangular' probe in Figure 2.9, the conversion factor can be determined with a precision of about ±20% by numerical techniques. For other probe designs, the uncertainties of the numerically determined conversion factors might be larger. However, the numerical approach gives a good validation of the frequency and media dependence of the conversion factor.

Discussion

The required sensitivity for compliance tests of 10 V/m can easily be met by electrical field measurement methods. The loss of phase and frequency information is no disadvantage for the dosimetric analysis of near-field exposure, since the signal characteristic is known *a priori*. Although the smallest achievable dimensions are still considerably larger than those of temperature probes, they are sufficiently small for the measurements inside human phantoms and for the frequencies used by mobile communications. A disadvantage is that special calibration data are required for each material. However, this is not a problem for routine measurements such as device certifications, which are always conducted with a limited number of different tissues.

Fiberoptic sensors are currently not a real alternative to the diode-loaded sensors, because of the lack of sensitivity and mainly because of the significantly larger dimensions of the sensors and more expensive technology.

2.6.5   Automated dosimetric scanners

The experimental assessment of the three-dimensional SAR distribution within a phantom easily involves measurements in several hundred points. Especially at higher frequencies, the locations of these points with respect to the phantom must be determined with the greatest precision in order to obtain repeatable measurements in the presence of rapid spatial attenuation and field variations. High precision is also required to accurately evaluate the spatial peak SAR values. It is obvious that the measurement process must be highly automated if such measurements must be performed routinely.

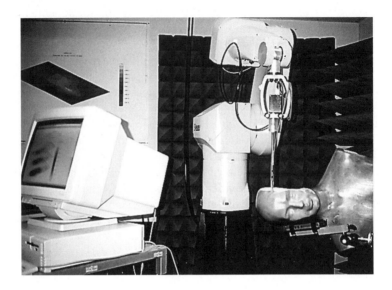

Fig. 2.10 Laboratory setup including robot, probe, data acquisition electronics, phantom and PC. Reproduced from Schmid *et al.* (1996).

This implies that those measurements are basically restricted to shell phantoms filled with a liquid simulating human tissue. However, as already discussed in Sections 2.3.1 and 2.5.4, this is no disadvantage with respect to certification procedures.

Although automated scanners based on temperature probes are possible, the maximum measurement speed would be unacceptably slow. Because of this and of the low sensitivity of temperature probes, only scanning systems based on E-field probes have been implemented so far. Systems developed in the 80s range from one-dimensional positioners (Cleveland and Athey, 1989) to three-axis scanners (Stuchly *et al.*, 1983) and on to six-axis robots (Balzano *et al.*, 1995). The first version of the latter goes back to the early 80s and has been continually improved and extended since then.

The first system designed for testing the compliance of MTE with safety limits is described in Schmid *et al.* (1996) and shown in Figure 2.10. It incorporates a high precision robot (working range greater than 0.9 m and a position repeatability of better than ±0.2 mm), isotropic E-field probes with diode loaded dipole sensors, an optical proximity sensor for automated positioning of the probe with respect to the phantom surface (precision better than ±0.2 mm) and sophisticated software for data processing and measurement control (Figure 2.11). The bandwidth ranges from 10 MHz to at least 3 GHz; the sensitivity is better than

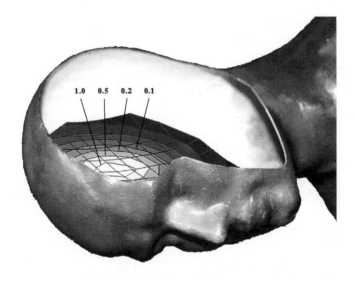

Fig. 2.11 SAR Distribution (mW/g) induced by a mobile phone measured with DASY2.

$1\,\mu\text{W/g}$. The dynamic range covers values up to $100\,\text{mW/g}$. Complex measurements, such as assessment of the spatial peak SAR value when starting with an unknown field distribution in the body, can be completed within 15 minutes. E-field probes and H-field probes for free space measurements have also been developed (Schmid and Kuster, 1997). The same system with improved performance and software capability has been made commercially available under the name DASY2 (DASY2, 1994). Another system based on a quite similar concept has recently been announced (IDX, 1996).

2.7   REVIEW OF NUMERICAL DOSIMETRY

2.7.1   Introduction

Theoretical approaches and numerical methods have provided important information on dosimetry in the frequency range of mobile communications since the early 60s. In the following an overview and assessment of various analytical and numerical methods are presented which have been applied to dosimetry and antenna design. For readers interested in the details of the methods, the most important references are given.

Analytical methods are restricted to very simple configurations. They nevertheless can provide valuable insights into the physical mechanisms and yield typical parameters.

Studies on complex-shaped nonhomogeneous bodies have been conducted using general-purpose codes for solving electromagnetic scattering problems. These codes are most reasonably classified into boundary and volume techniques. In boundary methods, space is divided into linear, homogeneous and isotropic domains, the boundaries of which are discretized. In volume techniques, on the other hand, the space is discretized directly. Depending on the method, this can entail problems with infinite domains. Boundary methods are obviously more efficient for geometrically simple configurations with a low surface/volume ratio, whereas volume methods are suitable for complex geometries and inhomogeneous materials.

2.7.2   Analytical and semi-analytical methods

Early findings on whole-body and locally enhanced absorption in biological bodies were obtained by studying homogeneous or layered spheres of tissue-like materials exposed to plane waves using the analytical Mie solution (Shapiro et al., 1971; Kritikos and Schwan, 1972;1975; Weil, 1975). The same approach has also been extended to prolate spheroids using spherical expansion (Ruppin, 1978).

The dependence of energy absorption on the polarization of an incident plane wave was studied using simple homogeneous prolate spheroids. Analytically based approximations were used, which were sometimes referred to as **long-wavelength analysis** based on perturbation theory (Durney, 1980). The frequency range for these homogeneous prolate spheroids was later expanded, using semi-analytical techniques, such as the **extended boundary condition method** (EBCM) and the **iterative extended boundary condition method** (IEBCM) (Iskander et al., 1983).

These studies on simple homogeneous prolate spheroids provided valuable insights into the absorption mechanism for plane wave exposure and helped to establish the exposure limits for the electric and magnetic fields that have found their way into all relevant safety standards. It is interesting to note that the investigations on simple structures have provided more useful dosimetric information than those done since the mid eighties on highly complex bodies.

The most complex analytical model for the dosimetry of mobile terminals has recently been presented by King (1995b).

It should be noted that theoretical methods sometimes require analytical approximations and may lead to integrals which can only be evaluated at high computational expense.

2.7.3   Method of moments (MoM)

The method of moments (MoM) was introduced in electrodynamics by Richmond (1965) and Harrington (1967) in the mid sixties. They originally presented MoM in a very general formulation for the solution of partial differential equations via a linear system of equations. The same approach is also known in other branches of numerical analysis under the names of method of weighted residuals, method of projection, Galerkin method, etc. Nowadays, the term MoM is restricted usually to those approaches that use an integral equation formulation, i.e. where charge and current distributions are discretized.

The method usually involves: (1) deriving the appropriate integral equation corresponding to the problem; (2) discretizing the unknown current distributions, usually with subsectional basis functions; (3) finding the moment equations, which entails derivation of the expansion functions via Green's function techniques, their numerical evaluation, and the evaluation of the testing integrals; (4) solving the linear system of equations, which usually has a dense symmetric matrix, in order to obtain the unknown parameters (e.g. current amplitudes).

Depending upon the particular application and the type of expansion functions, the numerical evaluation of the expansion functions and the singular behavior at the point of the expansion function itself can be quite expensive in terms of computational time.

MoM is especially popular for problems with perfectly conducting objects, such as antennas or scattering from other metal structures. Some external influences like a perfectly or finitely conducting ground, layered media, etc. can be introduced via the Green's functions, making their evaluation more difficult, but not increasing the number of unknowns.

A widely used MoM code is the Numerical Electromagnetic Code NEC, of which different versions and several commercial front-ends have been developed. NEC2 (NEC2, 1995) is currently publicly available, whereas the most recent version NEC4 is under strategic export limitations and not easily available outside the United States. A simpler but similar code is MiniNEC (MiniNEC, 1995). These, however, are not applicable for simulating MTE close to the human body, since lossy dielectric materials of arbitrary shape cannot be included.

A variant of MoM based on the tensor integral equation with volumetric discretization was applied in the mid-seventies to study the absorption in human-like phantoms (Livesay and Chen, 1974b). The body was subdivided into N blocks in which a constant volume current is expanded with one unknown for each spatial dimension. The electric field integral equation (EFIE) is evaluated in the centers of the cells. This leads to a system of equations with $3N$ unknowns and a dense matrix (Livesay and Chen, 1974a). Since the cost of the solution with a direct (i.e. non-iterative) method is roughly proportional to N^3, the problem size grows so fast that the method does not allow a reasonably fine discretization of the human body.

The boundary element method (BEM) can be considered either as a MoM or a finite element (FE) technique, if the surfaces of the scatterers are modeled with a finite element like surface mesh and finite element compatible basis functions. It is often used in conjunction with a space-discretizing finite element method (see Section 2.7.6) but can also be used as a standalone technique.

An implementation of a surface-discretization MoM which allows the modeling of arbitrary dielectrical and lossy domains uses – according to the equivalence principle – both electric and magnetic surface currents for each domain (Brüns et al., 1993). It has lately been successfully applied in the study of performance of antennas operating in the vicinity of homogeneous lossy bodies. The code CONCEPT is available in Brüns and Singer (1995)

As with many other methods, a difficulty of MoM is that error estimates for the uncertainty of the solution are difficult to obtain, since the solution is 'exact' within the approximation space, i.e. indirect error indicators have to be used.

Moment method matrix equations were originally solved by direct methods; iterative methods such as the conjugate gradient method have since been used. Recently, there have been some breakthroughs in iterative methods coupled with good preconditioners and a faster, approximate evaluation of the matrix-vector products that are used during the solution process. The resulting increase in calculation speed might again improve the competitiveness of the MoM approach.

There have been many publications on MoM. A classical reference is Harrington (1967); a newer and highly detailed book is Wang (1991); an overview with reprints of classical papers is given in Miller et al. (1991).

2.7.4   Generalized multipole technique (GMT)

During the eighties, several groups developed methods that were later unified under the name generalized multipole technique (GMT) (Ludwig, 1989). GMT refers to methods which approximate the unknown field in each domain by several sets of functions which, in contrast to MoM, do not have singularities within their respective domains or their boundaries. All of these functions are analytical solutions of Maxwell's equations for linear and homogeneous materials. As the name GMT implies, the most versatile and therefore dominant type of expansion functions are finite series of multipole solutions, although other types can be used as well, such as normal expansions, line multipoles, plane waves, waveguide modes, etc.

The expansions are matched in discrete points on the boundary of the domains, resulting in an overdetermined system of equations with a dense matrix. The overdetermination factor is typically between 2 and 10. This system is solved in the least squares sense, usually with QR-factorization methods (Golub and Van Loan, 1989).

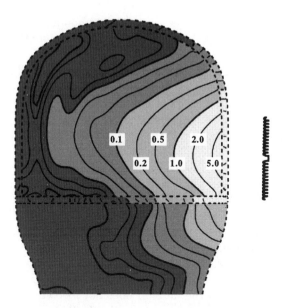

Fig. 2.12 Example of a dosimetric assessment performed by GMT. Illustrated is the SAR distribution in a simplified human head phantom exposed by a symmetrical helix (frequency: 900 MHz; total number of turns: 24; length = 60 mm; helix diameter: 4 mm; wire diameter = 0.5 mm) at a distance of 25 mm. The skull is 5 mm thick ($\epsilon_r = 4.9$, $\sigma = 0.15$ mho/m); the interior of the skull is filled with brain-simulating material ($\epsilon_r = 41$, $\sigma = 0.77$ mho/m); and the rest of the body is simulated as muscle tissue ($\epsilon_r = 55$, $\sigma = 1.45$ mho/m). Reproduced from Kuster (1993).

Since the global expansion functions of the GMT are very well behaved at the boundaries, the accuracy close to the boundaries is very high, which is important for dosimetric applications. A crucial advantage of the GMT, however, lies in the fact that the residual errors resulting from the least squares technique can be employed to validate the quality of the result (Kuster, 1993). Since the largest errors usually occur at the boundaries, the accuracy of the entire solution can be easily estimated (Regli, 1993). Furthermore, the error distribution is useful for improving the numerical model. The GMT therefore leads to very reliable dosimetric assessments. Since this method is closely related to analytical methods, accurate simulation of scattering problems ranging many orders of magnitudes of field strength are possible.

The severe limitation of GMT is its lack of robustness for simulating complex configurations. In contrast to MoM, in which subsectional basis functions are equivalent to a compact current, a GMT expansion is equivalent to a current distribution over the whole boundary of the domain. For geometrically complex bodies, the selection and placement of the expansion functions is not quite obvious and requires considerable expertise. Although automated approaches have been developed, the applicability of GMT remains limited to geometrically simple bodies (Figure 2.12).

The method is described in more detail in Hafner (1990). The software package 3D-MMP, which is based on the GMT, is commercially available (Hafner and Bomholt, 1993) with a graphic interface for the PC. The code has been successfully applied for dosimetric studies (Kuster and Balzano, 1992; Kuster, 1992b), as well as for antenna design (Tay and Kuster, 1994).

2.7.5   Finite-difference time-domain (FDTD)

Although the finite-difference approach can also be applied in the frequency domain, the finite-difference time-domain (FDTD) method is much more popular. Maxwell's equations are directly discretized in space as well as in time on a staggered Yee-grid (Yee, 1966) in an explicit scheme. Starting from an initial solution with zero field, the solution is directly computed in the time domain time-step by time-step, i.e. the method does not involve the solution of a matrix equation. Since the entire volume must be divided into cells, the number of unknowns is very large. However, the computational effort grows only linearly with the number of unknowns and the number of cells. Thus, the method scales much better to large problems than other techniques. The technique was first proposed by Yee (1966) and since then has been extensively studied and improved. The time-domain transmission-line matrix method (TD-TLM) (Hoefer, 1989) and the finite-integration technique (FIT) (Weiland, 1990) are conceptually slightly different methods which, however, lead to the same numerical scheme.

For a long time, the applications of the method were limited by the relatively large requirements for computational power in both memory size and processor performance. On the other hand, the algorithm is very easy to vectorize or parallelize.

Many other early limitations of the method have been eliminated. Several approaches for absorbing boundary conditions at the boundary of the computational domain have been developed (Mur, 1981; Berenger, 1994, Berntsen and Hornsleth, 1995), offering an excellent approximation of open space with a minimum of 'white space'. An approximation for the frequency dependent media water in the time domain has been reported in (Taflove, 1988), which allows results for a wide range of frequencies to be obtained from a single time domain solution.

A great advantage but also limiting factor is the extremely simple yet rigid and inflexible discretization of problems within the Yee-grid. Data conversion from CAD files to Yee-grids can be accomplished by simple routines, and even very complicated structures like biological bodies are relatively easy to discretize from magnetic resonant images (Figures 2.1 and 2.13). However, within

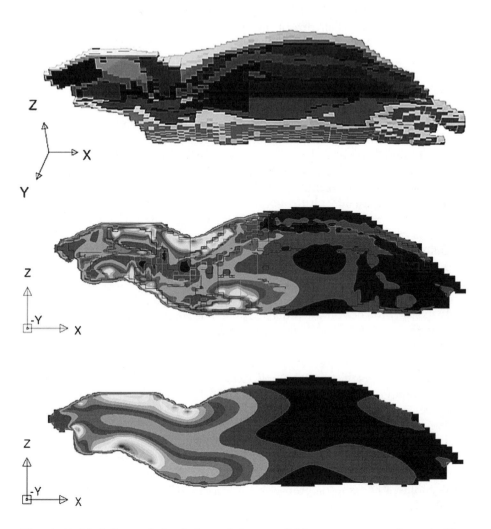

Fig. 2.13 Modeling and simulations of the near-field exposure setup shown in Figure 2.3 were performed to assess the field distribution induced in the brain tissue as well as the averaged whole-body SAR. The simulations were performed with the FIT code MAFIA. Top: discretization of the rat: 13 different tissues were identified; the voxel size was $1.5 \times 1 \times 1\,\mathrm{cm}^3$, yielding a total number of 300 000 voxels. Center: SAR distribution in the center sagittal plane. The maximum value is $3.2\,\mathrm{mW/cm}^3$ for an antenna input power of 1 W. The SAR distribution corresponds well with the experimentally determined values (see Figure 2.7). Bottom: simulation of the corresponding homogeneous model with the electromagnetic properties of brain tissue. The scale is linear. Reproduced from Burkhardt *et al.*, 1997.

this grid, local refinement, such as in finite-element meshes, is not possible, and all surfaces must be aligned with the grid orientation or modeled in a staircase approximation. Although several extensions of the method for circumventing these weaknesses have been studied, they are not generally applicable. They also complicate the modeling and reduce the numerical efficiency, accuracy and stability of the method.

Another weak point of the method is that there is no internal check for assessing the quality of the solution, i.e. the quantitative uncertainty of the resulting field distribution. Coarse discretization or overly small distances between scatterer and absorbing boundaries can cause errors which are difficult to detect. This is particularly vexing since FDTD is often applied to very complex configurations, where the significance of details or uncertainties due to modeling approximations are difficult to quantify *a priori*. In practice, apart from solving the problems with different discretization densities, calibration with canonical problems paired with a dose of faith is still the only validation technique used.

Taflove was the first to use FDTD for dosimetric problems (Umashankar and Taflove, 1975). Since the mid-eighties, Gandhi and his group (Gandhi, 1990) have extensively applied this technique to a wide range of dosimetric problems. Most recently, several groups have been using this technique specifically to study the dosimetric problems of mobile communications, e.g. Pedersen and Andersen (1994), Dimbylow and Mann (1994), Jensen and Rahmat-Samii (1995), Hombach *et al.* (1996).

The method is also used for antenna design and has produced excellent results, at least for geometrically simple structures which fit well into the Yee-grid. However, major difficulties are encountered if fine wire which does not align to the grid or structures smaller than the grid size, e.g. small helices to feed the antenna.

Recently, books on FDTD have been published that give a complete overview and have extensive further references (Taflove, 1995; Kunz and Luebbers, 1993). Several codes have been made commercially available. Among those which have been applied to dosimetric problems are MAFIA (CST, 1994), XFDTD (1996) and EMIT (1996).

2.7.6   Finite-element method (FE)

The method of finite elements was introduced to electromagnetics by Silvester and Ferrari (1996). Space is discretized in a finite-element mesh with linear or polynomial expansion functions within each element. The unknowns are associated with the field values in the nodes. A variational method or a method of weighted residuals is used to obtain a system of equations with a sparse matrix.

In wave propagation problems, the finite-element technique is generally used in the frequency domain. For quite some time, its applicability for solving the

Helmholtz equation was very limited because of problems with spurious modes (Sun *et al.*, 1995; Lynch *et al.*, 1985). Open domains were another limitation, since no efficient radiation boundary conditions were available. Therefore, the finite-element method was often paired with a boundary element method in a hybrid scheme (see next Section 2.7.7).

Although penalty methods can be used with the traditional finite-element technique in order to to avoid the corruption of results with spurious solutions (Lynch *et al.*, 1985), newer edge-element techniques, which prevent the possibility of spurious modes altogether (Bossavit, 1988; Jin, 1993), seem more promising. In the edge-element technique the unknowns are associated with the field tangential to the edges of the basic element, instead of the mesh vertices. The vector expansion functions that are used within the elements are tangential to all element surfaces which contain the edge and normal to all other surfaces. The edge-element technique is also much better suited to inhomogeneous problems, since no internal boundary conditions between elements with different electromagnetic properties need to be enforced. Furthermore, in contrast to the traditional finite-element technique, the edge-element technique possesses a direct way of controlling discretization errors in the solution by looking at the behavior of the normal components of the field between elements.

Recently, more efficient methods for open-space radiation boundary conditions have become available, and currently there is a lot of activity centered on the adaptation of Berenger-style boundary conditions (Berenger, 1994) to the finite-element technique. This makes hybrid combinations with the boundary element method for many applications obsolete, as discussed below.

The finite-element mesh is in principle highly flexible for discretizing almost arbitrary geometries. However, the generation of meshes in 3D is still a formidable task. While there are reasonably good techniques for the discretization of technical structures, the difficulty of generating finite-element models for the typically very inhomogeneous problems in dosimetry currently prevents widespread use. Nevertheless, the finite-element method has been used for 2D and 3D problems in hyperthermia treatment (Lynch *et al.*, 1985) and MRI dosimetry (Simunic *et al.*, 1995).

Since the introduction of absorbing boundary conditions, FE has also become a competitive method for antenna design, especially for antennas containing dielectric parts.

A good introductory textbook with many further references is Silvester and Ferrari (1996). Examples of commercial codes are Eminence (Ansoft, 1996), EMAS (MSC, 1996) and HFSS (1996).

2.7.7   Hybrid techniques

It becomes obvious from the above discussions that each of the various numerical methods has its particular strengths and limitations. Whereas a technique can be particularly efficient and well-suited for one kind of problem, it may have difficulties with others.

Many attempts have been made to combine different methods into a hybrid approach which has all the advantages and none of the disadvantages of the component methods.

The simplest hybrid simulation scheme is the unidirectional or explicit coupling of different methods. An example would be if the current distribution on a MTE simulated with a MoM code could be used as the excitation in dosimetry simulations performed with FDTD.

Many of the implicit hybrid techniques (i.e. where the methods are algorithmically coupled or unified) are combinations of the finite-element method with the boundary element method for simulating open space (Emson, 1988). Applications beyond the simple simulation of open space are rarely found. Many of these hybrid combinations were also 2D applications. In 3D, the absolute problem size is much larger and the relative sizes of the FE and the BEM problems shift, which makes the typical hybrid algorithm inefficient or impractical. Improvements in FE absorbing boundary conditions have made many of those hybrid codes obsolete.

A combination of FE with GMT has been presented in Bomholt (1994). This approach was subsequently generalized into a combination of MoM, GMT and FE within a iterative hybrid scheme (Bomholt, 1995). The advantage of this approach is that the solution of an explicitly combined matrix equation is avoided, which usually is the main obstacle for implementation and efficiency of hybrid techniques.

Further disadvantages of hybrid methods are that knowledge in several numerical methods is needed and that the coupling might lead to unexpected side-effects.

2.7.8   Discussion

FDTD is currently the most appropriate choice if highly inhomogeneous structures are to be analyzed for which boundary techniques have fundamental limitations. FE has the basic problem that there are no simple techniques for efficient 3D discretization of the complex structures as they occur in numerical dosimetry; its advantages can therefore not be exploited. Both methods have profited enormously from the advances in computer hardware; in the past supercomputers have been necessary to solve relevant problems.

On the other hand, simulations with strongly nonhomogeneous models are rarely necessary for most dosimetric computations. In fact, complexity not only makes the validation of the solution more difficult, but often reduces the general meaning and practical relevance of the results as well. For example, if the antenna in Figure 2.2 is shifted only slightly downwards, the spatial peak SAR would significantly change in the nonhomegeous phantom, whereas no changes will be observed for the homogeneous one. Another example illustrating the minor importance of simulating inhomogeneous bodies is the small change (<5%) of the SAR induced in the rat brain shown in Figure 2.13 when the rest of the body is homogeneously modeled. It should always be kept in mind that modeling of structure details which cause effects smaller than the assessable solution uncertainties is not only unnecessary, but also may mask major inaccuracies.

As a consequence, simple bodies, which can be considered as 'geometrically averaged' phantoms, are often superior for the study of physical effects and the derivation of absorption limits. Furthermore, validation is much easier for geometrically simple structures.

For the design of antennas with complex geometries, such as helix antennas, patch antennas, etc., MoM-based codes are still the most popular ones, although FDTD and FE are gaining ground. Fine details in the phantom are not necessary for the simulation of the radiation performance in the close vicinity of biological bodies, as they do not have significant influence on either the feed-point impedance of the antenna or the far field. A hybrid method using MoM for the antenna design and a different method for a simplified head phantom could be very competitive.

As illustrated in this chapter, the computational results published by different groups are difficult to compare. Since every group generates its own detailed phantoms, which are impossible to fully describe in publication, the cause of the differences is impossible to trace. Hence, a large improvement in the area of dosimetry would be achieved if a set of validated 'numerical phantoms' could be generated and made available. Apart from saving many people the expense of discretization and validation of the phantom, the cross-validation between several methods would also have a positive influence on the quality of the computational results.

2.8   CONCLUSIONS

Considerable progress has been achieved in experimental and numerical dosimetry during the last few years. Today a broad range of tools for dosimetric analysis for the frequency range of mobile communications is available.

Using existing tools, exposure setups for biological experiments can be dosimetrically evaluated, analyzed and optimized in great detail. However, an accurate analysis still requires a high level of expertise and should be performed by specialized groups.

The state of the art in experimental dosimetry provides all the instrumentation and knowhow necessary for the implementation of a certification procedure for handheld MTE. A procedure must now be defined by standardization agencies. Time is pressing, since an analysis of various MTE currently available on the market demonstrates that the spatial peak SAR values for some MTE used

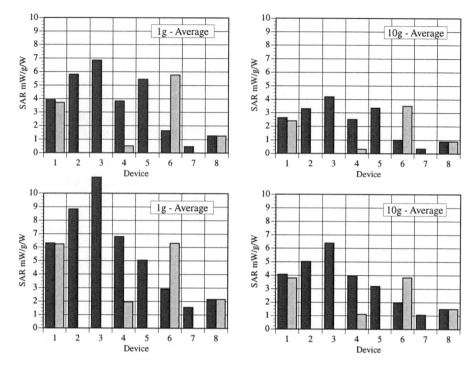

Fig. 2.14 Comparison of the 1 g and 10 g averaged spatial peak SAR exposures of commercially available devices operating in the frequency band of 900 MHz. Top: a position comparable to the intended use position. Bottom: a position in which the MTE was tilted until the antenna touched the shell of the phantom (in general the angle was considerably larger than the 100° suggest as the maximum angle in Section 2.5.3. The measurements were performed with DASY2 and a shell phantom filled with brain simulating liquid ($\epsilon_r = 42$, $\sigma = 0.9$ mho/m). Since the devices operate within different systems, the power was normalized to 1 W antenna input power. Dark grey: fully extended antenna; light grey: fully retracted antenna.

in cellular systems are close to the safety limits (Figures 2.14 and 2.15). The same figures show a strong dependence of the absorption upon MTE design. Hence, the manufacturers urgently need the basis on which they can optimize the devices in order to meet the exposure limits. Any further delay cannot be in the interest of manufacturers, service providers or consumers.

A reduction of the absorbed power would be even more beneficial for system performance. Under some conditions more than 50% of the input power is absorbed in the user and is lost for communications purposes (see Figure 2.4). Any improvement would reduce the battery size or extend the operational time of the device. Compared to the amount invested into battery technology, little

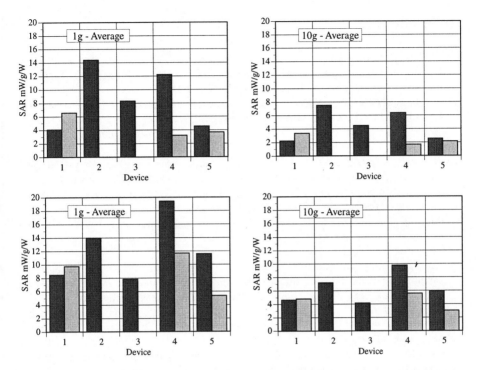

Fig. 2.15 Comparison of the 1 g and 10 g averaged spatial peak SAR exposures of commercially available devices operating in the frequency band of 1800 MHz. Top: a position comparable to the intended use position. Bottom: a position in which the MTE was tilted until the antenna touched the shell of the phantom (in general the angle was considerably larger than the 100° suggest as the maximum angle in Section 2.5.3. The measurements were performed with DASY2 and a shell phantom filled with brain simulating liquid ($\epsilon_r = 41$, $\sigma = 1.65$ mho/m). Since the devices operate within different systems, the power was normalized to 1 W antenna input power. Dark grey: fully extended antenna; light grey: fully retracted antenna.

has been done to utilize the great potential of optimizing the radiation efficiency of the device when operated close to the head. Improvements of several dBs are possible with appropriate design measures (also see Figures 2.14 and 2.15).

Although numerical simulation codes have been used to analyze different antennas (Pedersen and Andersen, 1994; Fuhl *et al.*, 1994), none of the codes available can be considered to be an effective CAD tool for antenna design. This is an area in which considerable progress in computational techniques is still needed.

REFERENCES

ANSI (1974) *ANSI C95.1-1974: An American National Standard; Safety Levels of Electromagnetic Radiation with Respect to Personnel.* The Institute of Electrical and Electronics Engineers, Inc., New York, NY 10017.

ANSI (1982) *ANSI C95.1-1982: American National Standard Safety Levels with Respect to Human Exposure to Radio Frequency Electromagnetic Fields, 300 kHz to 100 GHz.* The Institute of Electrical and Electronics Engineers, Inc., New York, NY 10017.

ANSI (1992) *ANSI/IEEE C95.1-1992: IEEE Standard for Safety Levels with Respect to Human Exposure to Radio Frequency Electromagnetic Fields, 3 kHz to 300 GHz.* The Institute of Electrical and Electronics Engineers, Inc., New York, NY 10017.

Ansoft (1996) *Maxwell Eminence.* Ansoft Corperation, Pittsburgh, USA.

Balzano, Q., Garay, O., and Manning, T.J. (1995) Electromagnetic energy exposure of simulated users of portable cellular telephones. *IEEE Transactions on Vehicular Technology,* 44(3), 390–403.

Balzano, Q., Garay, O., and Steel, F.R. (1977) Energy deposition in biological tissue near portable radio transmitters at VHF and UHF. *Conference Record of the 27th Conference of IEEE Transactions on Vehicular Technology Group,* pages 25–39.

Balzano, Q., Garay, O., and Steel, F.R. (1978a) Energy deposition in simulated human operators of 800 MHz portable transmitters. *IEEE Transactions on Vehicular Technology,* 27(4), 174–188.

Balzano, Q., Garay, O., and Steel, F.R. (1978b) Heating of biological tissue in the induction field of VHF portable radio transmitters. *IEEE Transactions on Vehicular Technology,* 27(2), 51–56.

Bassen, H.I. and Ross, R. (1978) An optically-linked telemetry system for use with electromagnetic field hazard probes. *IEEE Transactions on Electromagnetic Compatibility,* 20(5), 483–488.

Bassen, H.I. and Smith, G.S. (1983) Electric field probes – a review. *IEEE Transactions on Antennas and Propagation,* 31(5), 710–718.

Bassen, H.I., Swicord, M., and Abita, J. (1975) A miniature broad-band electric field probe. *Annals New York Academy of Science,* 20(5), 481–493.

Berenger, J. (1994) A perfectly matched layer for the absorption of electromagnetic waves. *Journal of Computational Physics,* 4, 185–200.

Berntsen, S. and Hornsleth, S. (1995) Retarded time absorbing boundary condition. *IEEE Transactions on Antennas and Propagation,* 42(8), pp. 1059–1064.

Bomholt, L.H. (1994) Coupling of the generalized multipole technique and the finite element method. *Applied Computational Electromagnetics Society Journal,* 9(3), 63–68.

Bomholt, L.H. (1995) A hybrid platform for computational electrodynamics integrating generalized multipole technique, method of moments and finite element technique. Zürich.

Bossavit, A. (1988) A rationale for 'edge elements' in 3-D fields computations. *IEEE Transactions on Magnetics,* 24, 74–79.

Bowman, R.R. (1976) A probe for measuring temperature in radio-frequency-heated material. *IEEE Transactions on Microwave Theory and Techniques,* 24(1), 43–45.

Brüns, H.-D. and Singer, H. (1995) Leistungsbeschreibung für das Rechenprogramm

Concept II. *Technical report, Technische Universität Hamburg-Harburg, W2100 Hamburg 90, Germany.*

Brüns, H.-D., Singer, H., and Mader, T. (1993) Field distributions of a handheld transmitter due to the influence of the human body. In *Proc. of the 9th Symposium on Electromagnetic Compatibility*, pages 0–14, Zürich.

Bundesamt für Gesundheit (1993) Gefährdet das moderne drahtlose Telefonieren die Gesundheit. *Technical report, Bundesamt für Gesundheit (BAG)*, Bulletin 22, Bern.

Burkhardt, M., Poković, K., Gnos, M. *et al.* (1996) Numerical and experimental dosimetry of petri dish exposure setups. *Journal of the Bioelectromagnetic Society* (in press).

Burkhardt, M., Spinelli, Y., and Kuster, N. Exposure setup to test CNS effects of wireless communications systems. *Health Physics* (submitted).

Cecelja, F., Balachandran, W., Berwick, M. *et al.* (1994) High precision, high frequency electromagnetic field optical sensors. *Proceeding of the COST244 Meetings*, XIII/J31/94-FR, pages 190–208.

CENELEC (1995) *CENELEC CLC/TC111B: European Prestandard (prENV 50166-2), Human Exposure to Electromagnetic Fields High-Frequency: 10 kHz – 300 GHz.* CENELEC, Brussels.

Cetas, T.C. (1978) Practical thermometry with a thermographic camera – calibration, and emittance measurements. *Rev. Sci. Instrum.*, **49**(2), 245–254.

Chatterjee, I., Gu, Y.-G., and Gandhi, O.P. (1985) Quantification of electromagnetic absorption in humans from body-mounted communication transceivers. *IEEE Transactions on Vehicular Technology*, **34**(2), 55–62.

Cleveland, R.F. and Athey, W.T. (1989) Specific absorption rate (SAR) in models of the human head exposed to handheld UHF portable radios. *Bioelectromagnetics*, **10**(1), 173–186.

CST (1994) *The MAFIA Collaboration, User's Guide Mafia Version 3.x.* CST GmbH, Lautenschlaegerstr. 38, D 64289 Darmstadt.

DASY2 (1994) Dosimetric Assessment System 2 (DASY2), Schmid & Partner Engineering AG, Staffelstrasse 8, 8045 Zurich, Switzerland.

Davis, C.C., Katona, G.A., Taylor, L.S. *et al.*(1996) *Dielectric Measurement of Tissues in the Mammalian Head at Cellular Telephone Frequencies.* Proceedings of the 18th Annual Meeting of the Bioelectromagnetic Society, pages 46–47, Victoria, B.C., Canada, June 9-14.

Dimbylow, P.J. and Mann, S. (1994) SAR calculations in an anatomically realistic model of the head for mobile communication transceivers at 900 MHz – 1.8 GHz. *Phys. Med. Biol.*, **39**(12), 1537–1553.

DIN/VDE (1984) *DIN 57 848 Teil 2/ VDE 0848 Teil 2: Sicherheit in elektromagnetischen Feldern – Schutz von Personen im Frequenzbereich von 30 kHz bis 300 GHz.* Deutsche Norm, VDE-Verlag GMBH, Berlin 12.

Durney, C.H. (1980) Electromagnetic dosimetry for models of humans and animals: a review of theoretical and numerical techniques. *Proceedings of the IEEE*, **68**(1), 33–40.

EMIT (1996) *EMI Toolbox.* SETH Corpration, Johnstown, PA 15905, USA.

Emson, C.R.I. (1988) Methods for the solution of open-boundary electromagnetic-field problems. *IEEE Proceeding*, **3**.

Foster K.R. (1995) Dielectric properties of tissues, in *The Biomedical Engineering*

Handbook, pages 1385–1394, CRC Press, Inc.

Fuhl, J., Nowak, P., and Bonek, E. (1994) Improved internal antenna for handheld terminals. *Electronics Letters*, **30**(22), 1816–1818.

Fujiwara, O., Higashihama, H., and Azzakami, T. (1990) Calculation of face-SAR due to portable transmitter. *Proc. International Wroclaw Symposium on Electromagnetic Compatibility.*

Gandhi, O.P. (1990) Numerical methods for specific absorption rate calculations, in *Biological Effects and Medical Applications of Electromagnetic Energy* (ed O. P. Gandhi), Prentice Hall Advanced Reference Seriespages, 113–140.

Golub, G.H. and Van Loan, C.F. (eds) (1989) *Matrix Computations.* Johns Hopkins University Press, 2nd edition.

Guy, A.W. (1971) Analyses of electromagnetic fields induced in biological tissue by thermographic studies on equivalent phantom models. *IEEE Transactions on Microwave Theory and Techniques*, **19**(2), 205–213.

Guy, A.W. (1984) Average SAR and SAR distribution in man exposed to 450 MHz radiofrequency radiation. *IEEE Transactions on Microwave Theory and Techniques*, **32**, 752–763.

Guy, A.W. and Chou, C.-K. (1986) Specific absorption rates of energy in man models exposed to cellular UHF mobile-antenna fields. *IEEE Transactions on Microwave Theory and Techniques*, **34**(6), 671–680.

Hafner, C. (1990) *The Generalized Multipole Technique for Computational Electromagnetics.* Artech House Books.

Hafner, C. and Bomholt, L.H. (eds) (1993) *The 3D Electrodynamic Wave Simulator.* New York: John Wiley & Sons Inc.

Harrington, R.F. (1967) Matrix methods for field problems. *Proc. IEEE*, volume **55**, pages 136–149.

Hartsgrove, G., Kraszewski, A., and Surowiec, A. (1987) Simulated biological materials for electromagnetic radiation absorption studies. *Bioelectromagnetics*, **8**(1), 29–36.

HFSS (1996). *High Frequency Structure Simulator.* Hewlett Packard, USA

Hill, D. (1982) Waveguide technique for the calibration of miniature implantable electric-field probes for use in microwave-bioeffects studies. *IEEE Transactions on Microwave Theory and Techniques*, **30**, 92–99.

Hoefer, W.J.R. (1989) *The Transmission Line Matrix (TLM) Method.* T. Itoh, John Wiley & Sons.

Hombach, V., Meier, K., Burkhardt, M. *et al.* (1996) The dependence of EM energy absorption upon human head modeling at 900 MHz. *IEEE Transactions on Microwave Theory and Techniques*, **44**(10) (in press).

IDX Systems Inc. (1996) *Near Field Measurement Systems*, 20 NE Granger Ave Bldg. B, Coryallis OR 97330.

IEEE (1992) *IEEE C95.3-1992: Recommended Practice for the Measurement of Potentially Hazardous Electromagnetic Fields – RF and Microwave.* The Institute of Electrical and Electronics Engineers, Inc., New York, NY 10017.

IRPA (1988) International non-ionizing radiation committee of the international radiation protection association: Guidelines on limits of exposure to radiofrequency electromagnetic fields in the frequency range from 100 kHz to 300 GHz. *Health Physics*, **54**(1), 115–123.

Iskander, M.F., Lakhtakia, A., and Durney, C.H. (1983) A new procedure for improving the solution stability and extending the frequency range of the EBCM. *IEEE Transactions on Antennas and Propagation*, **31**(2), 317–324.

Jensen, M.A. and Rahmat-Samii, Y. (1995) EM interaction of handset antennas and a human in personal communications. *Proceeding of the IEEE*, **83**(1), 7–17.

Jin, J. (1993) *The Finite Element Method in Electromagnetics*. Wiley.

Johnson, C. and Guy, A.W. (1972) Nonionizing electromagnetic wave effects in biological meterials and systems. *Proc. IEEE*, **60**, 692–718.

King, R.W.P. (1995) Electromagnetic field generated in model of human head by simplified telephone transceivers. *Radio Science*, **30**(1), 267–281.

Kritikos, H.N. and Schwan, H.P. (1972) Hot spots generated in conducting spheres by electromagnetic waves and biological implications. *IEEE Transactions on Biomedical Engineering*, **19**(1), 53–58.

Kritikos, H.N. and Schwan, H.P. (1975) The distribution of heating potential inside lossy spheres. *IEEE Transactions on Biomedical Engineering*, **22**(6), 457–463.

Kunz, K.S. and Luebbers, R.J. (1993) *The finite difference time domain method for electromagnetics*. CRC Press.

Kuster, N. (1992a) Messung und Berechnung zur absorbierten Hochfrequenzenergie bei körpernah betriebenen Antennen, in *Schutz vor elektromagnetischer Strahlung beim Mobilfunk* (ed SSK), Gustav Fischer Verlag, pages 107–125.

Kuster, N. (1992b) Multiple multipole method applied to an exposure safety study, in *ACES Special Issue on Bioelectromagnetic Computations* (eds A. Fleming and K. H. Joyner), Applied Computational Electromagnetics Society No. 2, volume **7**, pages 43–60.

Kuster, N. (1992c) Dosimetric Assessment of EM Sources Near Biological Bodies by Computer Simulations. *Diss. ETH Nr.9697*, Zurich.

Kuster, N. (1993) Multiple multipole method for simulating EM problems involving biological bodies. *IEEE Transactions on Biomedical Engineering*, **40**(7), 611–620.

Kuster, N. and Ballisti, R. (1989) MMP-method simulation of antennae with scattering objects in the closer nearfield. *IEEE Transactions on Magnetics*, **25**(4), 2881–2883. Third Biennial IEEE Conference on Electromagnetic Field Computation.

Kuster, N. and Balzano, Q. (1992) Energy absorption mechanism by biological bodies in the near field of dipole antennas above 300 MHz. *IEEE Transactions on Vehicular Technology*, **41**(1), 17–23.

Kuwabara, N., Kimihiro T. and Amemiya, F. (1992) Development and analysis of electric field sensor using $LiNbO_3$ optical modulator. *IEEE Transactions on Electromagnetic Compatibility*, **34**(4), 391–396.

Livesay, D.E. and Chen, K.-M. (1974a) Electromagnetic fields induced inside arbitrarily shaped biological bodies. *IEEE Transactions on Microwave Theory and Techniques*, **22**(9), 1273–1280.

Livesay, D.E. and Chen, K.M. (1974b) Electromagnetic fields induced inside arbitrary shaped biological bodies. *IEEE Transactions on Microwave Theory and Techniques*, **32**(12), 1273–1280.

Ludwig, A. (1989) A new technique for numerical electromagnetics. *IEEE AP-S Newsletter*, **31**, 40–41.

Lynch, D.R., Paulsen, K.D., and Strohbehn, J.W. (1985) Finite element solution of maxwell's equations for hyperthermia treatment planning. *Journal of Computa-*

tional Physics, **58**, 246–269.

MSC (1996) *EMAS*. MacNeal-Schwendler Corporation, Los Angeles, USA.

Meier, K. (1996) Scientific bases for dosimetric compliance tests of mobile telecommunications equipment. *Diss. ETH Nr.11722*, Zurich.

Meier, K., Burkhardt, M., Schmid, T. *et al.* (1996a) Broadband calibration of E-field probes in lossy media. *IEEE Transactions on Microwave Theory and Techniques*, **44**(10) (in press).

Meier, K., Egger, O., Schmid, T. *et al.* (1995) Dosimetric laboratory for mobile communications. In *Proc. of the 11th Symposium on Electromagnetic Compatibility*, pages 297–300, Zürich, Switzerland, March 7–9.

Meier, K., Kästle, R., Hombach, V. *et al.* (1997) The dependence of EM energy absorption upon human head modeling at 1800 MHz. *IEEE Transactions on Microwave Theory and Techniques* (submitted).

Meier, K., Kästle, R., and Schmid, T. (1996b) Abschlussbericht zum Projekt: Entwicklung von Phantomen zur standardisierten dosimetrischen Typenprüfung im Mobilfunk. Forschungsbericht Projekt Nr. 2-80-531-95, Institut für Feldtheorie und Höchstfrequenztechnik, ETH Zurich, 8092 Zurich, Switzerland.

Meier, K. and Kuster, N. (1995) Dosimetric measurements on various GSM-mobile telephones. *Proc. of the 17th Annual Meeting of the Bioelectromagnetics Society*, page 30, Boston, USA, June 18–22.

Microwave Consultants (1994) Dielectric database. *Microwave Consultants Ltd.*, London

Miller, E.K., Medgyesi-Mitschan, L., and Newmann, E.H. (eds) (1991) *Computational Electromagnetics – Frequency Domain Method of Moments*. IEEE Press.

MiniNEC (1995) MiniNEC Professional – EM Scientific Inc., 2533 N. Carson Street, Suite 2107, Carson City, NV 89706.

Mur, G. (1981) Absorbing boundary conditions for the finite-difference approximation of the time-domain electromagnetic field equations. *IEEE Transactions on Electromagnetic Compatibility*, **23**, 377–382.

NARDA (1995) E-Field Probe No. 8021B, The NARDA Microwave Corporation, 435 Moreland Road, Hauppauge, New York, NY 11788-3994.

NCRP (1986) National Council on Radiation Protection and Measurement: Biological effects and exposure criteria for radiofrequency electromagnetic fields. *NCRP Report No. 86*, 7910 Woodmont Avenue, Bethesda, MD. 20814.

NEC2 (1995) NEC2 – Developed at Lawrence Livermore National Laboratory, available by anonymous ftp from ftp.netcom.com.

Nojima, T., Kobayashi, T., Yamada, K. *et al.* (1991) Ceramic dry-phantom and its application to SAR estimation. In *IEEE MTT-S Digest*, pages OF–I–11.

NRPB (1986) *National Radiological Protection Board: Advice on the Protection of Workers and Members of the Public from Possible Hazards of Electric and Magnetic Fields with Frequencies Below 300 GHz*. NRPB, Chilton, Didcot, Oxon OX11 0RQ.

Pedersen, G.F. and Andersen, J.B. (1994) Integrated antennas for handheld telephones with low absorption. In *IEEE Vehicular Technology Conference 44rd*, pages 1537–1541, Stockholm, Sweden.

Pethig, P. (1984) Dielectric properties of biological materials: Biophysical and medical applications. *IEEE Transactions on Electrical Insulation*, **19**(5), 453–474.

Poković, K., Schmid, T., and Kuster, N. (1996) E-field probe with improved isotropy in brain simulating liquids. In *Proceedings of the ELMAR*, page 172–175, Zadar, Croatia, 23–25 June.

Regli, P. (1993) *Estimating the far field accuracy of MMP results*. Workshop Proceedings, 2nd Intern. Conference and Workshop on Approximations and Numerical Methods for the Solution of the Maxwell Equations, The George Washington University.

Richmond, J.H. (1965) Digital computer solutions of the rigorous equations for scattering problems. *Proc. IEEE*, **53**, pages 796–804.

Ruppin, R. (1978) Calculation of electromagnetic energy absorption in prolate spheroids by the point matching method. *IEEE Transactions on Microwave Theory and Techniques*, **26**(2), 87–90.

Schmid, T., Egger, O., and Kuster, N. (1996) Automated E-field scanning system for dosimetric assessments. *IEEE Transactions on Microwave Theory and Techniques*, **44**, 105–113.

Schmid, T. and Kuster, N. (1997) Novel E-field probes for close near field scanning, (submitted).

Shapiro, A.R., Lutomirski, R.F., and Yura, H.T. (1971) Induced fields and heating within a cranial structure irradiated by an electromagnetic plane wave. *IEEE Transactions on Biomedical Engineering*, **19**(2), 187–196.

Silvester, P.P. and Ferrari, R.F. (1996) *Finite Elements for Electrical Engineers*. Cambridge University Press, Cambridge UK.

Simunic, D., Wach, P., Renhart, W. *et al.* (1995) RF energy deposition in the human head during magnetic resonance imaging. *Electromagnetic Compatibility, 11th International Zurich Symposium*, pages 275–278.

Strahlenschutzkommission (1992) Empfehlung der Strahlenschutzkommission verabschiedet auf der 107. Sitzung am 12./13. Dezember 1991. *Schutz vor elektromagnetischer Strahlung beim Mobilfunk*, pages 3–18. Gustav Fischer Verlag.

Stuchly, M.A., Kraszewski, A., Stuchly, S.S. *et al.* (1987) RF energy deposition in a hetrogeneous model of man: Near- field exposures. *IEEE Transactions on Biomedical Engineering*, **34**(12), 944–950.

Stuchly, M.A., Spiegel, R.J., Stuchly, S.S. *et al.* (1986a) Exposure of man in the near-field of a resonant dipole: Comparison between theory and measurement. *IEEE Transactions on Microwave Theory and Techniques*, **34**(1), 27–31.

Stuchly, S.S., Barski, M., Tam, B. *et al.* (1983) Computer-based scanning system for electromagnetic scanning. *Rev. Sci. Instrum.*, **54**(11), 1547–1550.

Stuchly, S.S., Stuchly, M.A., Kraszewski, A. *et al.* (1986b) Energy deposition in a model of man: Frequency effects. *IEEE Transactions on Biomedical Engineering*, **33**(7), 702–711.

Sun, D., Manges, J., Yuan, X. *et al.* (1995) Spurious modes in finite-element methods. *IEEE Antennas and Propagation Magazine*, **37**(5), 12.

Taflove, A. (1988) Finite-difference time-domain (FDTD) modeling of electromagnetic wave scattering and interaction problems. *IEEE AP-S Newsletter*, pages 5–20.

Taflove, A. (1995) *Compuational Electrodynamics: The Finite-Difference Time-Domain Method*. Artech House.

Tay, R.Y. and Kuster, N. (1994) Performance of the generalized multipole technique (GMT/MMP) for antenna design and optimization. *Applied Computational Electromagnetics (ACES) journal*, **9**(3), 79–89.

TTC/MPT (1990) Protection guidelines for human exposure to radiofrequency electromagnetic waves. *A Report of Telecommunications Technology Council for the Ministry of Posts and Telecommunications, Deliberation No. 38.*

Umashankar, K. and Taflove, A. (1975) A novel method to analyze electromagnetic scattering of complex objects. *IEEE Transactions on Electromagnetic Compat.*, **25**(2), 623–660.

Wang, J.J.H. (1991) *Generalized Moment Methods in Electromagnetics.* Wiley.

Weil, C.M. (1975) Absorption characteristics of multilayered sphere models exposed to UHF/Microwave radiation. *IEEE Transactions on Biomedical Engineering*, **22**(6), 468–476.

Weiland, T. (1990) Maxwell's grid equations. *Frequenz*, **44**(1), 9–16.

Wickersheim, K.A. and Sun, M.H. (1987) Fiberoptic thermometry and its application. *Journal of Microwave Power*, pages 85–93.

XFDTD *XFDTD.* Remcom Inc., Calder Square, P.O. Box 10023, State College, PA 16805-0023, USA.

Yee, K.S. (1966) Numerical solution of initial boundary value problems involving Maxwell's equations in isotropic media. *IEEE Transactions on Antennas and Propagation*, **14**, 585–589.

3

RF interference (RFI) of medical devices by mobile communications transmitters

Howard I. Bassen

3.1 INTRODUCTION

In the early 1990s a significant increase in reports of medical device failures from electromagnetic interference (EMI) was noted worldwide (Silberberg, 1993; 1994; Segal *et al.*, 1995). A primary cause of this EMI was identified as radiated radiofrequency (RF) fields emitted by mobile communications transmitter/receivers (transceivers). The increase in reports of medical device failures was due to several factors. These factors included (1) a great increase in the number of electronically-controlled medical devices and (2) a significant increase in the number of sources of RF in the environment. Throughout hospitals and medical facilities ('the clinical environment') new medical devices utilizing electronics were installed. Outside the clinical environment, there was and continues to be a great increase in the use of electronically-controlled medical devices. These devices are used in the home, attached to patients, or implanted in their bodies. Often, the newer medical devices were more sensitive to radiofrequency interference (RFI). This was due to the increasing use of low-power integrated electronic circuitry in medical devices. This circuitry can be much more susceptible to electromagnetic fields than its electrical and electromechanical predecessors. The terminology associated with electromagnetic interference is presented in the appendix for this chapter.

A significant increase in the number of sources of RFI occurred recently in the environments where medical devices are used. Mobile communications devices comprise the largest portion of these sources of RFI. These include cellular phones, handheld transceivers, vehicle-mounted transceivers, and other wireless communication devices. These are increasing the background levels of radiofrequency electromagnetic fields in hospitals, homes, and workplaces. The number of land mobile transmitters in the U.S. alone exceeds 10 million. Cellular telephones and personal communications systems may well be in use by

Mobile Communications Safety
Edited by N. Kuster, Q. Balzano and J.C. Lin
Published in 1997 by Chapman & Hall, London. ISBN 0 412 75000 7.

a large fraction of the population, throughout the world. These portable communications devices can be brought into the close proximity of any medical device, without the knowledge of the medical personnel that operate the device or the user of the device. Modern digital mobile communications systems often utilize pulsed amplitude modulation. This modulation enhances the ability of the RF sources to interfere with medical device operation. For example, GSM cellular phones generate peak powers of up to 8 W and are modulated at 2 to 217 pulses per second. Many medical devices are designed to monitor the physiological frequencies of the human body. These frequencies range from about 0.5 Hz to several hundred Hz, and overlap the modulation frequencies of digital mobile communications systems.

Dozens of incidents of malfunctions of critical devices and injuries that were believed to be caused by RFI have been reported to the U. S. Food and Drug Administration (FDA) and other organizations that are responsible for regulating the safety of medical devices. Some of these reports have been collected, studied and summarized (Silberberg, 1993; Tan et al., 1995a). Many of these failures were believed to have been caused by RFI from mobile radio transmitters. The consequences of these failures ranged from inconveniences of medical device users (both medical personnel and patients) to serious injuries and deaths of patients. For example, in the early 1990s, in the United States, over 60 infants died over a period of a few years while being monitored for apnea (breathing cessation). The deaths were associated with unexplained failures of one model of apnea monitor to sound its audible alarm when patient breathing ceased. It was shown subsequently that this device was extremely susceptible to interference from RF fields produced by certain mobile communication base stations several hundred meters away, and by FM radio broadcast stations over one kilometer away (Ruggera et al., 1991). Therefore, RFI may well have contributed to some of these incidents. Many other models of apnea monitors from a number of different manufacturers were found to be dysfunctional when exposed to fields from nearby mobile RF transceivers. A voluntary recall of over 16 000 apnea monitors was performed by the manufacturer of the most RF-sensitive units after the FDA brought these test results to the manufacturer's attention.

Another problematic class of RFI-sensitive devices, electrically-powered wheelchairs, was discovered when problem reports came to the attention of the FDA. The FDA received a number of reports of unintended motion of electrically powered wheelchairs and scooters where the device and its user were involuntarily thrust into traffic or other dangerous situations. Several models produced by different manufacturers experienced these problems. FDA Laboratory and outdoor tests demonstrated that RFI from nearby emergency vehicle transceivers (such as police car radios) could induce severe episodes of unintended motion in several models of powered wheelchairs (Witters et al., 1994).

A third example of problematic RFI situation involved implanted cardiac pacemakers and defibrillators. Engineering groups in a number of countries performed independent studies of these devices in patients or in tissue-simulating models. These studies demonstrated that when digital cellular phones were held very close to the implanted device, undesirable effects were induced. These effects included the inhibition of electrical stimulation outputs from implanted cardiac pacemakers (Barbaro *et al.*, 1995; Eicher *et al.*, 1994; Carillo *et al.*, 1995) and the unintended firing of rescue shocks from implanted defibrillators (Bassen *et al.*, 1995).

There appears to be a significant amount of under-reporting of RFI-induced problems by clinical users of medical devices. A rough estimate is that for every report of a medical device failure due to RFI, ten to one hundred more RFI-induced problems are not reported. This is because most device users are not aware that a problem occurs while RF fields exist. Mobile RF transmitters can be brought into an area, transmit RF, and then taken out of the area, without the medical device user ever knowing that an RFI source was present. Also, because of the intermittent nature of RFI-induced failures, users and manufacturers of the affected medical devices do not know what to attribute these non-reproducible problems to.

3.2   WARNINGS AND RESTRICTIONS

A significant number of warnings have been published recently concerning the use of mobile radios in clinical settings where medical devices are used. Most of these concern the use of cellular telephones and handheld radios in clinical facilities.

- In 1991 a number of hospitals in Europe banned the use of cellular phones in certain areas of their facilities (Bostrum, 1991).
- In 1993 the Emergency Care Research Institute in the U.S. recommended prohibition of patient-owned transmitting devices (including cellular phones) in patient care areas (ECRI).
- In 1994 the Society of Biomedical Equipment Technicians (SBET, 1994) recommended banning the use of cellular phones in hospitals (Clemans, 1994).
- In 1994 the U.S. Army Medical Command initiated studies to evaluate the desirability of banning cellular phones from selected areas of all Army hospitals and certain other clinical facilities.
- In 1994 the Canadian Medical Devices Bureau recommended that the use of portable telecommunication devices be limited in hospitals. It recommended that cellular phones and two-way radios not be used in intensive care units, operating theaters, and patient rooms where critical-care medical equipment is in use. In addition, it recommended that patients using medical equipment at home should be cautioned about possible hazards from the use of portable wireless communication devices.
- In 1995 the Canadian Medical Devices Bureau issued an alert on digital cellular phone interference with implanted cardiac pacemakers. They

recommended that handheld digital cellular telephones not be kept in the breast pocket of a shirt or coat (Foster, 1995).

3.3   FACTORS THAT AFFECT THE OCCURRENCE OF RF INTERFERENCE

The operation of electronic circuits such as those in medical devices can be disrupted by RF electromagnetic fields only under certain conditions. The terminology associated with these conditions is presented, in detail, in the appendix for this chapter. To interfere, the RF fields immediately outside a device must have a relatively high field strength. If the field strength is strong enough to induce 'critical' voltages in the electronic circuit, the device's performance can be affected. Conversely, many weak RF fields that exist in the environment do not introduce interference in a medical device.

Many factors affect the severity of RF interference in medical devices. These factors include (1) the coupling between the source and the medical device, (2) the modulation imposed on the fields of the specific interference source, and (3) the distance between the interference source and the susceptible device.

Coupling refers to the interaction between the RF source (interference source) and the affected (susceptible) device. Special types of coupling occur when the susceptible device is in the close proximity (near field) of the source. Capacitive coupling occurs in a region near the source where the electric field from the source is dominant. This condition exists when the ratio of the electric to magnetic field is much greater than the 377 Ω value encountered in the far field. The electric field is dominant near the tip of a linear antenna, such as the monopole on a handheld radio. Inductive coupling occurs in a region near the source where the magnetic field is predominant, such as the base of a monopole on a handheld radio (Kuster *et al.*, 1992). Inductive coupling between cellular phones and implanted cardiac pacemakers was demonstrated by Carillo *et al.* (1995). The carrier frequency and modulation of a source of near or far-field RF radiation are critical factors in determining the induction of RFI in a medical device. Generally the frequencies with the greatest ability to induce RFI are those whose wavelengths are similar to the maximum dimension of a medical device's physical housing, or the length of its external cables and patient connected leads.

Several types of **modulation** can be imposed on the carrier of an RF transmitter. Amplitude modulation is usually the most significant parameter affecting the ability of a source of RF fields to induce interference. An RF carrier with amplitude modulation induces RF voltages in the signal processing and detection circuitry of a medical device. The modulation on the RF carrier is converted (rectified) to a low frequency voltage waveform by the many semiconductor junctions in the electronic circuitry. This enables the low frequencies of the

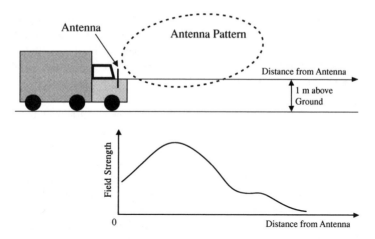

Fig. 3.1 Field strength vs. distance from a monopole antenna mounted on a truck.

amplitude modulation to enter the signal processing and detection circuitry of the device. If the amplitude modulation has frequency components in the 'physiological passband' of the medical device, significant interference occurs. Usually, the amplitude modulation that is on the RF carrier is intentionally imposed to carry communications information. However, unintentional AM can be induced on an unmodulated continuous wave (CW) carrier at the location of the susceptible device. This unintended modulation is created by motion-induced multipath effects. This occurs when a moving, conducting object passes between the CW source of RF and the device being exposed to the fields. Objects such as persons or vehicles near a medical device can create motion-induced multipath reflections. These reflections can combine with the original CW signal to produce amplitude modulation on the RF fields at the site of the medical device. If the amplitude modulation is at a frequency within the 'physiological passband' of the signals that the medical device is designed to detect, interference can occur.

The effects of the **distance** of the RF source from the medical device are highly significant with respect to RFI. Once in the far field of a transmitter, the field strength decays in direct proportion to increasing distance. In the far field, the ratio of the electric to the magnetic field is constant ($E/H = 377\,\Omega$). This occurs when the distance from the RF source is large compared to the size in wavelengths of the radiating antenna of the transmitter. There are exceptions to the general relationship of decreasing field strength occurring as distance from the RF source increases. First, the existence of reflections from conducting objects such as walls, cabinets, the ground, or wires and supports in the floor can create relatively high field strengths at certain locations. Reflections can create field strengths at one location that are higher than the field strengths existing at a closer distance to the RF source. Second, the field distribution produced by the antenna of an RF source may cause a decrease in field strength, when the source is brought closer to a medical device. For example, a monopole antenna mounted on the trunk or bumper of a truck can produce the following situation (Fig. 3.1). If a person measures the field strength at a height of one meter above the ground they may observe the following. While moving toward the truck from a distance of ten meters, the measured field strength will increase until a maximum value occurs. Then as the person continues to move toward the truck, the field strength will decrease. This is because the far-field radiation pattern of the monopole antenna on the truck is directed upward. At close distances, at a height of one meter, the field strength measuring instrument falls below the antenna's main lobe. This reduces the field strength significantly. At distances within a meter or so of the vehicle, the situation is more complex. Here, near-field conditions exist and the metal surfaces of the vehicles cause distortions of the field.

3.4   CHARACTERISTICS OF THE RF EMISSIONS FROM MOBILE SOURCES

Most medical device RFI situations involve small distances and complex spatial relationships between the RF source and the device being exposed. In 1994, Bassen *et al.* published data from extensive measurements of the field strengths produced by common RF sources in non-clinical environments. Measurements were performed in actual or simulated non-clinical environments where specific medical devices are used. Field strength measurements were performed on emissions from RF transceivers mounted in fire trucks, police cars, and other emergency vehicles such as ambulance vans, at an outdoor site. All measurements were made at a height of one meter above the ground. Electric field strengths were measured at distances of 10 m or less from each transceiver. Measurements of field strengths from cellular telephones were performed in an anechoic chamber. Isotropic, broadband field strength probes with three orthogonal, electrically-short antenna elements were used. Worst-case measurement uncertainties, including the sum of all errors in instrument calibration and usage were estimated as follows. These errors were less than ±3 dB (−29%, +41%). The field strengths of interest were those that equaled or exceeded the 3 V/m limits of the IEC 601-1-2 standard for medical device electromagnetic compatibility (IEC, 1992)

Measured data for each of the RF sources are presented in Table 3.1. The distance and the corresponding field strength measured at that point are listed for each situation. Also included in the table is information on the estimated time duration of RF transmissions throughout the day (termed duty factor).

Table 3.1 Maximum field strengths for commonly encountered RFI sources.

Source	Power W	Frequency MHz	Field strength V/m	Distance m	Duty factor
User handheld transmitters					
Cellular phone	0.6	840	5.3	1	medium
Cellular phone (held)	0.6	840	3.1	1	medium
VHF transceiver	5	150	3	2.6	low
VHF transceiver	4.3	460	3	3	low
Local transmitters					
Police car: bumper antenna*	100	39	8	6	low
Police car: roof antenna*	40	490	7	6	low
Ambulance van: roof antenna*	100	155	9	4.5	low
Fire truck: roof antenna*	40	155	6	6	low
Emergency jeep*	40	155	4	4.5	low
Cellular phone base station[†] (per channel with up to 100 channels per station)	500[‡]	860	4	30	high
Land mobile transmitter[‡]	2–300	30–936	10	30	high

* Measured one meter above ground. Distance is from nearest edge of vehicle to E-field sensor location.
† Effective radiated power (accounts for transmitting antenna gain).
‡ Calculated far-field data in main beam of antenna pattern.

This is meant to provide a means for estimating the likelihood of the transceiver being on when it is near an RF-susceptible device. A high duty factor is typical of an RF source that is transmitting almost continuously, throughout the day. A medium duty factor is defined as RF transmission by the source lasting about two to ten minutes, and occurring many times per day. A low duty factor is defined for the case where RF transmissions last for less than a minute, and occur no more than a few times per hour.

The power broadcast by cellular phone base stations is specified in Table 3.1 in terms of effective radiated power (ERP). ERP is the parameter that accounts for the directivity or focusing properties of a specific antenna used by a transmitter. Base station antennas have directivities or 'gains' of ten or more. The effective radiated power of these antennas is specified for the regions where the antenna pattern is aimed. Therefore, a base station antenna may have about 10 W of power delivered to it, but produce an effective radiated power of 500 W in certain directions.

3.5   CASE STUDIES OF MEDICAL DEVICE RFI CAUSED BY MOBILE COMMUNICATIONS SYSTEMS

3.5.1   Infant apnea monitors

In the introduction to this chapter it was pointed out that over 60 infant deaths went undetected by one model of an apnea (breathing cessation) monitor in the United States (Silberberg, 1993). This occurred over a period of a few years. It was shown subsequently that this model was extremely susceptible to interference from fields produced by mobile communication base stations up to 100 m away, and by FM radio broadcast stations over one kilometer away. Therefore, it is reasonable to assume that RFI may well have contributed to some of these incidents. Apnea monitors, as well as other medical devices, monitor low-level physiological signals via patient-connected electrodes. The circuitry used in these devices includes high gain, analog amplifiers with high-input impedances. The sensitive nature of this circuitry makes these devices susceptible to relatively low levels of RF fields. Laboratory testing by FDA was performed in TEM cells. This testing demonstrated that many different models of apnea monitors failed to operate properly when subjected to field strengths below 3 V/m. The most RFI-sensitive model failed in an unsafe manner when exposed to field strengths as low as 0.05 V/m in the 88–108 MHz FM radio broadcast band as follows. When amplitude modulation of 0.5 Hz was imposed on the RF carrier, the apnea monitor would fail to alarm when normal breathing had stopped. As a direct result of the RFI testing performed by FDA engineers, a voluntary recall of over 16 000 apnea monitors was performed by the manufacturer of the most RF-sensitive model.

3.5.2   Electrically-powered wheelchairs

Another class of devices that was identified as being susceptible to RFI from mobile transceivers was the electrically-powered wheelchair. The U. S. FDA received many reports of unintended motion of electrically powered wheelchairs and scooters that sometimes resulted in serious injury of the device's users. At the same time, FDA learned of wheelchair manufacturers testing their devices for RFI with mobile radio transmitters on emergency vehicles (e.g. fire trucks). Thus, RFI was suspected as a possible cause for these cases of unintended motion. FDA engineers developed a specialized RFI test method for powered wheelchairs. Initial testing in a laboratory exposure device, a GTEM cell, showed that certain wheelchair models were susceptible to RF interference from exposure field strengths of 10 V/m or less at certain frequencies (Alpert, 1994). The RFI caused several wheelchairs to release their electromechanical brakes, and activated their drive motors and wheels. From the data in Table 3.1,

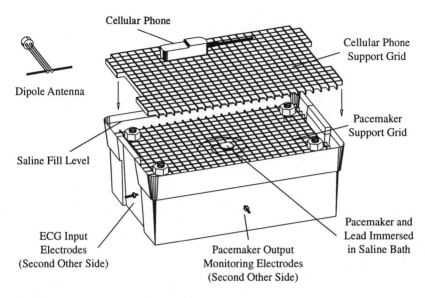

Fig. 3.2 A laboratory system for evaluating RFI in implantable cardiac pacemakers and defibrillators from cellular telephones.

FDA engineers knew that field strengths of 10 V/m existed at distances of 5 m or less from the antennas of police and fire vehicles' transceivers. Therefore, an association of some incidents of unintended motion could be made with RFI.

Once the RFI problem with powered wheelchairs and scooters was recognized, FDA began working with device manufacturers to address the problem (Witters *et al.*, 1994). FDA devised an RFI testing protocol that called for the wheelchairs to be exposed to uniform EM fields over the frequency range of 26 to 1000 MHz. Many manufacturers have tested their newest models to determine their devices' susceptibility to RF interference. Several manufacturers have modified their wheelchairs to be immune to at least 20 V/m. As a result of the FDA findings, voluntary standards organizations now recognize the need for electromagnetic compatibility testing of powered wheelchairs and scooters. The Rehabilitation Society of North America (RESNA, 1993) and the International Organization for Standardization have developed draft voluntary standards for wheelchair RFI immunity (ISO, 1994).

3.5.3 Interference of implanted cardiac pacemakers and defibrillators from digital cellular phones

Recently, several separate clinical studies have been performed using cellular phones held very close to pacemakers. The pacemakers were either implanted

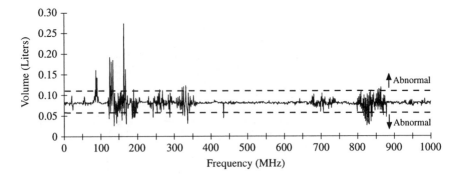

Fig. 3.3 Results of tests in a GTEM cell of one of the most popular models of ventilators, showing 10 V/m can cause failure. The output deviates significantly from the desired operating range (indicated by dashed horizontal lines) when exposed to 100–350 MHz fields.

in patients or placed one centimeter or less below the surface of a saline-filled plastic container (Eicher *et al.*, 1994; Barbaro *et al.*, 1995; Carillo *et al.*, 1995). These studies demonstrated that some of the pacemakers had their critical output pulses completely inhibited by certain digital cellular phones. This occurred when the phones were held up to 5 cm or more, from the pacemaker's pulse generator module. Tests were performed on implantable cardiac defibrillators (ICD) in a saline-filled torso simulator (Bassen *et al.*, 1995). Digital cellular phones can cause ICDs to discharge their high voltages into leads implanted in the heart of patients. In daily use, cellular phones can be expected to sometimes be placed as close as 5 to 10 cm from an implanted cardiac device. A user of a phone may turn the phone on while waiting for a call and place it in a shirt or jacket pocket, directly over the pulse generator module of an implanted cardiac device. In addition, a user may intentionally place the phone over their chest, when interrupting their phone conversation to speak to someone in their room.

Before about 1994, implantable cardiac pacemakers and implantable cardiac defibrillators were tested by their manufacturers for RF interference using the methods specified in the FDA/AAMI 1975 Draft Pacemaker Performance Standard (FDA, 1975). This standard specifies testing with far-field exposures at field strengths of 200 V/m at 450 MHz. The pacemaker pulse generator and its leads are immersed in a large plastic container filled with salt water (0.18% saline). The saline is used for two purposes. First, the saline is used to simulate the attenuating effects on RF fields caused by implantation of the pacemaker's pulse generator under the skin and fat of a patient's body, in the upper torso area. This salinity is much lower than the 0.9% mixture that is commonly used to simulate the electrical properties of muscle tissue. This 1975 test method does not require exposures to magnetic field strengths, especially at the high intensities produced by cellular phones within 10 cm of a pacemaker. Also, the RF frequency specified in the test method is not similar to the frequencies used by most cellular phones and other mobile transceivers. Therefore, a cardiac pacemaker can pass the 1975 standard's tests yet still be susceptible to interference from a nearby cellular phone.

In vitro test methods for implantable pacemakers and defibrillators have been developed specifically to address the cellular phone interference issue. Barbaro *et al.* (1995) used a human trunk simulator consisting of a thin-walled plastic box with dimensions of $30 \times 20 \times 15$ cm. The box was filled with 0.9% saline to simulate implantation in high-water-content tissue such as muscle. Two stainless steel plates were placed on the inside of opposite walls of the plastic box. This was done to apply electrocardiographic simulation signals to the pacemaker through the saline, while the pacemaker's output pulses were monitored with two other plates. In the U.S., the FDA and University of Oklahoma developed an *in-vitro* test method for pacemakers (Ruggera, 1996; Schlegal *et al.*, 1995). This test is similar to the method of Barbaro, except it uses a 26.5 liter plastic box with dimensions of $58.5 \times 42.5 \times 15.2$ cm and 0.18% saline solution. In this test system, the top surface of the simulator, on which the radiating source (cellular phone) rests, was a rigid plastic grid with many large square holes. A second grid, below, supports the pacemaker pulse generator and leads (Fig. 3.2). Also, a laboratory substitute for a cellular phone was developed. It consisted of a standard dipole antenna, fed with RF signals through a coaxial cable from an RF generator and linear amplifier. This laboratory substitute for a phone provides RF signals with known power, frequency, and modulation characteristics. These parameters can be varied to simulate the many different models of cellular phones and other wireless devices that could be placed close to the body of a person with an implanted pacemaker or defibrillator. In addition, powers higher than those radiated from a cellular phone can be used to determine thresholds of cardiac device failure for various carrier and modulation frequencies.

3.5.4   RFI problems with ventilators

Ventilators are medical devices that are used to control or assist the mechanical ventilation of a patient's lungs. These devices can be used to provide acute or chronic respiratory therapy to patients in the hospital, in their home, or even in an ambulance, a wheelchair, or a car. A patient that is dependent upon a ventilator will die or suffer serious injury after a few minutes of inadequate ventilation. Recently, reports were received of RF interference from handheld VHF radios and cellular phones affecting the proper operation of ventilators in hospitals (Biomedical Safety & Standards, 1995). Tests were performed by Canadian medical device researchers in hospitals (Tan *et al.*, 1995a; 1995b), and others. These tests confirmed that ventilators could be stopped when exposed to emissions from nearby transceivers. Further investigations demonstrated that the same modes of failure could be induced by exposures to RF field strengths of 3 to 10 V/m in an anechoic chamber (Tan *et al.*, 1995a). In the U. S., tests in a GTEM cell were performed over the 1–1000 MHz frequency range (Casamento, in press). Clinically-significant inappropriate performance was induced by a 10 V/m field strength at certain frequencies. The pair of dashed horizontal lines in Figure 3.3 indicates the upper and lower boundaries for acceptable ventilator performance. The FDA has developed recommendations for the minimum acceptable RFI immunity for respiratory devices. These are in the form of guidelines for FDA reviewers of premarket approval submissions from manufacturers of respiratory devices (CDRH, 1993).

3.5.5   RFI induced in hearing aids by digital cellular phones

The effectiveness of many models of hearing aids may be compromised by amplitude modulated RF fields. Joyner *et al.* (1993; 1994) used handheld and automobile-mounted digital cellular phones near various hearing aids. These phones radiated a maximum peak power of 8 W with the GSM pulse modulation scheme in the 900 MHz frequency range. Loud buzzing sounds were produced by the pulse modulation (217 Hz frame rate) of the RF carrier frequency. These sounds were perceived by hearing aid users with cellular phones located as far as 30 m from the most RFI-sensitive hearing aid. In-the-ear hearing aids were less sensitive than external, behind-the-ear units. In the U. S., one of the most popular digital cellular phone modulation schemes (North American Digital Cellular) operates with a pulse modulation frame rate of 50 Hz. These phones were shown to produce loud sounds in many models of hearing aids (Skopec, 1996). Other cellular phones that utilize frequency modulation (FM) rather than pulsed amplitude modulation produce minimal auditory interference. These include 'analog' cellular phones and digital cellular phones that utilize certain 'frequency hopping' code division multiple access (CDMA) modulation schemes.

3.6   MEDICAL DEVICE EMI TEST METHODS

A variety of test methods are recommended by international standards-setting groups to evaluate the RFI susceptibility of medical devices. These methods attempt to use special techniques to expose medical devices to spatially uniform, radiated RF fields. The techniques involve the use of a semi-anechoic chamber, a parallel plate exposure device, or an Open Area Test Site. A description of each system follows.

3.6.1   Semi-anechoic chamber

The semi-anechoic chamber is the exposure facility that is most highly recommended in the latest draft standard of International Electrotechnical Commission (IEC) for radiated RF immunity testing [IEC 1000-4-3]. This metal-lined
exposure system consists of a room at least 4–5 meters long, and several meters
high and wide. This indoor RF test facility is partially or completely lined with
RF absorbing material to minimize reflections that otherwise cause non-uniform
fields to exist in the chamber. This type of facility can be used to test the radiated RF immunity of devices at frequencies above a given lower frequency
limit. The lower frequency is determined by the quality of the RF absorber
and by the size of the chamber. Increasing the size of the chamber, and fully
lining it with high-performance absorber generally lowers the minimum usable
frequency. Generally, semi-anechoic chambers operate above 30–200 MHz depending on their construction. They have a useful upper frequency range of
several thousand MHz. Older style chambers are lined with electric-field absorbing material. This material consists of carbon-loaded plastic foam. This
absorber is designed for use above about 200 MHz. Using this type of chamber, and a 50 W transmitter, operating at frequencies of 200–1000 MHz, field
strengths of at least 40 V/m can be generated at a distance of one meter from a
log-periodic transmitting antenna. In the 900–3000 MHz range, a 10 W amplifier
can be used to generate 20 V/m at a distance of one meter from a log periodic
or a horn antenna. An alternate, wideband absorbing material consisting of
ferrite tiles has become available. New chambers using only ferrite tile absorber
can provide good anechoic performance over the 30 to 1000 MHz range. Using
a biconical antenna and a 100 W amplifier, field strengths of 20 V/m can be
generated in the 30–200 MHz range, one meter from the antenna. Chambers
lined with ferrite tiles that are covered with electric field absorber and excited
by appropriate antennas provide good performance from 30 MHz to 18 000 MHz
or higher.

3.6.2   Parallel plate exposure devices: TEM and GTEM cells

To overcome the inability of the anechoic chamber to operate effectively at
frequencies below about 30–100 MHz, a parallel plate exposure device is often
used. One type of parallel plate exposure device is the transverse electromagnetic (TEM) cell . This exposure system is completely enclosed by metal walls.
A device under test can be placed in a TEM cell and will be exposed to uniform, linearly-polarized RF electric and magnetic fields. The TEM cell has a
rectangular cross section and contains a flat center plate (septum), which is
parallel to, and slightly narrower than the outer metallic walls of the cell. A
cell suitable for testing small medical devices (e.g. a 20–30 cm cube) can generate uniform electric and magnetic fields from 0 to 150 MHz with a minimum

amount of RF power (e.g. 1.5 W). The frequency range over which the cell is capable of generating uniform TEM fields (similar to those encountered under far-field exposure conditions) is constrained by its size. As the size of the cell is increased (to allow testing of larger objects) the useful frequency range is lowered. Also, more RF power is necessary to produce a given field strength in a large cell than in a small cell.

A Gigahertz Transverse Electromagnetic (GTEM) cell is an exposure device that has been developed within the past ten years to combine the best features of TEM cells and anechoic chambers. GTEM cells have a frequency range of 0 to several GHz. The GTEM cell is in the shape of a pyramid, and the exposure signal is applied via a coaxial cable to a connector at the small end (Fig. 3.4). The GTEM cell used by FDA is 5.8 m long, 2.75 m wide and 2.3 m high. The maximum physical volume of the uniform exposure field region for testing devices in this cell is about 1 m wide by 0.8 m long by 0.5 m high. This limits the maximum size of a medical device that can be tested in this cell. Signal sources that produce about 10 W are required to expose devices to RF field strengths of at least 20 V/m. The GTEM cell is used in FDA with computer-automated signal sources and data acquisition systems to form a complete automated RFI exposure system. A GTEM cell that is approximately twice as large as the FDA's presently owned cell is commercially available. This larger cell enables testing medical devices with dimensions approximately twice the values cited above. However, significantly higher power is needed to generate the same field strengths in the larger cell.

3.6.3   Open area test site

The Open Area Test Site (OATS) is, in theory, the ultimate system for electromagnetic compatibility testing. An OATS consists of an outdoor site with a large ground plane made of electrically conductive material, such as wire mesh, buried a few centimeters below the surface of the ground. For radiated immunity testing, a transmitting antenna is placed above the ground plane to expose very large as well as small devices. With the proper antenna and separation distance, a uniform exposure field can be produced over the entire volume occupied by the device, even at low frequencies. However, the transmission of relatively intense electromagnetic fields into the open environment can be disruptive to nearby communications systems, such as radio and television broadcast receivers. Therefore, caution must be exercised to avoid transmitting at frequencies that could interfere with local, licensed wireless communications services. Some RFI test groups use an empty field or parking lot for an OATS. With an RF amplifier of 25–100 W, and using appropriate antennas, an OATS can be established that produces RF exposure fields of 10 V/m or more, at distances of one to three meters from the transmitting antenna.

The FDA used an OATS facility that was operated by the U.S. Army in

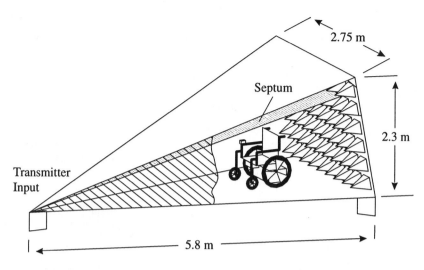

Fig. 3.4 GTEM cell containing a device under test.

Woodbridge, VA to test the RF immunity of infant apnea monitors. Here, a 305 m long, resistively-loaded, horizontal dipole antenna was elevated 15 m above the ground. It generated a spatially uniform electric field in a horizontal plane that had an area of more than 1 by 5 m. The area of uniform field strength was 1.5 m above the ground. A special structure of plastic pipe was constructed to support and position the device-under-test in this area. This OATS facility was then used to expose devices to field strengths of up to 1 V/m from 1 to 220 MHz.

3.6.4 Empirical *ad hoc* testing with mobile transceivers

Empirical testing is often used to assess the RF susceptibility of specific medical devices to particular mobile radios. This method involves testing the combination of a particular RF transceiver together with a specific model of a medical device. The tests can be performed at the site of the device's use, or in a laboratory environment. The transceiver is methodically placed at a variety of distances from the medical device under test, and the device's performance is observed. Several biomedical engineers and technicians have used actual hand-held transceivers in hospitals to test medical devices for RFI from these specific sources. Recently, surveys of a large variety of medical devices have been performed in hospitals (Tan *et al.*, 1995b), using *ad hoc* testing. Handheld VHF and UHF transceivers, and cellular phones were moved from different locations, over one meter away, to a few centimeters from each medical device under test.

Table 3.2 The relative advantages and limitations of each of the RFI exposure facilities.

Exposure facility	Volume of uniform fields	Frequency range MHz	RF power W*	Other factors
Semi-anechoic chamber	1 m³	40–200 200–3000	100 50	Preferred method in new RFI test standards
TEM cell	20×30×30 cm	0–150	1.5	Limited to low frequencies and small size test objects
GTEM cell	1×0.8×0.5 m	0–2500	10	Large physical size
Open area test site	Several m³	1–3000	10–40	Requires large, rural outdoor site, weather conditions limit operation
Empirical testing with mobile transceivers	Small, depends on separation of RF source and device	Limited to the frequencies emitted by the transceiver		Can identify source-specific problems with high intensity, near fields**

* RF Power required to produce 20 V/m.
** Not finding RFI may give false sense of security.

The tests indicated that the transceivers could cause most patient monitoring, therapeutic, and diagnostic medical devices to malfunction at close distances from transceivers. These tests indicated that a significant fraction of the devices that were tested malfunctioned when exposed to transceiver emissions with field strengths of 3 V/m.

Empirical testing with mobile transceivers offers unique advantages. This type of testing identifies source-specific problems with high intensity, near-field sources (handheld transceivers). It also enables the testing of large medical systems, *in-situ*. Testing of very large systems may not be possible in an anechoic chamber. However, empirical testing has several limitations. It limits the evaluation of RFI susceptibility to the specific frequencies, radiated powers, and modulation schemes of the transceivers that are used. This limited testing may indicate a lack of RFI and give a false sense of security to the users of the medical devices. *Ad hoc* (*in-situ*) testing for medical device RFI has been proposed for adoption by a subcommittee of the American National Standards Committee (ANSI C63.8, 1995).

3.6.5   A comparison of the characteristics of RFI exposure facilities

The relative advantages and limitations of common RFI exposure facilities are presented in Table 3.2. The total of the combined measurement uncertainties associated with any of these RFI testing facilities is ±3 to ±6 dB. A value of 6 dB represents a ratio of 2:1 between two E-field strengths. The costs of the various facilities are not compared, but the system using a TEM cell is significantly less expensive than the other systems listed. This is especially true when the prices of the necessary power amplifiers to be used with the exposure systems are considered. However, the TEM cell has severe limitations on the sample size it can accommodate at higher frequencies.

3.7   SPECIAL CONSIDERATIONS FOR RF SUSCEPTIBILITY OF MEDICAL DEVICES WITH INTERCONNECTING CABLES AND CONNECTIONS TO A PATIENT

Increased RFI susceptibility occurs when interconnecting cables are attached to a medical device. Cables are often connected from the device to AC power outlets. Also, devices with several separate electronics units have interconnecting cables to transfer data between units. An additional source of RFI enhancement in medical devices occurs if there is a connection to the body of the patient with cables. Each of these cables, as well as the body of the patient, acts as an antenna that increases the RF susceptibility of the medical device.

In the U.S., Food and Drug Administration engineers performed specialized tests of apnea monitor susceptibility at an OATS facility over the 1 to 220 MHz frequency range. This was done to assess the effects of RFI pickup from cables connected to the device (Bassen *et al.*, 1992). First, various arrangements of the patient-connection and power supply cables were tested. Full extension of the cables resulted in a higher sensitivity to RFI below 60 MHz, compared to the case where cables were not extended, but were bundled in a small coil. When the cables were extended and aligned with the E-field, the device's susceptibility increased by as much as 25 dB (18 times) at 40 MHz. Next, FDA engineers developed a compact 'serpentine' lead arrangement as shown in Figure 3.5. This configuration was designed to enable RFI testing of devices with the patient-connected leads only partially extended so exposures could be performed in a facility of limited size (such as a semi-anechoic chamber). An apnea monitor was tested at an OATS with the fully extended leads and with the leads configured in a serpentine cable configuration. The relative susceptibility of the device

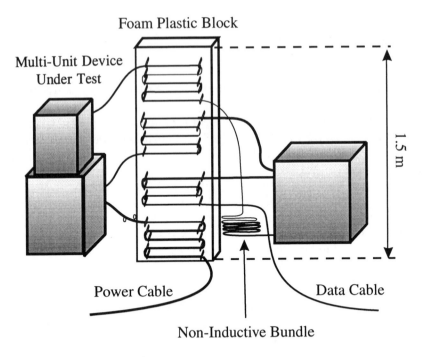

Fig. 3.5 Cables in a serpentine arrangement.

with each lead arrangement was compared. The RFI susceptibility of the two configurations was within ±7 dB over the frequency range of 1 to 220 MHz.

An additional source of enhancement of RFI in patient-connected devices is the body of a patient. It is well known that the body acts as an antenna when it resonates during exposure to electromagnetic fields in the 30–100 MHz range (Durney *et al.*, 1979). Bassen *et al.* (1992) made measurements of the relative RF voltages induced on a pair of standard, skin-mounted (cutaneous) electrodes and their connecting leads, attached to a human subject (Fig. 3.6). The electrodes were the type used with apnea and electrocardiographic monitors. An axial-lead diode was used as an RF detector by placing it across the proximal end of patient-connected leads. This was done while a human subject was connected to the distal end of the leads with the cutaneous electrodes. The human subject lay on a wooden bench, with the long axis of their body aligned with the electric field vector. The exposure field strength was 1 V/m. The bench was 0.8 m above the ground at the Woodbridge, VA OATS described previously in this chapter. The diode's DC voltage output was measured with a small battery-operated, analog, fiber optic data link. For the reference case, the electrodes were removed from the human subject and placed 5 cm above, and terminated in a 1000 Ω resistor. The detected voltage from the diode was

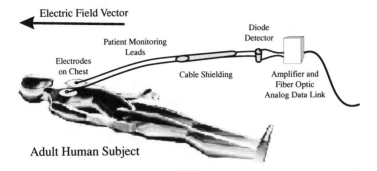

Fig. 3.6 Measurement setup for detecting the RF voltage induced at the end of a pair of leads connected to a human subject.

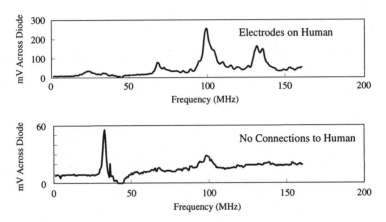

Fig. 3.7 Experimental data for patient-connected electrodes and leads. The upper trace shows the detected RF voltage versus frequency at the end of a pair of standard patient monitoring leads while the electrodes are connected to a human subject. The lower trace shows the voltage across the diode with the electrodes suspended 5 cm above the human subject, and connected to a 1000 Ω resistor, instead of the subject.

approximately proportional to RF electric field strength. The detected voltage was up to 5 times (14 dB) greater when the human subject was electrically attached to the leads, compared to the reference case (Fig. 3.7). This increase only occurred in the frequency range where human-body resonance occurred (100 MHz) for this set of leads and the particular person used in the test. These measurements proved that connection of a medical device, via standard electrodes and leads, to a human can increase the RFI susceptibility significantly at certain frequencies.

3.8   MEDICAL DEVICE RADIATED RFI SUSCEPTIBILITY STANDARDS

3.8.1   International standards

The predominant international standard for medical device radiated RF immunity is the International Electrotechnical Commission (IEC) standard 601-1-2, 1992. In general, to comply with this standard, a medical device must be immune to 3 V/m in the 26–1000 MHz frequency range. For non-life supporting devices, testing of immunity is only required at the specific frequencies of 27.12, 40.68, and 915 MHz. A draft revised version was prepared in 1996. It has been proposed that the lower frequency of this range be raised to 80 MHz, and that only conducted immunity tests be used below this frequency. Amplitude modulation of 80% is required with a sinusoidal signal. This modulation should be applied to the RF carrier at a single frequency that presents the most significant interference to the specific device under test. Test methods for radiated RFI are specified in the IEC 1000-4-3 standard (formerly IEC 801-3). The primary test method involves the use of a semi-anechoic chamber and a biconical, log periodic, or other linearly polarized transmitting antenna. Figure 3.8 illustrates the features of the IEC 1000-4-3 test configuration. Exposures of devices-under-test must be performed in a 'uniform area' of field strength that is 1.5 × 1.5 m. This area must be at least one meter from the exposure antenna. The front surface of the device under test and all wires and cables must be placed in the uniform area. This area should be at least 0.1 m above the floor, and preferably 0.8 meters. In addition, the planar area should be at least 0.8 m away from any RF-reflecting objects. To quantify the field strengths in the 'uniform area', measurements must be made at 16 evenly spaced points (including the four corners of the plane) with the device-under-test absent. The uniformity of the field must be within minus 0 and plus 6 dB for 12 of the 16 points. During testing, wires that are part of the medical device-under-test should be arranged in a manner that is consistent with any recommendations of the manufacturer. The first meter of each signal-carrying and power cable must be extended in the uniform area. The next two meters of the cable must be arranged in a non-inductive bundle. Exposures of four orientations of the device under test must be performed for both a horizontal and vertical polarization of the electric field. At least one exposure should be performed with the leads and cables aligned with the electric field vector.

In 1995, the IEC initiated a product-specific EMI performance standard for hearing aids (IEC, 1995). This draft standard requires an immunity of 3 V/m for frequencies of 800–960 MHz and 2 V/m for frequencies of 1400–2000 MHz. These include cellular phone frequency bands. Eighty percent, 1000 Hz, sinusoidal amplitude modulation is imposed on the RF carrier. The exposure must be performed in accordance with the proposed draft amendment 1 of IEC 1000-4-3.

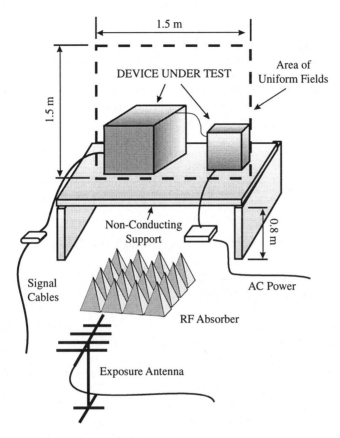

Fig. 3.8 The IEC 1000-4-3 test configuration.

3.8.2   U.S. FDAs draft reviewer guidance for anesthesiology and respiratory devices

The U.S. FDAs Center for Devices and Radiological Health (CDRH) issued a Draft Reviewer Guidance for Anesthesiology and Respiratory Devices (CDRH, 1993). It contains detailed requirements for testing a few specific classes of devices for immunity to all forms of EMI. One portion contains a Radiated Electromagnetic Fields Section. This document was developed to conform, as much as possible, with the IEC 601-1-2 and 1000-4-3 standards. The frequency range is 26–1000 MHz. Frequency steps of 1 MHz, or a frequency sweep rate of 0.1 MHz per second are used. Amplitude modulation must be imposed at a frequency within the 'physiological passband' of the signals that the device is designed to detect. Either square wave modulation (100%) or sine wave modulation (80%) may be used. As in the IEC 1000-4-3 standard, exposures of medical devices-under-test must be performed in a planar area of uniform field strength. One difference from the IEC test method is that the first 3 m of each of the cables must be arranged in the serpentine configuration shown in Figure 3.5. The remaining length of each cable is arranged to minimize coiling (non-inductive bundling). The CDRH Reviewer Guidance Document requires appropriate electric-field-strength instruments to be used to measure the field strength at each point. The instruments should have an isotropic response of ±1 dB. This ensures that measurements will be accurate, regardless of the E-field vector orientation. E-field measurements should have a total error of less than ±3 dB. The field sensors of the instrument must fit within a spherical volume having a diameter of 15 cm.

3.9   FAILURE PREVENTION AND RFI AVOIDANCE

It is clear from the data in Table 3.1 that medical devices that are used in medical facilities, as well as in the home and work environments, can be exposed to relatively strong RF fields from mobile communications devices. Therefore, it is necessary for manufacturers of all new medical devices to take steps to provide compatibility of their devices with this electromagnetic environment. The present environment should be considered as well as those that can be expected to exist during the useful life of a device. However, it will never be possible to incorporate enough immunity in a medical device to enable it to work in an electromagnetic field of unrestricted strengths, carrier frequencies, and modulation characteristics. Therefore it is also necessary to provide administrative or user controls and device usage warnings to accommodate severe RF environments. These controls and warnings are discussed later in this chapter.

3.9.1   Designing RFI compatibility into medical devices and mobile communications systems

For many years, military, aircraft, and automotive electronics systems have been required to meet severe RFI requirements (up to 200 V/m) because they could encounter these types of environments during their intended use. Therefore the technology was developed to 'harden' these devices to fields that are quite intense. Most RFI hardening techniques are not costly, if they are incorporated into the initial design of the electronics system. Standard RF immunity techniques involve shielding, grounding, and filtering of electronic circuitry. Shielding includes the use of metal boxes or non-conducting boxes coated with metallized paint. The use of RF-shielded cables is standard practice in home audio and video systems. Grounding of electronics circuitry and cable shields is a very inexpensive but necessary step in ensuring RFI immunity. All of the

RFI immunity techniques mentioned above can and have been incorporated in various medical devices. In light of the numerous reported RFI-induced failures of medical devices, it appears however that adequate immunity has not been incorporated in many devices.

RF filtering of signal-carrying conductors in sensitive patient-monitoring equipment should be performed carefully. This has been done rather success-fully in implanted cardiac pacemakers. Here weak electrophysiological voltages are monitored, yet immunity to over 200 V/m and 0.5 A/m at 850 MHz is ac-complished via the use of capacitive 'feed-thru' RF filters ahead of the input circuitry of the pacemaker (Carillo *et al.*, 1996). Patient-connected medical de-vices must accommodate the safety requirements for electrical leakage currents as well as RFI immunity requirements. Therefore, patient leads on devices that are connected to the AC powerline 'mains' must use special technologies to meet simultaneously both EMI and electrical safety requirements. Patient iso-lation techniques using optical or transformer coupling can provide electrical safety while not compromising RFI immunity. In addition to the standard EMI reduction techniques listed above, medical device designers can add interference recognition and fail-safe circuitry to their devices (Bassen, 1986). This is done in many cardiac pacemakers by limiting the maximum rate that a pacemaker can operate, under any circumstances.

Mobile RF systems and wireless communications systems can be optimized for compatibility with medical devices. Wireless networks that are intended for use in locations where medical devices are operated can be designed to ensure compatibility with medical electronics. Mobile RF transmitters can utilize mod-ulation schemes with frequencies that are out of the 'physiological passband' of most or all medical devices. Frequency modulation, or non-pulsed, spread spectrum techniques are highly preferred, compared to modulation schemes that use pulse-amplitude modulation. Another means for controlling RFI in facilities where medical devices are used involves systems design and planning by the facilities' managers. For example, the peak RF power transmitted by any handheld or portable cellular phone is controlled by the nearest base sta-tion. Thus, the radiated power of phones can be reduced to less than 10 mW instead of the maximum 600 to 3000 mW of radiated power if base stations are located near a health care facility. Care must be taken to avoid situations where high-power base stations are located too close to the health care facil-ity and produce RF ambient levels that can cause interference. Alternatively, low-power base stations (microcells) can be installed in a health care facility.

3.9.2   RFI administrative controls

Administrative controls to limit the exposure of medical devices to strong RF fields can be implemented in health care facilities. RFI sources can be restricted from certain areas of a hospital, such as an intensive care unit. In addition, RF transceivers can be required to be kept at least a specified minimum distance from any designated medical device. The concept of specifying a 'minimum separation distance' for each type of mobile transceiver has been proposed (Silberberg, 1994; Segal, 1996). For example, using the data in Table 3.1, handheld cellular phones that radiate a maximum of 0.6 W would be required to be kept at least one meter from a medical device that is immune to 3 V/m. A 5 W handheld transceiver would have to be kept 2.6 m from the same device. In practice, greater distances would be required to account for enhancement of signals by reflections of the fields from conducting objects such as the building's support structures and electrical wiring.

3.9.3   Device usage warnings and labeling

Warnings about potential medical device EMI problems can be placed on both the susceptible medical device and the potentially-interfering RF emitter. In addition, health care providers and users can be warned of the potential problem of RFI. These are concepts that have been implemented for many years, in a few special cases. Microwave ovens were believed to interfere with implanted cardiac pacemakers in the 1970s. As a result, signs were posted to warn pacemaker wearers that a microwave oven was in use in a self-service restaurant or cafeteria. Also, pacemaker manufacturers have included printed warnings about various sources of EMI, including microwave ovens, handheld transmitters, and devices such as electric razors that have field-emitting electric motors. These warnings are prominently displayed in the manual provided to the owner (patient), and the manual provided to the health care provider (cardiologist). Recently, warnings about EMI in implantable cardiac pacemakers due to nearby handheld cellular phones have been issued to owners and cardiologists by pacemaker manufacturers. Labels or warnings about EMI for medical devices other than pacemakers are rare, but are increasing in use. One example is the mailing by the U.S. FDA of letters to providers of electrically-powered wheelchairs (Alpert, 1994) and the posting of EMI susceptibility information labels on newly manufactured powered wheelchairs.

3.10   CONCLUSIONS

Presently, many medical devices that are tested for susceptibility to radio-frequency interference cannot meet the minimum immunity requirements of 3 V/m that are specified in the predominant international standards for these devices. At the same time, handheld cellular telephones produce field strengths that exceed 3 V/m at distances of 1 m. Higher-power transceivers produce 3 V/m fields at distances more than several meters. This situation has caused a number of serious failures of life-sustaining medical devices. Therefore, it is imperative for RF immunity to be designed into new medical devices. Even after this step is taken, other factors will have to be considered. The exact field strength that a device will be exposed to depends on many conditions that are beyond the control of the medical device designer. Due to their portable nature, most mobile transceivers can expose medical devices to field strengths of hundreds of volts per meter and several hundred milliamps per meter, when the transceiver is brought very close to the device. A worst-case example of RFI incompatibility of mobile transceivers with medical devices involves implantable cardiac pacemakers. Even though pacemakers have been designed to be immune to very intense electric fields (200 V/m) some of these devices still malfunction when a cellular phone is placed within a few centimeters of their pulse generator.

The lack of compatibility between existing medical devices and new mobile transceivers is likely to exist for 5–10 years beyond the date of manufacture of the medical device. Also, medical devices designed today may not be adequately protected against RFI from future wireless communication devices whose RF and modulation parameters are not even dreamt of today. Therefore, administrative controls may also have to be implemented. These include education of the medical device user on both the clinical and the home-use EMI environment. Accommodations must be made to adapt to the situation of incomplete RF compatibility between RF transceivers and medical devices. In health care facilities, mobile transceivers can be restricted to distances that are greater than a predefined value, in areas where critical devices are operated. Medical device users and patients with RFI susceptible implants or home use devices should, if possible, be educated to recognize mobile sources of RF, and to react appropriately to their use in clinical and non-clinical situations. Also, users of mobile RF transceivers must become more aware of the fact that their devices can adversely affect critical medical devices.

APPENDIX 3.A   RADIATED RF INTERFERENCE TERMINOLOGY

The following terms are important in the discussion of radiated radiofrequency interference of electronically-controlled medical devices.

- Coupling: The electromagnetic interaction between a source of RF fields and the affected medical device.
- Effective radiated power (ERP): The parameter that accounts for the effects on distant field strengths caused by the directivity or focusing properties of a specific antenna used by a transmitter. ERP is a useful parameter for calculating the field strength produced at a particular distant location by a transmitter with a directional antenna.

- Emissions: Electromagnetic fields produced by a source of RF energy. Emissions from a single source create a unique exposure field at each location of interest.
- Exposure: The ambient electric and magnetic fields at a point in space, generated by one or more RF emitters.
- Far field: A region of space that is removed sufficiently from a radiating RF source so that relatively uniform electric and magnetic field strengths exist. Far-field conditions occur when the distance from the RF source (antenna) is large compared to the size of the source, and large compared to the wavelength of the fields. Specifically, far-field conditions exist when the distance from the source of RF radiation is greater than

  $2D^2/\lambda$ where:

  D = the largest dimension of the antenna of an RF transmitter
  λ = wavelength of the RF carrier frequency

- Field strength: This parameter expresses the intensity of the electric fields and the magnetic fields that are produced at a given location, due to RF emissions from one or more RF sources. Usually field strengths at a point in space are measured in the absence of any objects, such as a device that is being tested for RF susceptibility. Electric rather than magnetic field strength is most commonly used to quantify radiated radiofrequency fields that can cause interference with electronic devices.
- Field strength unit: Electric field strengths are expressed in terms of volts per meter (V/m) or decibels (dB) below or above a given value, such as one microvolt per meter (μV/m). A ratio of 10:1 between two values of electric field strengths is 20 dB. For example, 1 V/m is equal to +120 dB μV/m. Magnetic field strength is usually expressed in units of Amperes per meter (A/m). A ratio of 10:1 between two values of magnetic field strength is 20 dB.
- Frequency: A measure of the cyclic repetitions per unit time of the instantaneous intensity of an electrical signal or electromagnetic wave. Frequency is expressed in units of Hertz (Hz), or cycles per second.
- Immunity (RF): The ability of a device to operate properly while being exposed to a certain intensity of external electromagnetic fields.
- Interference: A situation induced in an electronically-controlled device that results in its failure to operate in its intended manner. Interference may cause permanent or temporary failures of the device.
- Interference source: A source of RF interference fields.
- Modulation: Time variations of the characteristics of an RF field. The following types of modulation can be imposed on the carrier signal of an RF source:

  Amplitude modulation (AM) constitutes a time varying change in the field strength of an RF carrier. Pulsed amplitude modulation is a special type of AM that is often used in RF digital communications systems.

Pulsed modulation often involves 100% amplitude modulation of the RF carrier. Here, the carrier signal is turned on and off completely during the pulsing cycle.

Continuous wave (CW) RF fields are those that contain no imposed amplitude modulation.

Frequency modulation (FM) constitutes a time-varying change of the instantaneous frequency of an RF carrier. FM signals do not produce any amplitude modulation on the RF carrier.

- Near field: A region located close to a radiating RF source where the electric and magnetic fields vary considerably from point to point. Usually near-field conditions occur at distances that are less or equal to the size of the radiating antenna of an RF transmitter and closer than a wavelength from the antenna.
- Physiological passband: The range of frequencies associated with the events of a physiological process. Certain medical devices contain electronic circuitry that is designed to detect and process electrical signals only if they lie within a specific frequency range. For example, a heart rate monitor may be designed with a physiological passband of 0.5 to 3 Hz. This corresponds to a heart rate of 30 to 180 beats per minute.
- RF carrier: The primary radiofrequency signal that is generated by a source. The RF carrier must be modulated to convey the information that is intended to be communicated by a radio transmitter.
- Susceptibility: A condition where a device exhibits an unwanted reaction due to exposure to external electromagnetic fields with certain characteristics.
- Susceptible device: A electronically controlled device that is affected by interference fields.
- Transceiver: An RF communications device (transmitter/receiver) that both transmits information by imposing modulation on an RF carrier signal and receives information from another RF transmitter.
- Wavelength: The distance between instantaneous maxima in the electric fields of a radiating electromagnetic field. The wavelength of an RF carrier in air is equal to C/f, where f = frequency in Hz, and C = the speed of light $(3 \times 10^8 \text{ m/sec})$.

REFERENCES

Alpert, S. (1994) *Dear Powered Wheelchair/Scooter or Accessory Component Manufacturer*. Letter establishing minimum recommended immunity level to interfering electromagnetic energy, Food And Drug Administration, Center For Devices and Radiological Health, Rockville, MD 20850, U.S., May 26, 1994.

ANSI, American National Standards Institute C63.8 (1995) *Draft Ad-Hoc Test Method for Medical Device Testing*. ANSI, N.Y., U.S. November, 1995.

Barbaro, V., Bartolini, P., Militello, C. *et al.* (1995) Do European GSM mobile phones pose a potential risk to pacemaker patients? *In vitro* observations. *PACE*, **18**(6), 1218–1224.

Bassen, H. (1986) From problem reporting to technological solutions. *Med. Instrumentation*, **20**, 17–26.

Bassen, H., Ruggera, P. and Casamento, J. (1992) Changes in the susceptibility of a medical device resulting from connection to a full-size model of a human. *Proceedings of the 14th Annual International Conference of the IEEE Engineering in Medicine and Biology Society*, Nov. 1994, Baltimore MD, 2832–2834.

Bassen, H., Ruggera, P., Casamento, J. *et al.* (1994) Sources of radiofrequency interference for medical devices in the non-clinical environment. *Proceedings of the 16th Annual International Conference of the IEEE Engineering in Medicine and Biology Society*, Nov. 1994, Baltimore MD, 896–897.

Bassen, H. (1996) The FDA laboratory program, in Electromagnetic compatibility for medical device – issues and solutions (ed S. Sykes), *Conference Report Published by the Association for the Advancement of Medical Instrumentation*, Arlington VA, USA, 111–119.

Bassen, H., Moore, H. and Ruggera, P. (1995) Cellular phone interference testing of implantable cardiac defibrillators, *in vitro*. *Circulation*, **92**(8), 3547.

Biomedical Safety & Standards (1995) Ventilators Could Malfunction Under High EMI Exposure 25, 10: 1 and 75.

Bostrum, U. (1991) Interference from mobile telephones – a challenge for clinical engineers. *Clinical Engineering Update*, **10**.

CMDB, Canadian Medical Devices Bureau (1994) *Use of Portable Telecommunication Devices in Hospitals*. Policy statement from the Canadian Medical Devices Bureau, Health and Welfare, Ottawa, Ontario, Canada.

Carrillo, R., Saunkeah, B., Pickels, M. *et al.* (1995) Preliminary observations on cellular telephones and pacemakers. *PACE*, **18**(4), 863.

Carillo, R. *et al.* (1996) Electromagnetic filters impede adverse interference of pacemakers by digital cellular phones. *J. American College of Cardiology* (Supplement), **27**(2a), paper 901-22.

Casamento, J. Applying Standardized Electromagnetic Compatibility Testing Methods for Evaluating Radiofrequency Interference of Ventilators. *Med. Instrumentation* (in press).

CDRH, Center for Devices and Radiological Health (1993) *Reviewer Guidance for Premarket Notification Submissions*. Anesthesiology and Respiratory Devices Branch, Division of Cardiovascular, Respiratory, and Neurological Devices, November 1993.

Clemans, T. (1994) Electromagnetic compatibility. *Biomedical Instrumentation*, **28**, 13.

Durney, C., Iskander, M., Massoudi, H. *et al.* (1979) An empirical formula for broadband SAR calculations of prolate spheroidal models of humans and animals. *IEEE Trans. Microwave Theory and Tech.*, **27**, 758–762.

Eicher, B., Ryser, H., Knafl, U. *et al.* (1994) Effects of TDMA-modulated handheld telephones on pacemakers. *Abstracts of the 16th Annual Meeting of the Bioelectromagnetics Society*, Copenhagen, Denmark, June 1995, 67.

ECRI, Emergency Care Research Institute (1993) Guidance article: Cellular telephones and radio transmitters – interference with clinical equipment. *Health*

Devices, **22**(8–9), 416–418.

FDA Food and Drug Administration (1975) Draft: Pacemaker standard: Labeling requirements, performance requirements, and terminology for implantable artificial cardiac pacemakers. Association for the Advancement of Medical Instrumentation (AAMI). *Report FDA/HFK-76-38, Aug. 1975.*

Foster, K. (1995) *Digital Cellular Phone Interference with Cardiac Pacemakers.* Health Canada, Health Protection Branch Alert, Medical Devices Bureau, Ottawa, Ontario, Canada, Nov. 6, 1995.

IEC, International Electrotechnical Commission (1992) Medical Electrical Equipment, Part 1: General requirements for safety; Collateral Standard: Electromagnetic Compatibility, IEC 601-1-2.

IEC, International Electrotechnical Commission (1994) Electromagnetic Compatibility (EMC), Part 4: Testing and measurement techniques, Section 3: radiated, radio-frequency, electromagnetic field immunity test, IEC 1000-4-3.

IEC, International Electrotechnical Commission (1995) Draft: 1st Edition of IEC 118-13, Hearing Aids, Part 13: Electromagnetic Compatibility (EMC) product standard for Hearing Aids.

ISO, International Organization for Standardization (1994) Draft Revision of Standard 7176/1-1986, Wheelchairs, Part 1: Determination of Static Stability.

Joyner, K., Wood, M., Burwood, E. *et al.* (1993) *Interference to Hearing Aids by the New Digital Mobile Telephone System, Global System for Mobile (GSM) Communications Standard.* National Acoustic Laboratories, Australian Hearing Services, Sydney Australia.

Joyner, K., Anderson V. and Wood, M. (1994) Interference and energy deposition rates from digital mobile phones. *Abstracts of the 16th Annual Meeting of the Bioelectromagnetics Society,* Copenhagen, Denmark, June 1995, 67–68.

Kuster, N. and Balzano, Q. (1992) Energy deposition mechanism by biological bodies in the near field of a dipole antenna above 300 MHz. *IEEE Trans. on Vehicular Tech.,* **41**(1), 17–23.

RESNA, Rehabilitation Society of North America (1993) Draft Revision of Standard WC/01 Wheelchairs, Determination of Static Stability.

Ruggera, P. and O'Bryan, E. (1991) Studies of apnea monitor radiofrequency electromagnetic interference. *Proceedings of the 13th Annual International Conference of the IEEE Engineering in Medicine and Biology Society,* 1641–1643.

Ruggera, P. (1996) *In-vitro* testing of pacemakers for digital cellular phone electromagnetic interference. *Proc. of the 31st Annual Meeting and Exposition of the Association for the Advancement of Medical Instrumentation,* 92.

SBET, Society of Biomedical Equipment Technicians (1994) CMBE & SBET Recommend Cellular Phone Ban & RFI Standards Review. Society of Biomedical Equipment Technicians. *Biomedical Safety and Standards,* **24**(8), 1 and 59.

Schlegal, R. *et al.* (1995) *In-vitro* study of the interaction of cellular phones with cardiac pacemakers. *Proceedings of a Workshop on Electromagnetics, Health Care, and Health, 17th Annual International Conference of the IEEE Engineering in Medicine and Biology Society,* 33-36.

Segal, B., Skulic, B., Liu-Hinz, C. *et al.* (1995) Preliminary study of critical-care medical device susceptibility to portable radiofrequency sources. *Proc. Thirteenth Annual Meeting and Exposition of the Association for the Advancement of Medical*

Instrumentation, 83.

Segal, B. *et al.* (1996) Sources and victims: The potential magnitude of the electromagnetic interference problem. Conference report published by the Association for the Advancement of Medical Instrumentation, Arlington VA, USA, 24-39.

Silberberg, J. (1993) Performance degradation of electronic medical devices due to electromagnetic interference. *Compliance Engineering*, Fall 1993, 25–39.

Silberberg, J. (1994) Medical device electromagnetic interference issues, problem reports, standards, and recommendations. *Proceedings of the Health Canada Medical Devices Bureau, Round-Table Discussion on Electromagnetic Compatibility in Health Care*, Ottawa, Canada, September 22-23, 1994, 11-20.

Silberberg, J. and Witters, D. (1995) *Recommendations for Mitigation of EMI in Health Care Facilities*. American National Standards Institute, Committee C63, Subcommittee 8, May 20, 1995.

Skopec, M. (1996) *Hearing Aid Electromagnetic Interference from Digital Cellular Telephones*. Proceedings of the 18th Annual International Conference of the IEEE Engineering in Medicine and Biology (in press).

Tan, K.S. and Hinberg, I. (1995a) Malfunction in medical devices due to EMI from wireless telecommunication devices. *Proceedings Thirteenth Annual Meeting and Exposition of the Association for the Advancement of Medical Instrumentation*, 96.

Tan, K.S. and Hinberg, I. (1995b) Investigation of electromagnetic interference with medical devices in canadian hospitals. *Proceedings of a Workshop on Electromagnetics, Health Care and Health, held in association with the 17th Annual International Conference of the IEEE Engineering in Medicine and Biology Society*, 20–23.

Witters, D. and Ruggera, P. (1994) *Electromagnetic Compatibility (EMC) of Powered Wheelchairs and Scooters*. Proceedings of the 16th Annual International Conference of the IEEE Engineering in Medicine and Biology Society, 894–895.

4

Bioeffects of mobile communications fields: possible mechanisms for cumulative dose

W. Ross Adey

4.1 INTRODUCTION

Spectacular developments in radio engineering technology over the past decade have created striking new options in personal communication devices and systems. Through miniaturization born of computer chip technology, there has been a step function increment in device reliability and user convenience. User acceptance of these new technologies has been immediate and worldwide. In the perspective of human health, a population base of millions of daily users are now exposed to RF fields under near-field conditions, with expectations that these newly evolved behavioral patterns will continue on a lifelong basis.

There are important biomedical considerations associated with long-term exposure to any environmental factor capable of tissue interactions. These include effects specifically attributable to intermittency of exposure, frequency of recurrent exposure, interactions involving simultaneous exposure to multiple factors, age at onset of exposure, and even considerations of ethnicity that may determine individual susceptibility.

Moreover, these RF technologies continue to evolve, with new products differing significantly in the same application from one continent to another, as well as on a national basis. RF carrier frequencies strongly influence field coupling to the human body. Many instances of specificity in tissue interactions appear related to certain patterns of amplitude- or pulse-modulation at ELF frequencies.

With threshold phenomena based on sensitivity to modulation frequencies, much laboratory evidence is consistent with **athermal** models of these RF interactions. Indeed, through the use of a spectrum of electromagnetic fields as

Mobile Communications Safety
Edited by N. Kuster, Q. Balzano and J.C. Lin
Published in 1997 by Chapman & Hall, London. ISBN 0 412 75000 7.

fundamental tools, new concepts in organization of living matter have emerged. Gradually over the past twenty years, a quiet revolution has occurred (Adey, 1993a; 1993b; Liburdy, 1995). Increasingly, essential experimental evidence has met criteria of consistency and repeatability (Walleczek, 1994), across the hierarchy from ionic movements, through enzymatic responses, to regulatory mechanisms in cell growth. At the same time, physical and biophysical studies have evaluated sensitivities to ELF and ELF amplitude-modulated RF fields, with little or no evidence that observed responses relate directly or indirectly to cell or tissue heating (Adey, 1992a; 1992b).

The accepted existence of these athermal phenomena points to biological organization beyond limits set by chemical reactions in biomolecular systems. Their existence sets a far finer but largely unexplored realm in physical processes at the atomic level. If adverse (or even protective) health effects exist from exposures to the various cellular and other RF mobile phone fields, it is in athermal sensitivities that answers must be sought, since thermal effects are unlikely, although extensive modeling of energy absorption in the user's head has revealed that ANSI safety limits may be exceeded by a factor of two or more with an average antenna power of less than 0.6 W.

For ELF fields, substantial new knowledge at the cellular level describes major sequences in some of the key mechanisms that couple electromagnetic fields to biomolecular systems. A first goal has been to validate observations indicating biological sensitivity to fields with energies below the thermal collision energy (kT) of atomic and molecular structures exposed to such weak fields. These studies have filled major steps in an hierarchical sequence of signal transduction, beginning with evidence for physical mechanisms that might mediate first detection of weak electromagnetic fields at cell surfaces; and beyond this first transductive step, identification of a burgeoning sequence of amplification mechanisms coupling cell surface signals to the cell interior, inducing enzymatic cascades and ultimately to nuclear mechanisms mediating gene transcription (Adey, 1990a; 1992a).

In the last decade, because higher priorities have been assigned worldwide to research on possible health effects of ELF fields associated with electric power generation, distribution and use, funding for biomedical research on RF/microwave exposures research has been meager. No comparable body of knowledge exists on bioeffects of RF athermal exposures nor is it clear to what extent, if at all, findings in ELF research may be usefully extrapolated to exposures to AM or pulsed RF fields with similar ELF characteristics.

4.2   PHYSICAL ASPECTS OF RF ABSORPTION IN TISSUE

The human body has been studied as an antenna model, exhibiting whole and partial body resonances, with energy absorption based on physical dimensions and orientation of its parts with respect to planes of polarization of incident RF fields. In the upright position, the grounded body has a longitudinal resonance around 35 MHz (Gandhi, 1975). Ungrounded, this resonance is around 70 MHz. In the transverse and anteroposterior axes, maximum absorption occurs at frequencies from 135 to 163 MHz. Although these configurations may be consistently realized in far-field exposures, by contrast, near-field patterns of energy absorption, as in the user with the cellular phone near the head, will be dominated by regional peaks determined by proximity of the transmitting antenna to specific body parts. A pattern of secondary excitation of the remainder of the body will then probably follow far-field antenna models for the whole body noted above, but specific data for cellular phone frequencies is lacking.

4.2.1 Head resonant frequency

For the head, the resonant frequency is a function of head size, ranging from around 700 MHz in the infant to 400 MHz in adults (Gandhi *et al.*, 1977). Early studies using thermalizing far-field exposure levels described 'hot spots' of increased energy absorption within the head. These hot spots occur inside lossy spheres that model brain tissue with radii 8 cm<r>0.1 cm for frequencies between 300 MHz and 12 GHz (Kritikos *et al.*, 1975). However, at lower frequencies and at much higher frequencies, heating occurs primarily at the surface of the sphere facing the source. Heat conduction and convection from a central brain hot spot have been modeled, with inclusion of a factor for blood flow (Kritikos *et al.*, 1979). For a spherical head 10 cm in diameter, exposed to a 1.0 GHz, 10 mW/cm^2 field with a central hot spot 2 cm in diameter, the expected temperature rise would be 0.5°C with normal blood flow and heat conduction.

In this model, heat conduction and normal blood flow appear to contribute equally to heat removal from the hot spot. For a given incident field flux, the heating potential in the hot spot decreases rapidly with increasing head radius (Kritikos *et al.*, 1972; 1975; 1976). Thus, in man, the expected temperature rise would be lower at this 1.0 GHz field frequency than seen in the 10 cm model. There are strong differentials in convective capacities between cerebral gray and white matter, attributable to substantially higher densities of blood vessel capillary beds in cerebral cortical gray matter (Ranck, 1964). For the human head, simulated as a sphere 15 cm in diameter with three layers representing brain, fat and skin, a 2.45 GHz field is rapidly absorbed at the surface of the head (Kritikos *et al.*, 1972). There is a maximum SAR of 2.0 W/kg in the outer 1 cm of the phantom for an incident power density of 1.0 mW/cm^2, although the average SAR for the whole head is only 0.12 W/kg. But this picture changes sharply at the lower frequency of 918 MHz. Under the same exposure conditions, the SAR at the center of the head is 0.45 W/kg, significantly greater than the calculated surface SAR of 0.2 W/kg.

4.2.2   Intracranial fields induced by mobile phones

There have been numerous experimental assessments and numerical simulations of intracranial fields induced by mobile phones held against the head. These are extensively reported in Chapter 2. Initial studies were based on FM transmitters (Cleveland et al., 1989). The energy absorption mechanisms for lossy bodies in close proximity to antennas have been described (Gandhi et al., 1994; Kuster et al., 1992), although levels of energy deposition reported in these simulations differ significantly. This is a near-field situation, where energy deposition is largely induced by the magnetic component.

Most of the bioeffects already discussed make negligible contributions in comparison with this main interaction. In the latter, the most important parameter determining the amount of energy absorbed in the tissues of the head is the distance separating the antenna, or radiating structure, from the head. Absorption increases approximately as the inverse square of decreasing distance between the antenna or radiating structure and the tissues. Depth of penetration is basically determined by carrier frequency, with more rapid attenuation as the frequency increases. At frequencies of 10–20 GHz, typical attenuations are in the range of 20 dB/mm from the skin surface.

These near-field conditions differ sharply from far-field exposures, defined as occurring 20–30 wavelengths from a radiating source, where electric and magnetic vectors have well characterized orthogonal phase relationships. In conformity with near-field models having strong magnetic coupling to tissues immediately adjacent to the transmitting antenna, there is a consensus that maximum field levels occur in skin, subcutaneous tissues, bone and immediately subjacent brain tissue (for review, see Bach Andersen et al., 1995).

4.2.3   Layering resonances near the body surface

Layering resonances in the vicinity of the body surface emphasize the need for caution in the use of SAR in terms of averaged values. Absorbed energy has a spatial distribution over any real mammalian body that is quite sensitive to the layering of skin, fat, muscle and bone. This layering is associated with a resonance for three-dimensional bodies that is quite distinct from the geometrical resonance. Calculations for a multilayered prolate spheroidal model of man predicted a whole-body layering resonance at 1.8 GHz with an SAR 34% greater than predicted by a homogeneous model (Barber et al., 1979); but a related model for a specific skin-fat-muscle cylindrical model of man predicted a layering resonance frequency of 1.2 GHz, with an 'averaged' SAR double that calculated for the corresponding homogeneous model. The layering resonance frequency was the same for incident waves polarized parallel or perpendicular to the cylinder axis. The energy deposited in different body layers would clearly be different. Even with further modeling of this differential distribution with the body described as a series of small 'blocks', these differentials were submerged in the further calculation of a 'whole-body SAR' (Hagmann et al., 1979).

4.2.4   Millimeter wave attenuation at the body surface

For millimeter waves, attenuation in aqueous media is typically 20 dB/mm. Thus, penetration below the body surface will be limited. Nevertheless, extensive studies by Grundler et al. (1977; 1983; 1992) have pointed to the possibility of sharp resonances in effects of 41.5 GHz fields in modulation of yeast cell growth, with sensitivities extending down to incident field energies of 5 pW/cm^2.

4.2.5   Tissue thermoregulation during microwave exposures

There has been a careful evaluation of thermoregulatory and related tissue responses to high-intensity microwave fields. Increased vascular flow provides the basic physiological mechanism for sustaining a homeothermic state, in response to either increased metabolic heat production or to absorption of thermal energy from imposed fields.

Rats tolerate a 2.45 GHz field producing energy absorption at a rate of 22.5 W/kg for as long as 20 min before succumbing to hyperthermia (Phillips, 1970). This rate of energy absorption in a 400 g rat represents about 544 J/min, or about 5 times the reported basal metabolic rate for rats this size (Kleiber, 1947). The threshold for death during prolonged exposure, typically after 4–6 h, is about 2.5–3 times the basal metabolic rate (Philips et al., 1975). Rats exposed to 2.45 GHz fields for 30 min at an absorbed energy rate of 116 J/min showed an initial rise in colonic and skin temperature, but O_2 consumption, CO_2 production and heart rate were unaltered. Endocrinological functions are modified in rats by protracted irradiation with 2.45 GHz fields that raise body temperatures (Lu et al., 1977). With 4 h exposures, a threshold field intensity for raised colonic temperature was in the vicinity of 1 mW/cm^2 (for review, see Adey, 1981).

Studies of the microwave hearing phenomenon have suggested thermoelastic expansion in structures of the inner ear as the mechanism for perceiving the pulses (Frey, 1961; Lin, 1978; Chou et al., 1979). However, careful studies by Tyazhelov et al. (1979), with appropriate phasing of RF and acoustic pulses delivered simultaneously, have suggested inadequacies in the thermoacoustic model. Suppression of sensitivity to a 5 kHz RF signal by simultaneous acoustic stimulation at 10 kHz is 'at variance with the simplest principles of the thermoacoustic hypothesis, which can hardly explain a number of observed peculiarities of auditory sensation near threshold'; leading Tyazhelov and colleagues (Mirutenko *et al.*, 1977) to propose selective and differential heating of cell membrane ion channel proteins as the basis of microwave hearing.

4.3   RF/MICROWAVE INTERACTIONS AT THE MOLECULAR LEVEL

4.3.1   Collision-broadened vs. resonant spectra

At frequencies below the mm wave/far infrared spectral regions, theoretical considerations and experimental data (Illinger, 1981) support the concept of collision-broadened spectra in biomolecular interactions. Crucial to the form of the dielectric response function (complex permittivity) of a molecule at the field frequency is the duration of the collisional perturbation in relation to the period of the field, phenomena first addressed by Frohlich (1946) and by van Vleck and Weisskopf (1945).

Where the collisional perturbations are very brief for one period of the imposed RF field, every collision is effective in interrupting the absorption-emission process. Thus, in a fluid with many collisions per unit time relative to field frequency, every collision is effective and a collision-broadened relaxation spectrum results (Illinger, 1962). But where collisional perturbations are very long compared to the period of the RF field, there is a resonant-type spectrum. Since the duration of a typical collision in a molecular fluid is fixed at a given temperature and pressure, the field frequency determines whether there is a relaxation or resonance spectrum. Thus, there is no compelling evidence for resonant absorption in common molecular fluids below 3000 GHz. Attenuation of microwave fields in biological fluids is dominated by the ubiquitous presence of water. This broad attenuation due to water shields other biomolecular absorption processes, including quasi-lattice vibrations in biopolymers and the vibrations of hydrogen-bonded bridgeheads (Illinger, 1981).

4.3.2   Models of threshold effects

Heating and heat exchange have been viewed as the essential measure of living processes, and intrinsic thermal energy has been viewed as setting an immutable threshold for external stimulation. We will discuss a broad spectrum of biological phenomena incompatible with this concept. Through the use of imposed EM fields as tools, it is clear that heating is not the basis of these phenomena, and that understanding of biological thresholds requires a search for mechanisms effective at levels below intrinsic thermal collision energy (kT) of biomolecular substrates (Adey, 1993a; 1993b). No single model has general acceptance, nor does the gamut of experimental data yet suggest a single unifying hypothesis.

Multiple van der Pol oscillators

Frohlich (1968) hypothesized that electric vibrations at GHz frequencies would be excited coherently in the course of biological metabolic processes.

Excitations of this type may be significant as the basis of long-range biological interactions, but their experimental identification has posed considerable experimental difficulties. Positive experimental evidence has been reported in studies of cell growth conducted at 41.5 GHz, with rigorous control of field frequencies and intensities (Grundler *et al.*, 1992). In summary, 1) cell growth increased or decreased by 10–20% as a function of field frequency; 2) the frequency dependence exhibited a resonance-like structure; and 3) the shape of the resonance curve changed systematically with altered field intensities. The authors propose that only non-linear self-sustained oscillators coupled to cell growth would respond in this way. Extensive studies of a limit-cycle van der Pol oscillator system (Kaiser, 1983; 1984), sensitive to external perturbation and fitting the observed experimental behavior, would respond even at field intensities near zero.

Free radical mechanisms in biological thresholds

In an historical perspective, growth of knowledge in bioelectromagnetics has occurred in the face of pre-emptive views on the part of some physical scientists that athermal effects are in the realm of spurious or pathological science, because observed sensitivities relate to fields that lack sufficient energy to break chemical bonds. This perception that bond rupture represents a benchmark as an essential first step in biological transduction of electromagnetic fields is countered by growing theoretical and experimental evidence pointing to free radical mechanisms as one possible substrate. This model proposes that magnetic fields may interact with free radicals produced in on-going chemical reactions, rather than inducing their formation (Adey, 1993a).

Briefly, in chemical reactions, bonds break and re-form. Most chemical bonds between atoms consist of paired electrons with opposite spins, with one electron derived from each atomic partner to the union. In chemical reactions, the bond breaks, then each partner reclaims its electron from the bond and moves away to encounter a new partner. The atom is now a **free radical**, with a magnetic field generated by its spinning electron. Free radical lifetime is typically brief, in the nanosecond range. It is terminated by reforming a bond through meeting of two radicals with opposite electron spins, forming a **singlet pair**. Although this is the only way that a singlet pair can form, electrons with similar spins can unite in three ways, forming **triplet pairs**.

McLauchlan (1992) has proposed a role for free radicals in mediating biomolecular interactions with magnetic fields at 60 Hz electric power frequencies. These interactions would alter in the rate and amount of product of a chemical reaction. For fields around 8 mT, there would be 'an enormous effect of a small magnetic field on a chemical reaction, and the effect begins at the lowest applied field strength'. McLauchlan states that 'the all-important interaction has an energy very much less than the thermal energy of the system, and is effective exclusively through its influence on the kinetics; this is counter-intuitive to most scientists'.

In a detailed review, Grissom (1995) has set a perspective on his studies of the many enzymatic sensitivities to static magnetic fields in the millitesla-tesla range. But in the context of mobile phone users, interest centers on possible effects of much weaker fields oscillating at GHz frequencies. But even at these frequencies, interactions of tissue free radicals with cell phone fields during their typically brief nanosecond lifetimes may resemble those occurring in static fields. McLauchlan and Steiner (1991) attribute the highest level of free radical sensitivity to hyperfine-dependent singlet-triplet state mixing in radical pairs with a small number of hyperfine states (i.e. a small number of nuclear spins), or with a high degree of nuclear spin degeneracy, 'with the implication that even very low fields may have significant effects on radical reactions'.

Spin-mixing is suggested as a possible mechanistic basis for biosensitivities at extremely low magnetic field levels. Any process which changes the overall spin state of the radical pair can facilitate the reaction of the members of triplet-born pairs or inhibit the reaction of singlet-born pairs. Triplet states can be interconverted to singlets by **spin-lattice relaxation**, originating in fluctuating local magnetic fields at the electron, due to random motion. However, for organic radicals, their characteristic times in the microsecond range are far too slow to produce spin mixing before the probability of re-encounter of the geminate pair falls essentially to zero. These are **incoherent** processes and insignificant in most radical-pair interactions. On the other hand, **coherent** singlet-triplet interconversion can be sufficiently fast (in the nanosecond range) to occur before diffusion reduces radical re-encounter probability to negligible levels. It may happen when the electrons on the two radicals interacting with different local magnetic fields. These fields may originate in the applied field or in hyperfine coupling to nearby nuclei, with the implication that the applied field would be close to zero. Physiological evidence for magnetic field modulation of free radical-dependent brain mechanisms (Bawin *et al.*, 1994; 1995) will be discussed (Section 4.5.3).

Rf/microwave modulation-dependent tissue responses

Early studies in brain tissue showed that efflux of calcium from cerebral cortex is stimulated by RF fields in an ELF modulation frequency-dependent manner (Adey, 1980), with a maximal response at 16 Hz (Bawin *et al.*, 1975; Blackman *et al.*, 1979). A similar modulation dependence of calcium efflux was noted in isolated brain subcellular particles (synaptosomes) with dimensions under 1 μm (Lin-Liu *et al.*, 1982). Inside cells, modulation frequency-dependence occurs in activity of essential enzymes, including protein kinase messenger enzymes (Byus *et al.*, 1984) and a cell growth regulating enzyme system (ornithine decarboxylase) (Byus *et al.*, 1988). In attacking human tumor cells, cultured lymphocytes of the immune system are modulation frequency-dependent in their killing capacity (allogeneic cytotoxicity) (Lyle *et al.*, 1983). Early studies also reported correlated brain wave and behavioral responses in animal exposures to ELF-modulated RF fields at athermal levels (Bawin *et al.*, 1973).

The advent of digital mobile phone systems has focused current bioeffects research on an evaluation of possible modulation frequency-dependent tissue interactions. The current North American standard uses 50 packets/sec with time-division-multiple-access (TDMA) quadrature modulation. The GSM system in Europe and much of the rest of the world has a 217/sec packet rate. The pending North American iDEN system will use 22 packets/sec. The Iridium system of direct communication from handheld transmitters to orbiting satellites utilizes 11 packets/sec.

Communication between brain cells is mediated by a spectrum of chemical substances that both excite and inhibit transaction and transmission of information between them. These substances act by binding to their specific receptors on cell surfaces. This process is also sensitive to modulated microwave fields. Kolomytkin *et al.* (1994) studied specific receptor binding to rat brain synaptosomes of three neurotransmitters: gamma-aminobutyric acid (GABA), an inhibitory transmitter; and acetyl choline and glutamate, both excitatory. Microwave exposures used 880 MHz or 915 MHz fields at power densities from 10 to $1500 \, \mu W/cm^2$. With incident field densities of $1.5 \, mW/cm^2$, binding to GABA receptors decreased 30% at 16 pps, but differences were not significant at 3, 5, 7 or 30 pps. Conversely, 16 pps modulation induced a significant increase in glutamate receptor binding. For acetyl choline receptors, binding decreased 25% at 16 pps, with similar trends at higher and lower frequencies. As a function of field intensity, sensitivities of GABA and glutamate receptors persisted for field densities as low as $50 \, \mu W/cm^2$ at 16 pps with 915 MHz fields.

The question of comparability between ELF bioeffects and bioeffects of ELF-modulated RF fields

No single model yet explains observed bioeffects across the spectrum from ELF to millimeter waves. Indeed, emerging knowledge suggests a multiplicity of mechanisms, some dependent on RF field frequency, as in reported millimeter wave sensitivities (Grundler *et al.*, 1992). Illinger (1981) has concluded that there is no compelling evidence for resonant absorption below 3000 GHz in ordinary molecular fluids (see Section 4.3.1). Other sensitivities are virtually independent of RF frequency, but relate closely to frequency of ELF modulation of the RF field.

Specifically for the latter, at the same average field intensity as their modulated counterparts, unmodulated fields may be without any of the effects on a spectrum of biological activity attributable to the modulated signal. There is the challenging implication that detection of certain modulation components of RF/microwave fields may be an intrinsic property of tissue organization. Pointers to the probable cellular site of this RF demodulation sensitivity come from substantive findings in bioeffects of ELF fields, where models and experimental evidence first suggested that cell membrane surfaces offer an effective substrate (Adey, 1981; 1990a; 1990b; 1993; Luben, 1991; Liburdy, 1995). As will be discussed, the dense surface polyanionic negative charges located at the tips of glycoprotein strands attract a strongly positive atmosphere of hydrogen and calcium cations. With 'apparent' dielectric constants created by charge separation in this region in excess of 10^6 at frequencies below 1 kHz (Einolf et $al.$, 1971), it is hypothesized that this dynamic cell surface capacitance may be modulated by imposed ELF fields and mediate an envelope demodulation of amplitude-modulated RF fields (Adey, 1990a). Intrinsic and extrinsic electromagnetic fields in this zone induce a highly cooperative modification of calcium-glycoprotein binding along the cell membrane surface.

From the beginning of these studies in the 1970s, it was noted that there were similarities in responses of tissues and cultured cells to environmental fields that were either in the ELF spectrum, or were RF/microwave fields modulated at ELF frequencies. The major part of this ELF research has been conducted with fields simulating aspects of electric power transmission and distribution systems (50/60 Hz), and there is no comparable body of knowledge for amplitude-modulated or pulsed RF fields. Nevertheless, the available evidence has indicated similarities between certain cell ionic and biochemical responses to ELF fields, and to RF/microwave fields amplitude-modulated at these same ELF frequencies; suggesting that envelope demodulation of RF/microwave fields may be a critical determinant of ensuing biological responses.

In summary, similar sensitivities to both ELF and ELF-modulated RF fields have been reported in experiments at progressively more complex levels in the hierarchy of cellular organization. Calcium efflux from brain tissue responds to ELF exposures (Bawin et $al.$, 1976; Blackman et $al.$, 1985) and to ELF-modulated RF fields (Bawin et $al.$, 1975; Blackman et $al.$, 1979; 1985; Dutta et $al.$, 1984). In the same and different cell culture lines, the growth regulating enzyme ornithine decarboxylase (ODC) responds to ELF fields (Byus et $al.$, 1988; Litovitz et $al.$, 1993) and to ELF-modulated RF fields (Byus et $al.$, 1987; Litovitz et $al.$, 1993). Immune responses of lymphocytes targeted against human lymphoma tumor cells (allogeneic cytotoxicity) are sensitive to both ELF exposures (Lyle et $al.$, 1988) and to ELF-modulated fields, but not to unmodulated fields (Lyle et $al.$, 1983). Cerebral amino acid neurotransmitter mechanisms (glutamate, GABA and taurine) are influenced by ELF fields (Kaczmarek et $al.$, 1974) and ELF-modulated microwave fields, but not by unmodulated fields (Kolomytkin et $al.$, 1994).

Barnes (1996) has offered a novel concept for tissue demodulation of RF fields at weakly thermal levels. Low levels of electric and magnetic fields at low frequencies may affect chemical reaction rates by changing the encounter rate of reacting charged particles, rather than their energies. At radio frequencies, one mechanism by which these fields would affect chemical reaction rates is through thermal heating. For ELF-modulated fields, this thermal heating might serve to demodulate the signal and generate a small periodic chemical signal that would be of approximately the same size for typical human exposures to either ELF or modulated RF fields.

We have previously considered models of threshold phenomena that would be consistent with apparent biological thresholds for EM fields having incident energies at or below levels of thermal collision energy kT (Section 4.3.2). The possible role of van der Pol oscillators or free radicals has been proposed, both having relevance to RF/microwave interactions in the gigahertz range, but, as pointed out by Engstrom (1995a; 1995b), lacking a clear relationship to either ELF field bioeffects, or to ELF modulation-frequency-dependent sensitivities to RF/microwave fields.

Herein lies a major challenge to further understanding of one of the most fundamental aspects of bioelectromagnetic mechanisms. For that reason, Engstrom has proposed a concerted effort to determine whether the initial biological transductive step involves a 'fast' mechanisms on nanosecond time scales, with ELF sensitivities arising secondarily in biosystem poperties; or is the transductive step essentially a 'slow' event, perhaps involving phase transitions or Bose condensations in domain properties, as suggested by Grodsky (1977) Grodsky's approach offers a basis for ELF modulation-dependent effects in recent models attributing enhanced biological sensitivities to stochastic resonance as a property of cell aggregates (Astumian *et al.*, 1995) (see Section 4.3.2). Considerable theoretical and experimental effort has been directed to the mechanistic basis of resonant ELF biosystem phenomena.

Biophysical models of ionic resonance phenomena related to demodulation sensitivities

Human exposure guidelines for both ELF and RF fields await a clear understanding of a dose metric. As yet, there are only partial answers to such questions as the respective roles of the electric (E) or magnetic (B) components, or a combination of both, in eliciting a biological response. For magnetic fields, there are also possible tissue interactions between static and oscillating fields. Liburdy (1995) points out the importance of achieving exposure metrics in the light of differences between electric and magnetic field dosimetry in tissue and air, since magnetic fields penetrate tissue uniformly, whereas electric fields undergo a heterogeneous attenuation that is spatially determined by tissue anisotropy. With magnetic fields, electric fields are also induced along concomitant tissue current pathways in accordance with Faraday's laws of induction.

In the quest for biological ELF resonant responses, attention was first directed to possible joint actions of oscillating ELF magnetic fields with static fields by Blackman et al. (1985; 1988; 1990), Liboff et al. (1985; 1987), Rozak et al. (1987), and Smith et al. (1987). Blackman proposed a nuclear magnetic resonance model, based on an oscillating magnetic field oriented perpendicularly to a static field. Parallel orientation of these fields is consistent with a cyclotron resonance model, as proposed by Liboff. For a specific level of static magnetic field, a specific ion (of known mass and charge) will be associated with a characteristic cyclotron frequency. But a persisting difficulty in experimental testing of this relationship is that it does not specify the strength of the oscillating magnetic field. In the earth's geomagnetic field, cyclotron resonance frequencies for essential cations, such as Ca^{2+} and K^+, are in the ELF range, if the ions are stripped of their hydration shells.

In terms of cell ultrastructure, this requirement may only be met in the hydrophobic lipids in the interior of cell membranes. Moreover, the circular ion paths in the earth's magnetic field under cyclotron resonance conditions would be around 50 m. A major difficulty in assessing oscillating-static magnetic field combinations is the lack of a specific amplitude parameter for the oscillating field in the cyclotron equation, challenging the option to design experiments that would unequivocally test the theory.

From a quite different theoretical approach, Lednev (1991) characterized field exposure parameters with sufficient precision to test possible cellular interactions with specific combinations of oscillating and static magnetic fields. The Lednev *ion parametric resonance* model describes protein-bound ions as spatial oscillators with a series of vibrational frequencies that depend on the bond energy, and the charge and mass of the ligand-boundion. With the formation and breaking of coordination bonds between the protein and a chain of ions, the ions oscillate around a mean energy level, due to random thermal motion. The energy level of the bound ions split into two sublevels in the presence of a static magnetic field, and the splitting of the two levels occurs at a frequency equal to the cyclotron frequency. An oscillating magnetic field in the same axis as the static field may then modulate the two energy sublevels established by the static field. At the cyclotron frequency, this oscillating field modulates the probability of transitions between ion energy states according to a Bessel function argument, thus allowing calculation of intensity ratios of oscillating and static fields that satisfy experimental conditions (a damped sine wave with a first maximum (ratio 1.8), a zero crossing (ratio 3.8), and first minimum (ratio 5.3)). Modifications of the Lednev model purporting to correct it and aimed at satisfying certain experimental findings have been proposed (Blackman et al., 1994; Blanchard et al., 1994), but rejected by Lednev (1995). Evidence for sensitivity of biological systems under cyclotron conditions has been extensive but so far inconclusive, with inconsistencies that suggest action of uncontrolled intercurrent factors (see Liburdy, 1995 for review).

Stochastic resonance as a possible factor in enhancement of biological threshold sensitivities

There has been a revival of interest in the role of concurrent noise in coherent biological signal detection. Studies in the organization of brain tissue long ago raised the possibility that noise in a signal transduction system might enhance, rather than reduce its sensitivity, through phenomena in the category of **stochastic resonance** (Adey, 1972). This may underlie 'the extraordinary ability of some biological systems to amplify small signals in noisy environments' (Bezrukov *et al.*, 1995).

It is possible 'to envisage an information-processing system in which the very presence of an on-going noise-like activity produces no degradation in information-handling ability, and might even enhance it. Much would depend on the adaptive qualities, if any, of the noise-like activity, in response to afferent neural volleys, or to such factors as humoral fluxes of hormones and other chemical influences in the brain cell environment. We may envisage such a noisy system undergoing minor changes in the level of independence of its constituent wave generators and in their concomitant cell firing patterns' (Adey, 1972).

Bialek (1983; 1984) has addressed this biological problem in elegant detail in quantum mechanical terms, evaluating two distinct classes of quantum effects: first, a macroscopic quantum effect, typified by the ability of a sensory system to detect signals near the quantum limits to measurement; and second, a microscopic quantum effect, in which 'the dynamics of individual biological macromolecules depart from the predictions of a semi-classical theory'.

Bialek has concluded that: 1) Quantum-limited measurement occurs in several biological systems, including the displacement sensors of the inner ear, with thresholds below 10^{-11} m. Quantum limits to detection are reached in the ear in spite of a seemingly insurmountable level of thermal noise. 2) In order to reach the quantum limit, the receptor cells of the inner ear must possess amplifiers with noise performance approaching the limits posed by the uncertainty principle. Such 'perfect' amplifiers cannot be described by any chemical kineticmodel, nor by any quantum mechanical theory in which the random phase approximation is valid – the molecular dynamics of the amplifier must be such that quantum mechanical coherence is preserved for times comparable to the integration time of the detector. 3) In comparisons of two major quantum effects in molecular dynamics, viz., i) resonant dependence of electronic transition rates on vibrational frequencies, and ii) coherent evolution of the electronic states for times comparable to vibrational relaxation times, predicted consequences of quantum effects are observed in the case of heme proteins. 4) In systems with long vibrational relaxation times, the phonon modes can be pumped by chemical reactions (transitions among electronic states), and this leads to a phonon instability. In polymers (Schwarz, 1970), this instability resembles super-radiant emission of photons by an ensemble of excited atoms, and results in a coherent oscillation of the phonons throughout the polymer.

Limits imposed by thermal and 'excess' biological noise on threshold magnitudes and duration of weak E-fields at cell membranes have been considered by Astumian *et al.*, (1995). The model proposes rectification of oscillating E-fields by cell membrane proteins, with ensuing DC transport of ions offering a basis for signal averaging. Noise-induced enhancement signal transduction has been reported across voltage-dependent ion channels produced in lipid bilayers by the polypeptide alamethacin (Bezrukov *et al.*, 1995). Eichwald and Kaiser (1995) have modeled ELF intracellular calcium oscillations, based on the external field acting on the kinetics of signal transduction between activated cell membrane receptors and intracellular G proteins. The model and calculations are based on self-sustained, nonlinear oscillators, with entirely different responses to coherent signals and to noise perturbations, depending on specific combinations of cell internal biochemical and external physical parameters.

4.4   CELL SURFACE GLYCOPROTEINS AS A STRUCTURAL BASIS FOR EM FIELD INTERACTIONS

Experimental evidence (Liburdy, 1995) supports a role for electric fields as an effective stimulus at cell surfaces; a concept that gains support from engineering models (Misakian *et al.*, 1990; Bassen *et al.*, 1992). Evidence favoring the electric component of an EM field as an effective stimulus at cell surfaces, rather than a direct magnetic interaction, has come from studies of cell cultures in multiwell annular plates. These devices are constructed as a series of concentric rings, with cells grown at increasing distances from the center of the dish, allowing complete electrical isolation of cells in one ring from those in adjacent rings. In this system, calcium influx in mitogen-activated lymphocytes exposed to a 60 Hz magnetic field scaled with the induced E-field (Liburdy, 1992). Also, calcium uptake was indistinguishable between exposures to an E-field applied through electrodes, and a matching electric field induced by a magnetic field.

Cells in tissue are separated by narrow fluid channels, or 'gutters', typically not more than 150 Å wide, that act as windows on the electrochemical world surrounding each cell. These channels are also preferred pathways for intrinsic and environmental electromagnetic fields in tissue, since they offer a much lower electrical impedance than cell membranes. Functional measures of brain electrical impedance are thus an index of conductance in this extracellular space, and have been correlated with brain tissue physiological states in health and disease (Adey *et al.*, 1962; 1963; 1965; Porter *et al.*, 1965). These intercellular channels are also the site of electrochemical 'antennae' that protrude as protein strands from within the cell membrane. Relevant aspects of cell membrane structure have been reviewed elsewhere (Adey, 1990a; 1990b; 1992; 1993a; 1993b; Liburdy, 1995).

4.4.1   Establishment of cooperative protein-phospholipid domains in cell membranes

From the earliest studies by light microscopy in the 17th century, cell membranes were identified as sharply partitioning each cell from its neighbor, by reason of their high content of fat molecules (**phospholipids**). With the electron microscope, its structure is seen as a double layer of phospholipid molecules, the **plasma membrane**, approximately 40 Å thick. A steady **membrane potential** approximating 0.1 V exists across this thin membrane, translating to an enormous electric gradient of 100 kV/cm. In many respects, the cell membrane is thus a physical and an electric barrier. Since generally accepted physiological findings have revealed sensitivities to induced tissue electric gradients from ELF environmental fields and from ELF-modulated RF fields in the range $10^{-7} - 10^{-1}$ V/cm, we may anticipate powerful **amplification** mechanisms mediating transductive coupling of these weak stimuli from fluid surrounding cells to the cell interior.

This function of initial detection of low-level electromagnetic fields in fluid surrounding cells is attributed to glycoprotein strands protruding from the cell interior through the plasma membrane. They form a strongly negatively charged **glycocalyx** on the cell surface. They act as specific receptors for hormones, antibodies, neurotransmitter molecules and for certain chemical cancer promoters. They form, in conjunction with membrane phospholipids that surround them, essential pathways from cell surfaces for stimuli far weaker than the membrane potential. Their amplified signals to the cell interior elicit enzymatic responses regulating metabolism, messenger functions and cell growth.

In electron spin resonance studies with labeled tails of phospholipid molecules in an artificial phospholipid bilayer, McConnell (1975) noted that intrusion of a protein strand into this bilayer induces coherent states between charges on the tails of adjoining phospholipid molecules for considerable distances away from the protein strand. At the same time, motions of the phospholipid tails are constrained and they behave more rigidly. These interactions suggest establishment of energetic domains determined by joint states of intramembranous proteins and surrounding phospholipid molecules (Adey, 1992a).

4.4.2   Biophysical models of transmembrane signals: inward signaling along transmembrane receptor proteins

States of dielectric strain associated with these phospholipid-protein interactions are likely to determine optical properties within their cooperative domains. As in fiber optic systems (Christiansen, 1989), dependence of these optical properties on membrane excitation states may determine stability of dark soliton propagation as a means of transmembrane signaling.

Dark solitons suggest analogies with the sharp changes in optical properties of living vertebrate and invertebrate axons accompanying polarizing currents (Tobias *et al.*,1950), and the highly cooperative movements of about 18 Å reported with laser interferometry at the axon surface within 1 msec of excitation (Hill *et al.*, 1977).

Highly cooperative electron transfer along receptor proteins has been suggested as the basis for electromagnetic field interactions. Pioneering studies by Chance (DeVault *et al.*, 1966) disclosed the physical nature of the first steps in activation of cytochrome c-bacteriochlorophyll complex by millisecond electron transfer. Since the transfer was temperature-independent from 120°K to 4°K, they deduced that the reaction proceeded through a quantum mechanical tunneling mechanism, perhaps taking place over distances as large as 30 Å. Their studies coincided with Mitchell's development of his Nobel award winning chemiosmotic model, which proposed that the key electron-transfer steps of respiration operated across the full 35 Å width of the cell membrane.

Extension of these early concepts (Moser *et al.*, 1992) has suggested options for future research on detection and coupling of electromagnetic fields at cell membranes. For example, a variation of 20 Å in the distance between donors and acceptors may change the electron-transfer rate by 10^{12}-fold. In the time domain, the model also suggests a strong dependence on distance. Thus, in considering electron-transfer across the full thickness of the cell membrane, with edge-to-edge distances between 25 and 35 Å, the optimal electron transfer rate for the shorter distance is in the range of seconds, shifting to a scale of days for the longer distance. Under these conditions, protein behaves like an organic glass, presenting a uniform electronic barrier to electron tunneling and a uniform nuclear frequency. If used in the study of biological membranes, it would be sufficient to select distance, free energy and reorganizational energy, in order to define rate and directional specificity of biological electron-transfer, and thus, to meet physiological requirements in a wide range of cytochrome (respiration enzyme) systems.

4.5   HIERARCHICAL SEQUENCE IN SIGNALING EVENTS: AUTOREGULATION OF RF SENSING AT CELL SURFACES

Studies in the biochemistry of cell membrane transductive coupling suggest a sequence in activation of cell membrane receptors and related enzymes in regulating a variety of cell functions, ranging from growth of connective tissue cells to the ordering of the electroencephalogram (EEG) in brain tissue. There is evidence that ELF and ELF-modulated RF fields modulate key steps in these sequences.

4.5.1 Activation of ornithine decarboxylase (ODC)

Ornithine decarboxylase (ODC) is an enzyme essential for cell growth and DNA synthesis. It synthesizes **polyamines** from the amino acid ornithine. Polyamines (putrescine, spermadine, spermine, cadaverine) are long chain molecules that are highly positively charged (polycationic). They have the highest charge/mass ratio of any biomolecule. High ODC activity occurs in the unregulated growth of tumor cells, as in the malignancy of prostate cancer. Elevated levels of polyamines trigger transcription of the proto-oncogenes c-*myc* and c-*fos* by c-*ras*. Thus, polyamines may participate in a cascade of events leading to communication between membrane-bound and nuclear oncogene products (Tabib *et al.*, 1994).

Moderate increases in ODC activity have been reported in a variety of cell cultures in response to ELF (60 Hz) electromagnetic fields, and to ELF-modulated RF fields (Byus *et al.*, 1987; 1988).

Litovitz *et al.* (1993) have examined the modulation-frequency dependence of ODC activity in cultured cells (fibroblasts), determining the minimal duration that a single ELF modulation frequency must be sustained (**coherence time**) in order to elicit an ODC response. Using a 915 MHz field, switching modulation frequencies from 55 to 65 Hz at coherence times of 1 sec or less abolished enhancement of ODC responses, while coherence times of 10 s or longer produced full enhancement. These microwave coherence effects were 'remarkably similar to those observed in ELF fields'.

Byus and colleagues (Tjandrawinata *et al.*, 1994) have shown that polyamines synthesized within cells are also exported to cell surfaces. There may be at least two major results of this polyamine export to the intercellular gutters. 1) As highly charged cationic molecules, they enter a polyanionic atmosphere established by the stranded protruding terminals of glycoproteins. By coulombic attraction, they may thus modulate levels of the net cell surface fixed negative charge. Modulation of this cell surface fixed charge has been reported to directly influence drug interactions, as for example, between acetyl choline and curare (Van der Kloot *et al.*, 1979). 2) In more specific interactions, exported polyamines have been shown to modulate excitability of specific cell surface receptors.

4.5.2 Polyamine regulation of glutamate receptors at cell membranes

Cell membrane receptors for the amino acid L-glutamate contribute to excitatory transmission throughout the brain and spinal cord (for review, see McBain *et al.*, 1994). There is a well established modulatory role for polyamines in regulation of the glutamate receptor. These effects are complex, in part because polyamines appear to act via multiple mechanisms. The polyamines spermine and spermidine simultaneously potentiate and inhibit responses at glutamate receptors (Benveniste *et al.*, 1993; McGurk *et al.*, 1990; Rock *et al.*, 1992). The effects are not mutually exclusive, and may relate to either an action within the pore of the receptor channel, or to binding to sites within the vestibule of the channel, producing a reduction in ion channel conductance due to charge-screening effects.

4.5.3   The glutamate receptor and normal/pathological synthesis of nitric oxide: sensitivity to magnetic fields

An enzymatic cascade is initiated within cells when glutamate receptors are activated, leading to the synthesis of nitric oxide (NO). Receptor activation initiates an influx of calcium, triggering the enzyme nitric oxide synthase to produce nitric oxide from the amino acid arginine. As a gaseous molecule, NO readily diffuses into cells surrounding its cell of origin. It has been identified as a widely distributed neuroregulator and neurotransmitter in many body tissues (Izumi *et al.*, 1993). Its chemical actions in brain tissue appear to involve production of the chemical cGMP (cyclic-guanosine monophosphate) from GTP (guanosine triphosphate). The pathophysiology of NO links its free radical molecular configuration to **oxidative stress**, with a role in Alzheimer's and Parkinson's disease, and in certain types of epilepsy. Magnetic resonance spectroscopy (MRS) has suggested decreased levels of N-acetylaspartate, an activator of the glutamate receptor, in the striatum of the brains of patients with Parkinson's disease (Holshouser *et al.*, 1995).

Studies of the role of NO in controlling the regularity of patterns of EEG waves in rat brain hippocampal tissue have shown that inhibition of its synthesis is associated with shorter and more stable intervals between successive bursts of rhythmic waves. Conversely, donors of NO and cGMP analogs applied during blockade of NO synthesis lengthen and destabilize intervals between successive rhythmic wave bursts (Bawin *et al.*, 1995a; 1995b).

The rate of occurrence of these rhythmic EEG wave bursts in rat brain hippocampal tissue is also disrupted by exposure to weak (peak amplitudes 0.8 and 8.0 gauss), 1 Hz sinusoidal magnetic fields (Bawin *et al.*, 1995a; 1995b). These field effects depend on synthesis of NO in the tissue. They are consistent with reports of altered EEG patterns in man and laboratory animals by ELF magnetic fields (Bell *et al.*, 1992a; 1992b; Lyskov *et al.*, 1993).

In summary, the evidence supports a model of sequential interactions between ELF and ELF-modulated RF fields and certain cellular regulatory mechanisms: ODC activation leads to polyamine synthesis within cells; highly cationic polyamines are exported to polyanionic cell surfaces; at cell surfaces, polyamines regulate excitability of glutamate receptors; activation of glutamate receptors initiates NO synthesis; as a highly diffusible free radical, NO is active in the cell of origin and in adjacent cells; and in brain tissue, NO is sensitive as a free radical to ELF magnetic fields in modulation of patterns of EEG rhythms.

4.6   CELL GROWTH REGULATION THROUGH INTERCELLULAR COMMUNICATION: MODULATION BY MICROWAVE FIELDS

Cells in normal tissue may be considered an organized society, 'whispering together' in a faint and private language. They communicate with their neighbors through chemical stimuli, and through electrical fields far weaker than the huge electrical barrier of the membrane potential. **Gap-junctions**, specialized plaques of protein placed between neighboring cell membranes, provide electrical and chemical coupling between them (Loewenstein, 1981). By contrast, 'cancer can be regarded as a rebellion in an orderly society of cells. Cancer cells neglect their neighbors and grow autonomously over surrounding normal cells. Since intercellular communication plays an important role in maintaining an orderly society, it must be disturbed during the process of carcinogenesis' (Yamasaki, 1987; 1990).

Disruption of gap-junction communication can lead to unregulated cell growth (for review, see Adey, 1992b). Experimental evidence supports a role for electromagnetic fields in modulation of this gap-junction communication in cell (Cain *et al.*, 1993) and animal (McLean *et al.*, 1991) studies of joint actions of chemical tumor promoters and fields at cell membranes. The most widely used experimental tumor promoter, the phorbol ester TPA, causes a dramatic inhibition of gap-junction assembly, but does not alter channel gating nor enhance disassembly of pre-existing gap-junction structures (Lampe, 1994).

A possible role for nonionizing electromagnetic fields in human cancer has been frequently denied, based on the simplistic contention that these fields lack sufficient energy to rupture chemical bonds in nuclear DNA. This incompatibility is not at issue. More importantly, over the past 20 years, models of tumor formation and supporting experimental evidence have focused on nuclear regulation of cell division through signaling sequences initiated at cell membranes. Through **cell membrane amplification**, including enzyme activation, signaling energetics in cell nuclei may be millions of times greater than in initial transductive steps.

4.6.1   Genotoxic carcinogenesis

Deeply rooted in the history of research in carcinogenesis and tumor formation has been the concept that damage to DNA in cell nuclei is a necessary and sufficient basis for tumor formation. It describes the essence of models of **genotoxic**

carcinogenesis, or multistage carcinogenesis, with successive stages of initiation, promotion and progression. There is a consensus that tumor formation involves at least two steps; an early step of initiation, and a later promotion effect. A single agent may cause both initiation and promotion, or two or more agents may be necessary, working together in the proper sequence. The interval between exposure to an initiator and appearance of the disease (latent period) is often 20 years or more.

Initiation Initiation involves damage to genetic stores of DNA in cell nuclei, but the changes are not expressed, i.e. a tumor does not result unless one or more promoting agents act repeatedly at a later time. Initiation may be a single event, as in exposure to ionizing radiation, or to certain chemicals, including coal tar derivatives. Initiated cells are **transformed** (mutated). They are cancer cells, but remain quiescent if not stimulated by a promoter.

Promotion Promotion results from agents having little or no initiating action when tested alone, but they markedly enhance tumor yield when applied repeatedly and intermittently following a low dose of an initiator (Slaga *et al.*, 1978; Berridge *et al.*, 1988; Nishizuka, 1984). They do not act on nuclear DNA, and many are known to act by binding to receptors at cell membranes (Weinstein, 1988).

Progression Cells that have been initiated, then promoted repeatedly and intermittently, undergo progression to fully transformed cells. They then have the ability to form tumors.

4.6.2   Epigenetic (non-genotoxic) carcinogenesis: evidence for electromagnetic field actions in tumor formation

New lines of research in tumor formation reflect identification of a growing number of agents, tumor promoters, that appear to play a causal role in human cancer, without direct action on DNA stores. Pitot and Dragan (1991) have summarized this approach in relation to current and future cancer research. Epigenetic models focus on action of tumor-promoting agents, many in primary interactions with membrane-associated receptors.

In experimental cancer studies, the most widely used chemical promoter is the phorbol ester TPA. Its cell membrane receptor is the membrane-bound messenger enzyme **protein kinase C** (PKC) (Castagna *et al.*, 1982). Intracellular signals initiated by PKC at cell membranes play a key role in nuclear DNA mechanisms in cell division (Nishizuka, 1983; 1984). Experimental evidence from cell and animal studies supports a model of joint actions of chemical tumor promoters and electromagnetic fields at cell membranes (Cain *et al.*, 1993; McLean *et al.*, 1991).

Experimental cell studies of tumor promotion models

Cain *et al.* (1993) have tested the separate and joint actions of the tumor promoter TPA and 60 Hz magnetic fields on the growth of two types of cells (fibroblasts) grown together in the same culture dish (co-culture). One cell type was normal; the other was a line of daughter cells previously mutated with ultraviolet light and behaving as cancer cells with uncontrolled growth. When grown together, contact with the parent cells inhibited the unregulated growth of the mutant daughter cells. The tumour promoter TPA unbalanced this contact equilibrium, allowing return of the unregulated growth of mutant daughter cells and formation of tiny tumors (foci) in the culture dish. A 60 Hz magnetic field (0.1 mT, 1 h exposure 4 times daily) increased by 60% the number of TPA-induced foci ($p < 0.001$), with an approximate doubling of the size and cell density of the foci. Fields alone had no effect.

In this system, cells grow to confluence in 10–14 days, and to a mature monolayer in 28 days. Thus, the intermittent exposures occurred while the cells were growing, in the presence of TPA; suggesting that 60 Hz magnetic fields act in conjunction with chemical tumor promoters to enhance development and expression of the cancerous daughter cells scattered amongst normal parent cells, a phenomenon defined as **co-promotion**.

There is also evidence that 60 Hz magnetic fields may act at cancer cell membranes to inhibit the normal oncostatic (cancer stopping) influence of hormones. Blask (1990) reported that growth of MCF-7 human breast cancer cells is inhibited by the hormone melatonin, produced in the pineal gland of the brain. It is a growth inhibitor of estrogen-positive breast cancer cells and circulates in the blood with a diurnal cycle that peaks at night. Blood levels of melatonin have been reported depressed in animals by 60 Hz magnetic fields (Wilson *et al.*, 1990; Reiter *et al.*, 1990; Lerchl *et al.*, 1991; Stevens *et al.*, 1992). Exposure to 60 Hz magnetic fields has also been hypothesized as a factor in human breast cancer (Stevens, 1987; Tynes *et al.*, 1990; Demers *et al.*, 1991; Matanoski *et al.*, 1991).

Confirming Blask's original observation, Liburdy *et al.* (1993) found that when MCF-7 cells were grown in physiological concentrations of melatonin (10^{-11} M), and exposed to an 0.24 μT, 60 Hz magnetic field that simulated a typical environmental background field, melatonin inhibited cell growth about 30% over a 7-day cycle. However, at a higher 1.1 μT field level, the oncostatic action of melatonin was completely blocked.

Animal models of tumor promotion

Relatively few animal studies have been reported on possible tumor-promoting actions of either ELF or RF/microwave fields.

Szmigielski *et al.* (1982) exposed two strains of mice, one with a high incidence of spontaneous breast cancer and the other with skin painted with the carcinogen 3,4-benzpyrene (BP), to CW 2.45 GHz microwave fields (5 or 15 mW/cm², 2 h daily, 6 sessions per week). Mice susceptible to breast cancer were irradiated from age 6 weeks to age 12 months. Breast tumors appeared earlier than in controls. A similar acceleration was observed for skin tumors in the BP-painted mice. In other groups of mice stressed by confinement, chronic microwave exposure at 5 mW/cm² for 3 months lowered natural anti-neoplastic resistance, resulting in a significantly higher rate of lung cancers (controls, tumor numbers 2.8 ±1.6 SD; exposed, tumor numbers 6.1 ±1.8).

In an ELF initiation-promotion study of skin cancer in mice (McLean *et al.*, 1991), the skin of the back was initiated with a single subthreshold dose of the carcinogen dimethylbenzanthrene (DMBA). The mice were then exposed to a 2 mT 60 Hz magnetic field for 21 weeks, to test whether the field would act as a tumor promoter. No tumors developed in either sham- or field-exposed animals. Two additional groups were then treated weekly with the tumor promoter TPA. The time to tumor appearance was shorter (but not statistically so), in the group exposed to magnetic fields and TPA. This study, which was limited by small sample size, also suggests reduced immune surveillance by natural killer (NK) cell activity, which might otherwise prevent or retard tumor cell growth.

Loscher and colleagues (Loscher *et al.*, 1995; Mevissen *et al.*, 1995) have reported that dimethylbenzanthrene (DMBA)-treated female rats exposed to 50 Hz magnetic fields for 13 weeks exhibited enhanced growth of mammary tumors. The magnitude of the co-promoting effect was linearly related to flux density. Significantly enhanced tumor growth occurred at fluxed densities of 50 and 100 μT, while 0.3 μT was ineffective, and 10 μT induced an intermediate (nonsignificant) response. They have modeled this response on the 'melatonin hypothesis', relating hormone-sensitive cancers to magnetic field exposure. A significant reduction in nocturnal serum melatonin levels occurred with exposures at 0.3 or 10 μT, i.e. at levels below those associated with significant tumor co-promotion in the DMBA model. At 50 μT, ornithine decarboxylase (ODC) activity, associated with cell growth and tumor promotion, was significantly enhanced in the mammary glands without DMBA dosage, but not in other tissues, suggesting that the magnetic field exposure had increased stem cell proliferation. As an index of reduced immune surveillance, T cell activation was significantly reduced in exposures at 50 μT.

Brain tumor incidence in rats chronically exposed to digital cellular phone fields in an initiation-promotion model

Digital phone systems that have replaced older FM technology operate in a packet mode, producing pulsed fields at the user's head. The North American Digital Cellular (NADC) standard produces 50 packets/sec, using 3:1 multiplexed Time-Division-Multiple-Access (TDMA) modulation with a 33% duty cycle.

Evidence of brain tumor promotion from exposure to these TDMA fields has been sought in rats exposed to a single dose of the short-lived carcinogen ENU (ethylnitrosourea) *in utero*, and thereafter, intermittently exposed to digital phone fields for 23 months (Adey *et al.*, 1996). The mean life span of Fischer rats used in this study is 26 months. A low dose of ENU (4 mg/kg on day 18 of pregnancy) was selected to give maximum sensitivity to possible tumor promotion by phone fields over the lifetime of the animals. Far-field irradiation with an 836 MHz circularly-polarized field began on day 19 and continued after parturition until weaning of offspring at 23 days of age. Near-field exposure of offspring began at 35 days, and continued for the next 22 months, 4 days weekly. Exposures were for 2 h daily, field-on 7.5 min, field-off 7.5 min. Modeled far-field time-averaged SARs were: pregnant dam (uterus) 0.3 W/kg; fetus (brain) 0.29 W/kg; isolated pup (brain) 0.035 W/kg; young rat ((brain) 0.13 W/kg). Time-averaged near-field thermographic SARs were: larger males 0.75 W/kg (localized maximum 1.0 W/kg); smaller females 0.58 W/kg (localized maximum 0.75 W/kg). Survivors (n= 182, 77%) of the original 236 rats were sacrificed at age 709–712 days.

The TDMA field had no enhancing effect on incidence, type or location of spontaneous nervous system tumors. At experiment termination, the TDMA field appeared to reduce incidence of malignant glial cell tumors in rats that had received the ENU drug when compared with rats receiving ENU and no field exposure (4 vs 13). The TDMA field also appeared to reduce the incidence of spontaneous glial tumors occurring in rats not receiving the ENU drug when they were compared with control animals (2 vs 7). Tumors in exposed rats were smaller in volume. There were no gender differences in tumor incidence. In rats not surviving to experiment termination (n= 54, 22%), the TDMA field appeared to prolong latency of appearance of both spontaneous and ENU-induced glial cell tumors, but did not alter histological criteria of tumor types. Consistent non-significant differences in survival rates were noted between the four rat groups, with higher death rates in a progression: sham/field;sham/sham;ENU/field;ENU/sham.

Small experimental rat numbers emphasize caution in interpreting these data, although findings were consistent in showing no tumor-enhancing field effect. Since the experiment design and low ENU dosage were predicated on a promotional field effect, apparent 'protective' field effects do not gain statistical support. ENU has a short brain half-life of 8–10 min. In that time, it causes irreversible alkylation of the enzyme DNA O-6 guanine, essential in DNA synthesis.

These observations of an apparent protective effect are not isolated. Low dosage with X-rays of rats at the time of ENU dosage has been reported to sharply reduce subsequent incidence of induced brain glial tumors (Warkany *et al.*, 1976), through activation of AT enzymes that participate in DNA repair (Stammberger *et al.*, 1990). Consistent with that model, an interpretation of this study may suggest an action of TDMA fields in mechanisms of DNA repair.

4.7 DNA DAMAGE AND DNA REPAIR: DISORDERED REPAIR MECHANISMS AND THE POSSIBLE ROLE OF LONG-TERM, LOW-LEVEL MICROWAVE EXPOSURE IN CANCER MECHANISMS

Recent research has come full circle in the quest for unifying hypotheses that might offer a more general synthesis in the pathophysiology of tumor formation. The renewed search has centered on models and mechanisms that go beyond the traditional emphasis on DNA damage as the sole and sufficent cause of tumor formation, or even as a primary precipitating factor.

4.7.1 Clinical studies of DNA repair mechanisms in cancer models

Clinical evidence points to the significance of DNA repair mechanisms in tumor prevention and tumor initiation. Even the most trivial metabolic intervention, such as consumption of coffee, is known to produce numerous but transient breaks in nuclear DNA that are normally completely repaired in a matter of hours. What evidence suggests a role for defects in DNA repair mechanisms in carcinogenesis?

Defects in cloned DNA repair genes have been recently associated with a predisposition to some cancers and other disorders (Taylor et al., 1994). Moreover, free radicals of the oxygen and nitrogen species may act as complete carcinogens, the outcome depending on interactions between DNA damage, antioxidant levels and DNA repair systems (Wiseman et al., 1995). Studies of a familial cluster of breast cancer cases in one generation offer a model in which possible interaction between DNA repair proficiency and exposure to ionizing radiation in childhood (Helzlsouer et al., 1995), supports the hypothesis that a deficiency in repair of X-irradiation DNA damage may increase susceptibility to breast cancer.

The most common form of childhood cancer is acute lymphoblastic leukemia (ALL). Studies by the Swedish National Institute for Occupational Health have reported that children chronically exposed to powerline magnetic fields exhibit a 3-fold increase in incidence of leukemia (Feychting et al., 1992), and similar data have been reported by other investigators. Uckun and Luben and their collaborators (1995) present evidence that exposure of precursors cells in the B-lymphocyte lineage to 60 Hz, 1 G magnetic fields activates the Lyn protein tyrosine kinases, initiating an enzyme cascade that culminates in activation of the powerful messenger enzyme protein kinase C (PKC). Activation of Lyn kinase is sufficient and mandatory for the PKC response in these B-lineage cells. No directly genotoxic action of these fields is known, and there is wide agreement that exposure of cells to these fields does not produce mutations or chromosome damage. The authors conclude that 'any participation by EMF in leukemogenesis of B-lineage ALL is likely to be by influencing survival, proliferation, and/or differentiation of B-lineage lymphoid cells, rather than by producing the primary mutational or initiation event'; and that a delicate growth regulatory balance might be altered in B-lineage lymphoid cells by EMF-induced activation of Lyn.

4.7.2   Animal studies of DNA single-strand breaks

Particular significance may therefore attach to reports of extensive DNA single-strand breaks in animals chronically exposed to low-level microwave fields. Sarkar *et al.* (1994) first reported band patterns of DNA fragments from brain and testis tissue in the size range 6–8 kilobases following protracted microwave exposure in mice. Exposures ranged from 120 to 200 days in 2.45 GHz CW fields at densities of 1 mW/cm^2 (SAR 1.18 W/kg) for 2 h/day. DNA assays used gel electrophoresis and autoradiography.

This rearrangement of DNA has been further tested for both CW and pulsed microwave fields, using a fluorescence microscopy technique capable of detecting 1 break per 2×10^{10} daltons of DNA (Lai *et al.*, 1995). Immediately after a 2 h exposure to pulsed microwaves (2.45 GHz, pulse width 2 μs, pulse repetition frequency 500/s), no effects were noted, but a dose rate-dependent increase in DNA single-strand breaks (0.6 vs. 1.2 W/kg whole body SAR) was found in rat brain cells at 4 h post-exposure. By contrast, in rats exposed to 2.45 GHz CW fields for 2 h (SAR 1.2 W/kg), increased single-strand breaks were observed immediately, as well as at 4 h post-exposure.

4.8   THE QUESTION OF CUMULATIVE DOSE: TEMPORAL SEQUENCES IN TISSUE RESPONSES AND THE APPARENT ROLE OF INTERMITTENCY

In the most general terms, epidemiological data have suggested a relationship between duration of exposure to environmental electromagnetic fields, typically measured over years, and the onset of a disease process. Inherently, these long-term exposures are intermittent, whether measured on a diurnal basis or on a longer time scale. However, use of a time-weighted-average (TWA) as an exposure metric has been of limited value in seeking a precise correlate with disease risk, nor have other measures of the electromagnetic environment, such as ambient field levels, established a reliable measure of dose-dependence. Though not yet offering a solution, some laboratory studies may now point the way to future research.

4.8.1   Natural field potentials and synchronization of cell firing in brain tissue

In the cerebral cortex, fields generated by localized firing of nerve cells have been shown to contribute significantly to the synchronization of inactive neighboring cells during epileptiform activity (Jefferys *et al.*, 1982; Richardson *et al.*, 1984). Bawin *et al.* (1984; 1986) found that sinusoidal electric fields (5 and 60 Hz, amplitudes 5–50 mV/cm in tissue) considered too weak to directly modulate neuronal excitability could nevertheless induce progressive long-lasting increases in population spikes (synchronous firing of many nerve cells in one region of brain tissue as a response to a single stimulating pulse) in non-epileptic brain tissue. These are **ephaptic interactions** occurring directly through ELF field influences, in the absence of generally accepted chemical **synaptic transmission** that occurs through endings of nerve fibers that terminate on another brain nerve cell (Taylor *et al.*, 1984). Stimulation of nervous tissue with brief trains of high frequency pulses (200–500 Hz), defined as a **tetanic stimulus**, is also followed by long-lasting increases in population spikes. This phenomenon of **post-tetanic potentiation** has been equated with elemental aspects of memory mechanisms in information storage and retrieval in brain tissue.

4.8.2   ON- and OFF-responses as factors in estimation of cumulative tissue dose for nonionizing electromagnetic fields

In exposures to ionizing radiation, tissue dose involves an essentially simple calculation based on the product of field intensity and exposure duration. For nonionizing fields, the essential exposure parameters are far more complex.

As yet, there is no clear tissue metric for nonionizing fields, but a recurring aspect of laboratory studies has been observations of ON- and OFF-effects. As ON-effects, cell responses to EM fields may be transient, even though the exposure is sustained. This was noted in protein kinase responses in human lymphocytes to ELF-modulated RF fields; an initial rapid decrease in activity of 60% within 15–30 min was followed by a return to control levels within an hour (Byus *et al.*, 1984).

In bone cells exposed to pulsed 72 Hz magnetic fields used in fracture therapy, Luben *et al.* (1982) noted that bone cells are desensitized to the effects of parathyroid hormone (PTH) during exposure, but regained sensitivity as an OFF-effect. Luben *et al.* (1994) have proposed that interference with membrane-mediated signal transduction is a plausible mechanism by which low energy magnetic fields may influence intracellular processes. Their study compared actions of 60 Hz, 0.1 mT sinusoidal magnetic fields with actions of the tumor promoter TPA. The fields and the chemical promoter both rapidly but transiently increased cell membrane levels of the messenger enzyme protein kinase C (PKC), but reduced its activity in the cell cytoplasm. Specifically, turning off the field led to a recovery of PKC activity, as determined by a 4–5-fold increase in total cell PKC activity over a 4 h period; during this period, there was a maximum desensitization of the cell membrane PTH receptor.

In a different time frame, epidemiological studies have raised questions about potential health effects of large magnetic transients and heavy starting loads asociated with initial operation of domestic and industrial equipment. We have discussed the **coherence time** during which amplitude modulation of an ELF-modulated RF field must sustain modulation at a specific ELF frequency, before switching to a different but closely related frequency, in order to initiate an enzyme response (Litovitz *et al.*, 1993). For the enzyme ornithine decarboxylase (ODC), the minimum coherence time is between 1 and 10 sec to reliably elicit an enzymatic response.

Long-term effects of low-level microwaves on human lymphocyte DNA

Garaj-Vrhovac *et al.* (1990; 1992) have examined the incidence of micronuclei in blood lymphocytes of a small series of microwave workers with long-term exposures. Ten workers at a radar station and ten workers occupationally exposed to polyvinyl chloride were compared with controls not exposed to either agent. The mean duration of exposures was 15 years (range 8–25 years). Microwave field levels in the work place ranged between 10 and 50 μW/cm^2. Both agents induced qualitative and quantitative chromosome changes, more severe with vinyl chloride than microwaves. Abnormal micronuclei (detached portions of nuclear DNA) were more numerous in workers with microwaves than with vinyl chloride. Conversely, anaphase bridges were constantly present in chromosomes of vinyl chloride workers but rare in microwave workers. These effects have been associated with neoplastic transformations (Miller *et al.*, 1983).

4.8.3   Time-dependent brain tumor risk in RF/microwave occupational exposures

A case-control study by the U. S. National Cancer Institute of brain tumor incidence in RF/microwave occupational exposures (Thomas *et al.*, 1987) in the states of New Jersey, Pennsylvania and Louisiana concluded that all excess risk for primary brain tumors in white males aged over 30 years derived from jobs involving design, manufacture, installation or repair of electronic equipment (Risk Ratio= 2.3, 95% CI= 1.3, 4.2). Cases were divided into cohorts with 5, 10, 15 and 20+ years of exposure. Risks of these malignant tumors (astrocytomas) increased ten-fold for those employed 20 years or more. RRs were not increased in men exposed to RF/microwave fields but who never worked in electrical or electronics jobs, leading the authors to emphasize concurrent chemical exposures to soldering fumes, solvents and a variety of chemicals as possible co-factors with RF/microwave fields in tumor promotion.

4.9   SUMMARY AND CONCLUSIONS: THE COMPLEXITY OF THE HUMAN SITUATION

Over the past 15 years, there have been emergent concerns that the great and growing use of electric power, of incalculable value in opening doors to a myriad electrical and electronic systems and devices essential in the home and in the workplace, may carry a burden of adverse health effects. In this same era, bioelectromagnetic research worldwide has been driven by this pressing social mandate to arrive at valid estimates of levels of risk. This hazard research has followed a dual course, with epidemiological and laboratory studies proceeding in parallel, but with few options for coordination.

Despite its overt initial role as handmaiden to hazard assessment, bioelectromagnetic research has independently laid foundations pointing to a quite new understanding of living matter, based on physical processes at the atomic level, far beyond the realm of chemical reactions in a biomolecular fabric. Appropriate models describing these bioeffects are based in nonequilibrium thermodynamics, with nonlinear electrodynamics at the atomic level as integral features. Tissue heating, modeled in equilibrium thermodynamics, fails to offer suitable models for an impressive spectrum of observed electromagnetic field bioeffects. Indeed, bioelectromagnetic research appears to have swept beyond immediate goals in hazard research.

Laboratory studies have identified cell membranes as probably the major primary tissue site of interaction with environmental ELF and ELF-modulated RF/microwave fields. They have determined major sequences in the coupling of cell surface signals to a cascade of high energy enzymatic mechanisms inside cells. Major effects of these fields have been noted in 1) regulation of the immune system; 2) in modulation of brain and central nervous system functions, including regulation of the pineal gland and its hormone melatonin, which regulate the body's 24 h daily rhythm, and are indirectly involved in other hormonal mechanisms, including normal estrogen receptor formation in the breast; 3) in regulation of cell growth, through enzymatic mechanisms mediating DNA synthesis and repair, and 4) in apparently acting at cell membranes with chemical cancer promoters, or with the body's intrinsic hormonal mechanisms, as co-factors in tumor formation.

Epidemiological studies have drawn attention to ELF and ELF-modulated RF fields as possible risk factors in leukemia, lymphoma, breast tumors, skin melanoma and brain tumors. It is clear that these studies are merely pointers to much needed information on an exposure metric for health effects in man. Nevertheless, they emphasize the profound complexity of tissue effects of nonionizing EM fields. Unlike ionizing radiation, the nonionizing metric must take account of profound tissue effects attributable to intermittency of exposure, and the frequently transient character of the ensuing biological response.

In our civilized society, the human condition inherently involves a vast mix of electromagnetic field exposures, most transient, some long-lasting. Thus, use of a cellular telephone must be seen as part of a ceaseless panorama of endlessly changing exposures. Typically, we may expect concurrent exposures to a spectrum of static and ELF 50/60 Hz fields, some or all interacting with the phone's RF/microwave fields in body tissues. In civilized society, man's chemical environment is similarly mixed and poorly defined. Laboratory evidence supports the possibility that environmental electromagnetic fields may interact with chemical pollutants to enhance their tumor-promoting actions (Adey, 1990b). On the one hand, this new laboratory knowledge emphasizes emergence of bioelectromagnetics as an interdisciplinary field at the frontier of both physical and life sciences, holding prospects for major new advances in understanding functions of the human body in health and disease. On the other, without much further fundamental research, there are few prospects of developing a metric for tissue dose in EM field exposure; and without a metric, further epidemiological studies may hold little prospect of major progress.

REFERENCES

Adey, W.R. (1972) Organization of brain tissue: is the brain a noisy processor? *Internat. J. Neurosci.*, **49**, 271–284.

Adey, W.R. (1980) Frequency and power windowing in tissue interactions with weak electromagnetic fields. *Proc. IEEE*, **68**, 119-125.

Adey, W.R. (1981) Tissue interactions with nonionizing electromagnetic fields. *Physiol. Rev.*, **61**, 435–514.

Adey, W.R. (1990a) Electromagnetic fields and the essence of living systems, in *Modern Radio Science* (ed J. B. Andersen), University Press, Oxford, pp. 1–36.

Adey, W.R. (1990b) Joint actions of nonionizing environmental electromagnetic fields and chemical pollution in cancer promotion. *Environmental Health Perspectives*, **86**, 297–305.

Adey, W.R. (1992a) Collective properties of cell membranes, in *Interaction Mechanisms of Low-Level Electromagnetic Fields in Living Systems* (eds B. Norden and C. Ramel), University Press, Oxford, pp. 47–77.

Adey, W.R. (1992b) ELF magnetic fields and promotion of cancer: experimental studies, in *Interaction Mechanisms of Low-Level Electromagnetic Fields in Living Systems* (eds B. Norden and C. Ramel), University Press, Oxford, pp. 23–46.

Adey, W.R. (1993a) Electromagnetics in biology and medicine, in *Modern Radio Science* (ed H. Matsumoto), University Press, Oxford, pp. 231–249.

Adey, W.R. (1993b) Biological effects of electromagnetic fields. *J. Cell. Biochem.*, **51**, 410–416.

Adey, W.R., Kado, J. and Didio, J. (1962) Impedance measurements in brain tissue of animals using microvolt signals. *Exptl. Neurol.*, **5**, 47–66.

Adey, W.R., Kado, J., Didio, J. *et al.* (1963) Impedance changes in cerebral tissue accompanying a learned discriminative performance in the cat. *Exptl. Neurol.*, **7**, 259–281.

Adey, W.R., Kado, R.T. and Walter, D.O. (1965) Impedance characteristics of cortical and subcortical structures; evaluation of regional specificity in hypercapnea ad hypothermia. *Exptl. Neurol.*, **11**, 190–216.

Adey, W.R., Byus, C.V., Haggren, W. *et al.* (1996) *Brain tumor incidence in rats chronically exposed to digital cellular telephone fields in an initiation-promotion model.* Bioelectromagnetics Society, 18th Annual Meeting, Proceedings, Abstract A-7-3.

Astumian, R.D., Weaver, J.C. and Adair, R.K. (1995) Rectification and signal averaging of weak electric fields by biological signals. *Proc. Nat. Acad. Sci. USA*, **92**, 3740–3743.

Bach Andersen, J., Johansen, C., Pedersen, G.F. *et al.* (1995) *On the Possible Health Effects Related to GSM and DECT Transmissions.* A tutorial study. Center for Personkommunikation, Institute of Electronic Systems, Aalborg University, Denmark. 60 pp.

Barber, P.W., Gandhi, O.P., Hagmann, M.J. *et al.* (1979) I. Electromagnetic absorption in a multilayer model of man. *IEEE Trans. Biomed. Eng.*, **26**, 400–405.

Barnes, F.S. (1996) The effects of ELF on chemical reaction rates in biological systems, in *Biological Effects of Magnetic and Electromagnetic Fields* (ed S. Ueno), Plenum Press, New York, pp. 37–44.

Bassen, H., Litovitz, T., Penafiel, M. *et al.* (1992) *In vitro* exposure systems for inducing uniform electric and magnetic fields in cell culture. *Bioelectromagnetics*, **13**, 183–198.

Bawin, S.M., Gavalas-Medici, R. and Adey, W.R. (1973) Effects of modulated very high frequency fields on specific brain rhythms in cats. *Brain Res.*, **58**, 365–384.

Bawin, S.M., Kaczmarek, L.K. and Adey, W.R. (1975) Effects of modulated VHF fields on the central nervous system. *Ann. NY Acad. Sci.*, **247**, 74–81.

Bawin, S.M., Sheppard, A.R., Mahoney, M.D. *et al.* (1986a) Influences of sinusoidal electric fields on excitability in the rat hippocampal slice. *Brain Res.*, **323**, 227–237.

Bawin, S.M., Sheppard, A.R., Mahoney, M.D. *et al.* (1986b) Comparison between the effects of extracellular direct and sinusoidal currents on excitability in hippocampal slices. *Brain Res.*, **362**, 350–354.

Bawin, S.M., Satmary, W.M. and Adey, W.R. (1994) Nitric oxide modulates rhythmic slow activity in rat hippocampal slices. *NeuroReport*, **5**, 1869–1872.

Bawin, S.M., Satmary, W.M., Jones, R.A. *et al.* (1995a) *Interactions Between ELF Magnetic Fields and Brain Processes Require Synthesis of Nitric Oxide.* Proceedings of the Bioelectromagnetics Society, 17th Annual Meeting, p. 83.

Bawin, S.M., Satmary, W.M., Jones, R.A. *et al.* (1995b) Extremely low frequency magnetic fields disrupt rhythmic slow activity in rat hippocampal slices (in press).

Bell, G.B., Marino, A.A. and Chesson, A.L. (1992) Alteration in brain electrical activity caused by magnetic fields: detecting the detection process. *Electroenceph. Clin. Neurophysiol.*, **83**, 389–397.

Bell, G.B., Marino, A.A., Chesson, A.L. *et al.* (1992) Electrical states in the rabbit brain can be altered by light and electromagnetic fields. *Brain Res.*, **570**, 307–315.

Benveniste, M. and Mayer, M.L. (1993) Multiple effects of spermine on N-methyl-D-aspartic acid receptor responses of rat cultured hippocampal neurones. *J. Physiol. Lond.*, **464**, 131–163.

Berridge, M.J., Cobbold, P.H. and Cuthbertson, K.S.R. (1988) Spatial and temporal aspects of cell signalling. *Phil. Trans. Roy. Soc.*, **320**, 325–343.

Bezrukov, S.M. and Vodyanoy, I. (1995) Noise-induced enhancement of signal transduction across voltage-dependent ion channels. *Nature*, **378**, 362–364.

Bialek, W. (1983) Macroquantum effects in biology; the evidence. Ph.D. Thesis, Department of Chemistry, University of California, Berkeley, 250 pp.

Bialek, W. and Wit, H.P. (1984) Quantum limits to oscillator stability: theory and experiments on acoustic emissions from the human ear. *Phys. Lett.*, **104A**, 173–178.

Blackman, C.F., Elder, J.A., Weil, C.M. *et al.* (1979) Induction of calcium ion efflux from brain tissue by radio frequency radiation: effects of modulation frequency and field strength. *Radio Sci.*, **14**, 93–98.

Blackman, C.F., Benane, S.G., House, D.E. *et al.* (1985) Effects of ELF (1–120 Hz) and modulated (50 Hz) RF fields on the efflux of calcium ions from brain tissue *in vitro*. *Bioelectromagnetics*, **6**, 327–338..

Blackman, C.F., Benane, S.G., Elliot, D.J. *et al.* (1988) Influence of electromagnetic fields on the efflux of calcium ions from brain tissue *in vitro*: a three-model analysis consistent with the frequency response up to 510 Hz. *Bioelectromagnetics*, **9**, 215–227.

Blackman, C.F., Benane,S.G., House, D.E. *et al.* (1990) Importance of alignment between local DC magnetic field and an oscillating magnetic fields in responses of brain tissue *in vitro* and *in vivo*. *Bioelectromagnetics*, **11**, 159–167.

Blackman, C.F., Blanchard, J.P., Benane, S.G. *et al.* (1994) Empirical test of an ion parametric resonance model for magnetic field interactions with PC-12 cells. *Bioelectromagnetics*, **15**, 239–260.

Blanchard, J.P. and Blackman, C.F. (1994) Clarification and application of an ion parametric resonance model for magnetic field interactions with biological systems. *Bioelectromagnetics*, **15**, 217–238.

Byus, C.V., Lundak, R.L., Fletcher, R.M. *et al.* (1984) Alterations in protein kinase activity following exposure of cultured lymphocytes to modulated microwave fields. *Bioelectromagnetics*, **5**, 34–51.

Byus, C.V., Pieper, S. and Adey, W.R. (1987) The effect of low-energy 60 Hz environmental electromagnetic fields upon the growth related enzyme ornithine decarboxylase. *Carcinogenesis*, **8**, 1385–1389.

Byus, C.V., Kartun, K.S., Pieper, S.E. *et al.* (1988) Increased ornithine decarboxylase activity in cultured cells exposed to low energy microwave fields and phorbol ester tumor promoters. *Cancer Res.*, **48**, 4222–26.

Cain, C.D., Thomas, D.L. and Adey, W.R. (1993) 60 Hz magnetic field acts as co-promoter in focus formation of $C3H10T^1/_2$ cells. *Carcinogenesis*, **14**, 955–960.

Castagna, M., Takai, Y., Kaibuchi, K. *et al.* (1982) Direct activation of calcium-activated phospholipid-dependent protein kinase by tumor-promoting phorbol esters. *J. Biol. Chem.*, **257**, 7847–51.

Christiansen, P.L. (1989) Shocking optical solitons. *Nature*, **339**, 17–18.

Cleveland, R.F. and Athey, T.W. (1989) Specific absorption rate (SAR) in models of the human head exposed to handheld portable radios. *Bioelectromagnetics*, **10**, 173–186.

Demers, P.A. *et al.* (1991) Occupational exposure to electromagnetic fields and breast cancer in men. *Am. J. Epidemiol.*, **132**, 775–776..

DeVault, D. and Chance, B. (1966) Studies of photosynthesis using a pulsed laser. I. Temperature dependence of cytochrome oxidation rate in chromatium. Evidence of tunneling. *Biophys. J.*, **6**, 825–847.

Dutta, S.K., Subramoniam, A., Ghosh, B. *et al.* (1984) Microwave radiation-induced calcium efflux from brain tissue, *in vitro. Bioelectromagnetics*, **5**, 71–78.

Eichwald, C. and Kaiser, F. (1995) Model for external influences on cellular signal transduction pathways including cytosolic calcium oscillations. *Bioelectromagnetics*, **16**, 75-85.

Einolf, C.W. and Carstensen, E.L. (1971) Low-frequency dielectric dispersion in suspension of ion-exchange resins. *J. Phys. Chem.*, **75**, 1091–1099.

Engstrom, S. (1995a) *What is the Locus of ELF Magnetic Field Interaction?* Bioelectromagnetic Society, Proceedings 17th Annual Meeting, Boston MA, p. 114.

Engstrom, S. (1995b) *An Experiment to Determine the Natural Timescale of Magnetic Field Interaction with Biological Systems.* Annual Review of Research on Biological Effects of Electric and Magnetic Fields from Generation, Delivery and Use of Electricity, U.S. Department of Energy, Office of Energy Management. Proceedings, p. 19.

Feychting, M. and Ahlbom, A. (1992) Magnetic fields and cancer in people residing near Swedish high voltage power lines. Karolinska Institute, Stockholm. *IMM-Report 6/92*, 67 pp.

Frohlich, H. (1946) Shape of collision-broadened spectral lines. *Nature*, **157**, 468.

Frohlich, H. (1968) Long-range coherence and energy storage in biological systems. *Internat. J. Quant. Chem.*, **2**, 641-659.

Gandhi, O.P. (1975) Strong dependence of whole animal absorption on polarization and frequency of radio frequency energy. *Ann. NY Acad. Sci.*, **247**, 532–538.

Gandhi, O.P. and Hagmann, M.J. (1977) Some recent results on deposition of electromagnetic energy in animals and models of man, in *The Physical Basis of Electromagnetic Interactions with Biological Systems* (eds L. S. Taylor and A. Y. Cheung), University of Maryland, College Park, pp. 243–260.

Gandhi, O.P. *et al.* (1994) *Electromagnetic Absorption in the Human Head for Cellular Telephones.* Bioelectromagnetics Society, 16th Annual Meeting, Proceedings, pp. 64–65.

Garaj-Vhrovac, V., Fucic, A. and Horvat, D. (1990) Comparison of chromosome aberration and micronuclei induction in human lymphocytes after occupational exposure to vinyl chloride monomer and microwave radiation. *Periodicum Biologorium*, **92**, 411-416.

Garaj-Vhrovac, V., Fucic, A. and Horvat, D. (1992) The correlation between the frequency of micronuclei and specific chromosome aberrations in human lymphocytes exposed to microwave radiation *in vitro. Mutat. Res.*, **281**, 181–186.

Grissom, C.B. (1995) Magnetic field effects in biology: a survey of possible mechanisms with emphasis on radical-pair recombination. *Chem Rev.*, **95**, 3–24.

Grodsky, I.T. (1977) Neuronal membranes: a physical synthesis. *Math. Biosci.*, **28**, 191–219.

Grundler, W., Keilmann, F. and Frohlich. H. (1977) Resonant growth rate response of yeast cells irradiated by weak microwaves. *Phys. Lett.*, **62A**, 463–466.

Grundler, W. and Kaiser, F. (1992) Experimental evidence for coherent excitations correlated with cell growth. *Nanobiology*, **1**, 163-176.

Grundler, W., Keilmann, F., Putterlik, V. *et al.* (1983) Nonthermal resonant effects of 42 GHz microwaves on the growth of yeast cultures, in *Coherent Excitations in Biological Systems* (eds H. Frohlich and F. Kremer), Springer, Berlin, pp. 21–37.

Grundler, W., Kaiser, F., Keilmann, F. *et al.* (1992) Mechanics of electromagnetic interaction with cellular systems. *Naturwissenschaften*, **79**, 551–559.

Hagmann, M.J., Gandhi, O.P. and Durney, C.H. (1979) Numerical calculation of electromagnetic enrgy deposition for a realistic model of man. *IEEE Trans. Microwave Theory Tech.*, **27**, 804–809.

Helzlsouer, K.J., Harris, E.L., Parshad, R. *et al.* (1995) Familial clustering of breast cancer: possible interaction between DNA repair proficiency and radiation exposure in the development of breast cancer. *Int. J. Cancer*, **64**, 14–17.

Hill, B.C., Schubert, E.D., Nokes, M.A. *et al.* (1977) Laser interferometer measurements of changes in crayfish axon diameter concurrent with action potential. *Science*, **196**, 426–428.

Holshouser, B.A., Komu, M., Moller, H.A. *et al.* (1995) Localized proton NMR spectroscopy in the striatum of patients with idiopathic Parkinson's disease: a multicenter pilot study. *Magnetic Resonance in Medicine*, **33**, 589–594.

Illinger, K.H. (1962) Dispersion of microwaves in gases and liquids. *Progr. Dielect.*, **4**, 37–100.

Illinger, K.H. (1981) *Biological Effects of Ionizing Radiation.* American Chemical Society Symposium Series, No. 157, 342 pp.

Izumi, Y. and Zorumski, C.F. (1993) Nitric oxide and long-term synaptic depression in the rat hippocampus. *NeuroReport*, **4**, 1131-1134.

Jefferys, J.G.R. and Haas, H.L. (1982) Synchronized bursting of CA1 hippocampal pyramidal cells in the absence of synaptic trransmission. *Nature*, **300**, 448–450.

Kaczmarek, L.K. and Adey, W.R. (1974) Some chemical and electrophysiological effects of glutamate in cerebral cortex. *J. Neurobiol.*, **5**, 231–241.

Kaiser, F. (1983) Theory of resonant effects of RF and microwave energy, in *Biological Effects and Dosimetry of Nonionizing Radiation* (eds M. Grandolfo, F. Michaelson and A. Rindi), Plenum Press, New York, pp. 251–282

Kaiser, F. (1984) Entrainment, quasi-periodicity-chaos-collapse: bifurcation routes of externally driven self-sustained oscillating systems, in *Nonlinear Electrodynamics in Biological Systems* (eds W. R. Adey and A. F. Lawrence), Plenum Press, New York, pp. 393–412.

Kolomytkin, O., Yurinska, M., Zharikov, S. *et al.* (1994) Response of brain receptor systems to microwave energy exposure, in *On the Nature of Electromagnetic Field Interactions with Biological Systems* (ed A. H. Frey), R. G. Landes, Austin, Texas, pp. 195–206.

Kritikos, H.N. and Schwan, H.P. (1972) Hot spots generated in conducting spheres by electromagnetic waves and biological implications. *IEEE Trans. Biomed. Eng.*, **19**, 53–58.

Kritikos, H.N. and Schwan, H.P. (1975) The distribution of heating potential inside lossy spheres. *IEEE Trans. Biomed. Eng.*, **22**, 457–463.

Kritikos, H.N. and Schwan, H.P. (1976) Formation of hot spots in multilayered spheres. *IEEE Trans. Biomed. Eng.*, **23**, 168–172.

Kritikos, H.N. and Schwan, H.P. (1979) Potential temperature rise induced by electromagnetic field in brain tissue. *IEEE Trans. Biomed. Eng.*, **26**, 123–124.

Kuster, N. and Balzano, Q. (1995) Experimental and numerical dosimetry. This volume.

Lai, H. and Singh, N. (1995) Acute low-density microoawave exposure increases DNA single-strand breaks in rat brain cells. *Bioelectromagnetics*, **16**, 207–210.

Lampe, P.D. (1994) Analyzing phorbol ester effects on gap junctional communication: a dramatic inhibition of assembly. *J. Cell. Biol.*, **127**, 1895–1905.

Lednev, V.V. (1991) Possible mechanism for the influence of weak magnetic fields on biological systems. *Bioelectromagnetics*, **12**, 71–75.

Lednev, V.V. (1995) Comments on 'Clarification and application of ion parametric resonance model for magnetic field interactions with biological systems' by Blanchard and Blackman. *Bioelectromagnetics*, **16**, 268–269.

Lerchl, A., Reiter, R.J., Howes, K.A. *et al.* (1991) Evidence that extremely low frequency Ca^{2+}-cyclotron resonance depresses pineal melatonin synthesis *in vitro*. *Neurosci. Lett.*, **124**, 213–215.

Liboff, A.R. (1985) Cyclotron resonance in membrane transport, in *Interactions Between Electromagnetic Fields and Cells* (eds A. Chiabrera, C. Nicolini and H. P. Schwan), Plenum Press, New York, pp. 281–296.

Liboff, A.R., Rozak, R.J., Sherman, M.L. *et al.* (1987) Calcium-45 cyclotron resonance in human lymphocytes. *J. Bioelectr.*, **6**, 13–22.

Liburdy, R.P. (1992) Biological interactions of cellular sytems with time-varying magnetic fields. *Ann. N.Y. Acad. Sci.*, **649**, 74–95.

Liburdy, R.P. (1995) Cellular studies and interaction mechanisms of extremely low frequency fields. *Radio Sci.*, **30**, 179–203.

Lin-Liu, S. and Adey, W.R. (1982) Low frequency amplitude-modulated microwave fields change calciumc efflux rates from synaptosomes. *Bioelectromagnetics*, **3**, 309–322.

Litovitz, T., Krause, D., Penafiel, M. *et al.* (1993) The role of coherence time in the effect of microwaves on ornithine decarboxylase activity. *Bioelectromagnetics*, **14**, 395–404.

Loewenstein, W. () Junctional intercellular communication: the cell-to-cell communication channel. *Physiol. Rev.*, **61**, 829–913.

Loscher, W. and Mevissen M. (1995) *Linear Relationship Between Flux Density and Tumor Copromoting Effect of Magnetic Field in Rat Breast Cancer Model.* Bioelectromagnetics Society, 17th Annual Meeting, Proceedings, p. 78.

Luben, R.A. (1991) Effects of low energy electromagnetic fields (pulsed and DC) on membrane signal transduction processes in biological systems. *Health Phys.*, **61**, 15–28.

Luben, R.A., Morgan, A.P., Carlson, A. *et al.* (1994) *One Gauss 60 Hz Magnetic Fields Modulate Protein Kinase Activity by a Mechanism Similar to That of Tumor Promoting Phorbol Esters.* Bioelectromagnetics Society, 16th Annual Meeting. Proceedings, p. 74.

Lyle, D.B., Schechter, P., Adey, W.R. *et al.* (1983) Suppression of T lymphocyte cytoxicity following exposure to sinusoidally amplitude-modulated fields. *Bioelectromagnetics*, **4**, 281–292.

Lyle, D.B., Ayotte, R.D., Sheppard, A.R. *et al.* (1988) Suppression of T lymphocyte cytotoxicity following exposure to 60 Hz sinusoidal electric fields. *Bioelectromagnetics*, **9**, 303–313.

Lyskov, E.B., Juutilainen, J., Jousmaki, V. *et al.* (1993) Effects of 45 Hz magnetic fields on the functional state of the human brain. *Bioelectromagnetics*, **14**, 87–95.

Matanoski, G.M., Breyese, P.N. and Elliot, E.A. (1991) Electromagnetic field exposure and male breast cancer. *Lancet*, **33**, 737.

McBain, C.J. and Mayer, M.L. (1994) N-methyl-D-aspartic acid receptor structure and function. *Physiol. Rev.*, **74**, 723–760.

McConnell. H.M. (1975) Coupling between lateral and perpendicular motion in biological membranes, in *Functional Linkage in Biomolecular Systems* (eds F. O. Schmitt, D. M. Schneider and D. M. Crothers), Raven Press, New York, pp. 123–131.

McGurk, J.F., Bennett, M.V. and Zukin, R.S. (1990) Polyamines potentiate responses of *N*-methyl-D-aspartate receptors expressed in *Xenopus* oocytes. *Proc. Natl. Acad. Sci. USA*, **87**, 9971–9974.

McLauchlan, K. (1992) Are environmental electromagnetic fields dangerous? *Physics World*, pp. 41-45, January.

McLauchlan, K. and Steiner, U.E. (1991) The spin-correlated radical pair as a reaction intermediate. *Molec. Physics*, **73**, 241–263.

McLean, J.R.N., Stuchly, M.A., Mitchel, R.E.J. *et al.* (1991) Cancer promotion in a mouse-skin model by a 60 Hz magnetic field: II. Tumor development and immune response. *Bioelectromagnetics*, **12**, 273–288.

Mevissen, M., Loscher, W., Lerchl, A. *et al.* (1995) *Possible mechanisms of the tumor copromoting effect of magnetic field exposure in a rat breast cancer model.* Bioelectromagnetics Society, 17th Annual Meeting, Proceedings, p. 50.

Miller, D.A. and Miller, O.J. (1983) Chromosomes and cancer in the mouse: studies in tumors established cell lines and cell hybrids. *Advances Cancer Res.*, **39**, 153–183.

Mirutenko, V.I. and Bogach, P.C. (1977) Participation of Na-ions in the mechanisms of microwave effect on the nonstriated muscle cell membrane potential. *Molecular Genetics and Biophysics*, **2**, 102–104.

Misakian, M. and Kaune, W.T. (1990) Optimal experimental design for *in vitro* studies with ELF magnetic fields. *Bioelectromagnetics*, **11**, 251–255.

Moser, C.C., Keske, J.M., Warncke, K. *et al.* (1990) Nature of biological electron transfer. *Nature*, **355**, 796–802.

Nishizuka, Y. (1983) Protein kinase C as a possible receptor protein of tumor-promoting phorbol esters. *J. Biol. Chem.*, **258**, 11442-6.

Nishizuka, Y. (1984) The role of protein kinase C in cell surface signal transduction and tumour promotion. *Nature*, **308**, 693–698.

Pitot, H.C. and Dragan, Y.P. (1991) Facts and theories concerning the mechanisms of carcinogenesis. *FASEB J.*, **5**, 2280-8.

Porter, R., Adey, W.R. and Kado, R.T. (1965) Measurement of electrical impedance in the human brain: some preliminary observations. *Neurology*, **14**, 1002–1012.

Ranck, J.B. (1964) Specific impedance of cerebral cortex during spreading depression and an analysis of neuronal, neuroglial and interstitial contributions. *Exp. Neurol.*, **9**, 1–16.

Reiter, R.J. and Richardson, B.A. (1990) Magnetic field effects on pineal indoleamine metabolism and possible biological consequences. *FASEB J.*, **6**, 2283-7.

Richardson, T.L., Turner, R.W. and Miller, J.J. (1984) Extracellular fields influence transmembrane potentials, and synchronization of hippocampal neuronal activity. *Brain Res.*, **294**, 255–262.

Rock, D.M. and MacDonald, R.L. (1992) Spermine and related polyamines produce a voltage-dependent reduction of *N*-methyl-D-aspartate receptor single-channel conductance. *Mol. Pharmacol.*, **42**,157–164.

Rozak, R.J., Sherman, M.L., Liboff, A.R. *et al.* (1987) Nifedipine is an antagonist to cyclotron resonance enhancement of ^{45}Ca incorporation in human lymphocytes. *Cell Calcium*, **8**, 413–427.

Sarkar, S., Ali, S. and Behari, J. (1994) Effect of low power microwave on the mouse genome: a direct DNA analysis. *Mutation Res.*, **320**, 141–147.

Schwarz, G. (1970) Cooperative binding to linear biopolymers. II. Fundamental static and dynamic properties. *Eur. J. Biochem.*, **12**, 442–453.

Slaga, T.J., Sivak, A. and Boutwell, R.K. (eds) (1978) *Mechanisms of Tumor Promotion and Carcinogenesis*, Vol. 2, Raven Press, New York.

Smith, S.D., McLeod, B.R., Liboff, A.R. *et al.* (1987) Cyclotron resonance and diatom mobility. *Bioelectromagnetics*, **8**, 215–227.

Stammberger, J., Schmahl, W. and Nice, L. (1990) The effects of X-irradiation, *N*-ethyl-*N*-nitrosourea or combined treatment on O^6-alkylguanine-DNA alkyltransferase activity in fetal rat brain and liver and the induction of CNS tumors. *Carcinogenesis*, **11**, 219–222.

Stevens, R.G. (1987) Electric power use and breast cancer: a hypothesis. *Am. J. Epidemiol.*, **125**, 556–561.

Stevens, R.G., Davis, S., Thomas, D.B. *et al.* (1992) Electric power, pineal function and the risk of breast cancer. *FASEB J.*, **6**, 853–860.

Szmigielski, S., Svdinski, A., Piatrasek, A. *et al.* (1982) Accelerated development of spontaneous and benzpyrene-induced skin cancer in mice exposed to 2450 MHz microwave radiation. *Bioelectromagnetics*, **3**, 179–192.

Tabib, A. and Bachrach, U. (1994) Activation of the proto-oncogene c-*myc* and c-*fos* by c-*ras*: involvement of polyamines. *Biochem. Biophys. Res. Communications*, **202**, 720–727.

Taylor, C.P. and Dudek, F.E. (1984) Excitation of hippocampal pyramidal cells by an electrical field effect. *J. Neurophysiol.*, **52**, 126–142.

Taylor, A.M.R., McConville, C.M. and Byrd, P.J. (1994) Cancer and DNA processing disorders. *Brit. Med. Bull.*, **50**, 708–717.

Thomas, T.L., Stolley, P.D., Stemhagen, A. *et al.* (1987) Brain tumor mortality risk among men with electrical and electronics jobs: a case control study. *J. Nat. Cancer Inst.*, **79**, 233–238.

Tjandrawinata, R.R., Hawel, L. 3rd and Byus, C.V. (1994) Regulation of putrescine export in lipopolysaccharide or IFN-gamma-activated murine monocytic leukemic RAW264 cells. *J. Immunol.*, **152**, 3039–52.

Tynes, T. and Andersen, A. (1990) Electromagnetic fields and male breast cancer. *Lancet*, **336**, 1596.

Uckun, F.M., Kurosaki, T., Jin, J. *et al.* (1995) Exposure of B-lineage lymphoid cells to low energy electromagnetic fields stimulates Lyn kinase. *J. Biol. Chem.*, **270**, 27666–70.

Van der Kloot, W.G. and Cohen, I. (1979) Membrane surface potential changes may alter drug interactions: an example, acetyl choline and curare. *Science*, **203**, 1351–52.

Van Vleck, J.H. and Weisskopf, V.F. (1945) Survey of the theory of ferromagnetics. *Rev. Mod. Phys.*, **17**, 27–47.

Walleczek, J. (1994) Immune cell interactions with extremely low frequency magnetic fields: experimental verification and free radical mechanisms, in *On the Nature of Electromagneitc Field Interactions with Biological Systems* (ed A. H. Frey), R. G. Landes Company, Austin TX, pp. 167–180.

Walleczek, J. and Liburdy, R.P. (1990) Nonthermal 60 Hz sinusoidal magnetic field exposure enhances $^{45}Ca^{2+}$ uptake in rat thymocytes: dependence on mitogen activation. *FEBS Lett.*, **271**, 157-160.

Warkany, J., Mandebur, T.I. and Kalter, H. (1976) Oncogenic response of rats with X-ray induced microencephaly to transplacental ethylnitrosourea. *J. Natl.Cancer Inst.*, **56**, 59–64.

Weinstein, I.B. (1988) The origins of human cancer: molecular mechanisms of carcinogenesis and their implications for cancer treatment and prevention. *Cancer Res.*, **48**, 4135-43.

Wilson, B.W., Wright, C.W., Morris, J.E. *et al.* (1990) Evidence for an effect of ELF electromagnetic fields on human pineal gland function. *J. Pineal Res.*, **9**, 259–269.

Wiseman, H., Kaur, H. and Halliwell, B. (1995) DNA dmage and cancer: measurement and mechanism. *Cancer Lett.*, **93**, 113–120.

Yamasaki, H. (1987) The role of cell-to-cell communication in tumor promotion, in *Nongenotoxic Mechanisms in Carcinogenesis* (eds T. E. Butterworth and T. J. Slaga), 25th Banbury Report, Cold Spring Harbor Laboratory.

Yamasaki, H. (1991) Aberrant expression and function of gap junctions during carcinogenesis. *Envir. Health Perspectives*, **16**, 136-144.

5

Additional considerations about the bioeffects of mobile communications

Craig V. Byus and Leo Hawel, III

5.1 INTRODUCTION

There are two major questions undergoing considerable discussion regarding the potential biological effects elicited by exposure to electromagnetic fields. The first question is 'Can biological systems at the subcellular or cellular level sense and respond to any of a number of environmentally relevant electromagnetic fields?' By defining a measurable and reproducible molecular effect of exposure of a biological system to low-energy electromagnetic fields, it is hoped that the existence of a physical mechanism involved in mediating this response could be firmly established and ultimately understood. The second question of considerable interest is 'Does exposure of the human population to these low-energy "environmentally relevant" fields pose any kind of health risk?' The answer to this question has become particularly important due to the greater emphasis which is placed now upon the prevention rather than the treatment of disease. If, however, biological systems are incapable of sensing or responding to these fields, then there could be no health risk associated with this exposure. Furthermore, the establishment of a biological effect elicited by electromagnetic field exposure does not necessarily imply that there is any adverse effect upon the health of animals or humans.

The purpose of the information given here is to present one approach to determine whether a biological system is capable of responding or sensing exposure to one environmentally-relevant field, i.e. amplitude-modulated radio frequency fields. In this regard, we have performed a detailed series of experiments assessing the ability of amplitude-modulated RF fields to alter the activity of the enzyme ornithine decarboxylase (ODC), as well as ODC messenger RNA levels and polyamine export in a number of cultured cell lines. While some of this information has been presented previously (Byus *et al.*, 1988; 1987), new

Mobile Communications Safety
Edited by N. Kuster, Q. Balzano and J.C. Lin
Published in 1997 by Chapman & Hall, London. ISBN 0 412 75000 7.

evidence in this context will hopefully provide additional information concerning the understanding of the interaction of these fields with biological systems. In addition, a discussion is presented concerning the difficulties and limitations of animal studies designed to assess the ability of low-energy electromagnetic fields to cause or modulate cancer in animal models. The design and interpretation of these animal experiments needs to be made in a unique way. This is due to the differences which exist between the study of low-energy electromagnetic fields effects in relation to cancer in comparison to the more conventional study of ionizing radiation and chemicals.

5.2   SPECIFIC ENZYME INTERACTION

5.2.1   Polyamine metabolism – background

The polyamines putrescine, spermidine and spermine are small aliphatic amines which contain 2, 3 and 4 positive charges, respectively, at physiological pH (for review of the topic see Pegg, 1986; Tabor *et al.*, 1984; Heby *et al.*, 1990; van Daalen *et al.*, 1989; Porter *et al.*, 1990). These compounds have the highest net charge-to-mass ratio of any biosynthetic compound and are found ubiquitously in prokaryotic and eukaryotic cells. The biosynthesis of polyamines has been shown to be essential for the normal growth, proliferation, and differentiation of eukaryotes and prokaryotes as well. If, for example, the synthesis of polyamines is interrupted or inhibited by selective enzymatic inhibitors of the polyamine biosynthetic pathways, the growth and differentiation of eukaryotic cells fails to proceed normally. Polyamines are believed to play an important role in the stabilization of the three-dimensional structure of macromolecules due to the tight ionic binding to negative charges which exists on these macromolecules under physiological conditions. As such, polyamines have been shown to bind tightly to sialic acid residues on membranes, to RNA, DNA, and proteins. The requirement of some macromolecules for the precisely spaced cationic charges present on the polyamines cannot be replaced by other naturally-occurring cations such as magnesium.

The biosynthesis of the polyamines has been shown to be a highly regulated process in eukaryotes involving primarily the regulation of the rate-limiting enzyme ornithine decarboxylase (ODC) in polyamine biosynthesis (Byus *et al.*, 1987). The amino acid ornithine is decarboxylated by ODC, a pyridoxal phosphate requiring enzyme yielding the product diaminobutane or putrescine. Putrescine is then further converted to spermidine and spermine by sequential decarboxylation of S-adenosyl methionine (SAM) and the transfer of a propylamine moiety from the SAM to putrescine and to spermidine to form spermidine and spermine. The regulation of ornithine decarboxylase activity has been shown to involve both transcriptional regulation of the gene, alterations in the half-life of the ODC mRNA, translational regulation of the ODC mRNA, as well as post-translational regulation of the ODC protein through interaction with another protein called the ODC antizyme (Heby et al., 1990). Changes in ornithine decarboxylase activity are reported to occur rapidly within 30–60 min of the stimulation of cells to grow or divide by any of a number of hormones and growth factors (Pegg, 1986; Tabor et al., 1984; Heby et al., 1990; van Daalen et al., 1989; Porter et al., 1990; Wu et al., 1981; 1984; Byus, 1990; Byus et al., 1991). While the absolute amount of ornithine decarboxylase present inside of quiescent cells is quite small (on the order of several thousand molecules per cell), the amount of ODC enzyme can change markedly, sometimes up to 500-fold following appropriate stimulus to the system. Given the ease and sensitivity of the assay for ornithine decarboxylase, its overall importance in the potential growth and differentiation of the cell, and its the potential involvement of polyamines in a number of disease processes including cancer, we decided to study the ability of low-energy electromagnetic fields to alter ornithine decarboxylase activity in cultured cell systems.

5.2.2   Results

In the experiments described below, cultured mammalian cells were exposed to a 450 MHz sinusoidally amplitude-modulated RF field in a Crawford cell as described in detail previously (Byus et al., 1988). An input of 1.7 W peak envelope power (PEP) to the cell produced a peak field intensity of $1.0 \, \text{mW/cm}^2$. The SAR under these exposure conditions was 0.08 W/kg. The Crawford cell was housed in a large constant-temperature incubator maintained at 35 °C. Temperature in the culture cell media during exposure did not change by more than $\pm \, 0.1$ °C. The activity of ornithine decarboxylase was measured in supernatant preparations and was representative of the amount of $^{14}CO_2$ liberated from ^{14}C L-ornithine during a 60-minute incubation under standard conditions at 37 °C as described in detail (Byus et al., 1988; 1987; 1991; Wu et al., 1984). The cultured cells were exposed to the field for one hour, after which they were removed and the various biochemical parameters assayed at the times indicated post exposure.

For both cultured Chinese Hamster Ovary cells (CHO) and 294T human melanoma cells cultured in monolayer, ODC activity was observed to increase by 50–80% within the first hour of exposure to the 16 Hz amplitude-modulated RF field (Figure 5.1). For both cell lines, ODC activity remained elevated for at least 1 hour after removing the cells from the field, and returned to near control levels of activity within 2–3 hours of field exposure. Similar alterations in the activity of ODC in Reuber H35 hepatoma cells to that reported in Figure 5.1 were also observed (Byus et al., 1988).

In an attempt to further define the potential mechanism involved in the ability of the amplitude-modulated RF field to increase ODC activity in this

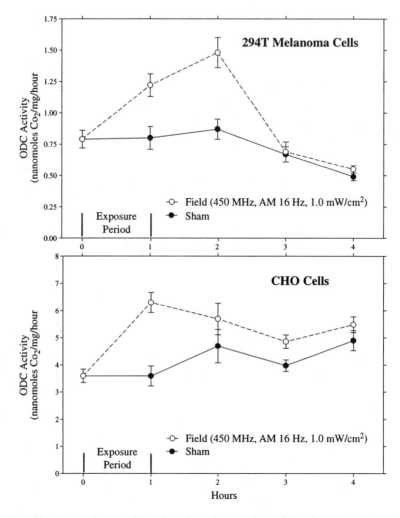

Fig. 5.1 Alterations in ornithine decarboxylase activity following exposure to 16 Hz AM RF field.

cultured cell system, the frequency dependence of the sinusoidal, amplitude modulation frequency of the RF field was determined following a 1-hour exposure of the cells the field (Figure 5.2). The unmodulated 450 MHz carrier field produced no measurable changes in ODC activity in comparison to sham or unexposed cells. However, as the modulation frequency increased, it was observed that modulation frequencies of between 10–20 Hz were capable of causing an increase in ODC activity above the sham control values. Higher modulation frequencies in the order of 40 and 120 Hz did not result in a measurable increase

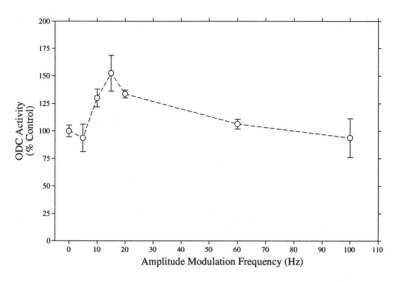

Fig. 5.2 Effect of low frequency amplitude modulation on ornithine decarboxylase activity.

in ODC activity compared to the sham exposed cells. Thus, it would appear that there is something about the low frequency amplitude modulation which allows the RF field to couple to a biological system, eliciting a measurable and reproducible response in this cell (an increase in ODC activity) as has been described for other parameters such as calcium efflux (Adey, 1981).

A number of laboratories have reported alterations in ODC activity in cultured cells (Byus et al., 1988; 1987; Somjen et al., 1983; Cain et al., 1986; 1993; Litovitz et al., 1991; 1994; Mattsson et al., 1992; Valtersson et al., 1995) following exposure to a number of varieties of electromagnetic fields including amplitude-modulated RF, 60 Hz electric, and 50–60 Hz magnetic fields. In virtually all of these studies, short-term exposure to low-energy electromagnetic fields have resulted in small but measurable and reproducible changes in ODC activity. The general observations made by these investigators was that a relatively low-energy athermal field was required to cause the changes in the activity of this enzyme and that exposure required a relatively short time to elicit the response (on the order of 1–12 hours). It also appears that there is a low frequency component which is required of the electromagentic field in order to elicit the response of increase in ODC activity. While the RF-field amplitude-modulated at 60 Hz did not alter ODC activity as shown above, 50–60 MHz magnetic fields have been reported by a number of laboratories to reproducibly alter the activity of ODC (Litovitz et al., 1991; 1994; Mattsson et al., 1992; Valtersson et al., 1995; Cain et al., 1993). Litovitz et al. (1991;

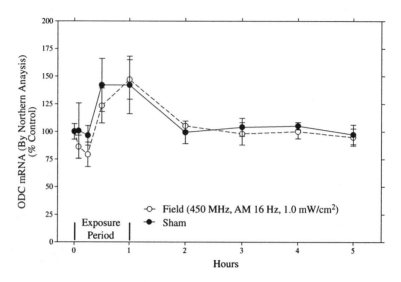

Fig. 5.3 Alterations in ODC mRNA in H35 rat hepatoma cells following exposure to 450 MHz AM field.

1994) have continued to study the parameters of the field which are capable of eliciting ODC activity in their model system. These investigators determined that an extremely low frequency (60 Hz) magnetic field must be coherent for some minimal length of time (on the order of 10 seconds), in order to affect the alteration of the enzyme in their L929 mouse cell system. Their investigation into the requirement of temporal coherence in the field continues to be highly innovative in nature and should continue to provide valuable new information concerning the mechanisms of cellular detection of weak low-frequency EM fields in the presence of endogenous thermal noise fields.

There has been much discussion concerning the ability of low-energy electromagnetic fields to cause alterations in gene transcription (Wei *et al.*, 1990; Goodman *et al.*, 1992; Phillips *et al.*, 1992). Since ODC is an enzyme which has been shown to be highly regulated at the level of mRNA coding for this enzyme, the ability of the amplitude-modulated RF field to alter ODC mRNA levels were determined using total RNA isolated as described previously (Chomzcynski *et al.*, 1987). The RNA was separated by electrophoresis and transferred to a nylon membrane, and the membrane was probed with a randomly primed ^{32}P labeled ODC probe for a period of 3 hours at 42 °C. When hybridization was complete, the filter was washed and subjected to autoradiography at 70 °C for 48 hours. The autoradiogram was scanned with a densitometer and the density of the bands compared as an indication of the relative amounts of ODC mRNA present in the various samples. Northern analysis performed in this manner revealed only the typical 2 bands of 2.2 and 2.4 Kb indicative

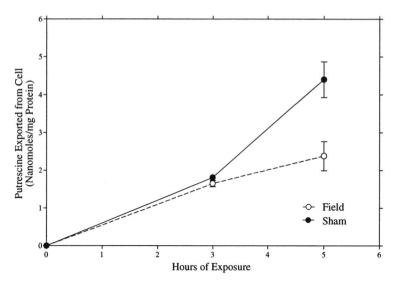

Fig. 5.4 Effect of modulated RF field on putrescine export in H35 rat hepatoma cells.

of ODC mRNA. Since ODC activity was increasing during the initial hour of exposure as shown in Figure 5.1, ODC mRNA levels were measured at 4 times during the initial hour of exposure as well as for 4 hours following exposure to the 450 MHz field amplitude-modulated at 16 Hz. No measurable increase in ODC mRNA was detected at any of the time periods tested during and following exposure to the amplitude-modulated RF field (Figure 5.3). Under these same conditions, insulin and TPA (a phorbol ester tumor promoter) results in an 8-10-fold increase in ODC mRNA within a 4-hour period. It is conceivable that small increases in steady-state ODC mRNA levels were occurring during and/or following field exposure but were not detectable due to the variation of ±5 to 15% ODC mRNA which occurs in this Northern analysis procedure. It is also conceivable that small changes in steady-state ODC mRNA could be important in the maintenance of the overall level of the enzyme, as well as the effects upon polyamine biosynthesis and, ultimately, cell growth and proliferation. However, no statistically significant measurable increase in ODC mRNA was observed under these assay and exposure conditions in which the activity of the enzyme did increase.

It has been determined that the polyamines, particularly putrescine, in relatively large amounts, is exported from inside the cell to outside the cell (Hawel *et al.*, 1994a; 1994b; Tjandrawinata *et al.*, 1995; Wallace *et al.*, 1981; McCormick, 1978). The relevance of this process to the overall maintenance of polyamines inside the cell cannot be overemphasized. In this regard, cells were exposed to the 16 Hz amplitude-modulated field as described previously and the level of putrescine in the media was measured throughout a 5-hour period. Under these conditions, significant inhibition in the level of putrescine export was observed in the presence of the field in comparison to the sham-exposed cells (Figure 5.4). Other laboratories have also measured alteration in the level of putrescine export in the presence of magnetic field exposure (Cain *et al.*, 1995) and at least one other group has shown that low-frequency magnetic field exposure has also resulted in a significant effect on another export protein, the multiple drug-resistant protein system (Hannan *et al.*, 1995). We are particularly interested in the manner in which field exposure alters the level of export of putrescine from the cell, an explanation of the overall increases in ODC activity which is observed. We continue to investigate putrescine export as a potential direct mediator of field effects.

5.3   LIMITATIONS OF CELLS AND ANIMAL MODELS

5.3.1   Analysis of limitations of animal cancer models in relation to the study of EMF effects

In order to assess the potential health effects of an environmental agent, often-times animal toxicology experiments are performed. The advantage of this type of approach for assessing the potential risk of a given agent or chemical is that experiments can be performed in a highly-controlled environment where the exposure parameters can be well-controlled and quantified, and the potential deleterious outcome to the health of the animal (i.e. cancer), can be accurately measured. Conventional chemical toxicology has developed a rigorous set of criteria for the performance of animal experiments in order that accurate conclusions about the particular chemical can be drawn (U. S. Congress, 1987; National Institute of Health, 1993). While a number of the premises upon which the methods are based have been criticized in recent years by some (Cranor, 1993), they are currently in use and the level of risk calculated from such experiments has been used to regulate chemical release into the environment by the city, state, and federal governments.

Currently, there are several experiments being performed designed to assess the effects of RF and low-energy electromagnetic fields in various animal cancer models. For the most part these studies are very well conceived and are being performed to the highest currently accepted standards employed in the assessment of chemical toxicology and chemical carcinogenesis. However, they have several basic limitations which minimize their relevance in the assessment of the potential cancer risk of environmentally relevant electromagnetic fields.

In assessing the potential cancer effect of a chemical that may be found in the environment, the general approach which is followed is to determine the maximally tolerated dose of this chemical which can be chronically given to an animal over a period of time in which the cancer or tumor endpoint is to be studied in a given animal. This can be many months or up to 1 to 2 years. Once this dose is determined, 50–80% of this dose is used as the highest amount of chemical to be given in an animal carcinogenesis experiment. Several other lower doses are then determined in a log manner, in order to establish the dose-response relationship between the administered dose of the chemical and the cancer outcome (i.e. numbers of tumors, tumor incidence, effects on latency, etc.). A dose-response curve is then generated from which the quantitative relationship between degree of carcinogenicity and chemical dose is established. This relationship is extrapolated in a linear manner down to the levels at which environmental exposure for humans occur in order to calculate a risk value. For most chemical carcinogens tested in animal models it is required to extrapolate many orders of magnitude (sometimes up to 5 orders of magnitude), below the lowest dose observed to alter the cancer endpoint in the animal experiments to reach 'environmentally relevant' levels of the chemical.

While this high- to low-dose extrapolation has been the topic of considerable discussion by numerous groups through many years, it is the generally accepted method for calculating risk values of chemicals from animal data (U. S. Congress, 1987; National Institute of Health, 1993). This extrapolation approach is scientifically valid for chemical initiating or mutational agents since the ability of a carcinogen to cause mutations in DNA (or DNA adduct formation) is linearly proportional to the concentration of chemical with minimal upper or lower limit nonlinearity. The use of relatively large doses of chemicals followed by high- to low-dose extrapolation is employed experimentally in order that relatively small numbers of animals (100 or less per group) can be used to observe statistically significant increases in tumor incidence or number following exposure to a given concentration of chemical. Few animal experiments are ever performed with more than 100 animals per group, due to the large expense in carrying out such experiments.

In the case of electromagnetic field experiments in relation to animal carcinogenesis, it is difficult, if not impossible to determine a maximally tolerated dose, and to perform a relevant high-dose to low-environmental dose extrapolation. The reason for this limitation is that if one increases the dose/intensity of electromagnetic field exposure, it is far from clear that the mechanism by which a cell or tissue senses and responds to low level EMF is the same as the mechanisms following higher EMF intensities. For example, RF or microwave fields at high intensities would cause significant heating of a cell or tissue with well known consequences. Yet, at low intensity exposure there may be other interactive processes resulting in a cellular response in the absence of a measurable temperarture rise. The physical stimulus of EMF itself might be sensed differently at high concentrations or high dosages by the animal and the determination of a 'maximally tolerated' dose as the upper limit of administration is not relevant in this case. Thus, it is likely that even if one is giving considerably more dose of electromagnetic field than is present in the environment (either ascertained by the length of time of exposure or by some measure of field intensity), that the highest concentration or amount of electromagnetic fields given may not cause a statistically measurable increase in tumorigenicity in the animal model chosen.

No animal carcinogenesis model is capable of detecting an increase of more than 1 excess cancer in 10–20 animals, i.e. a 5–10% increase in tumor incidence or tumor number. If a group of animals is exposed to an electromagnetic field which causes no statistically measurable increase in tumor incidence or tumor number compared to the control animals, the conclusion is not that there was no increase, but that there was no measurable increase greater than 5–10%. However, if electromagnetic fields caused even a 1% increase in tumor incidence or number, this would be enormously significant in terms of the population at risk for cancer. In this regard, it would take thousands of animals to measure a 1% increase in tumor incidence or tumorigenicity. It would be unfeasible for practical considerations to design an animal experiment having thousands of animals per group*.

For these reasons, the power of a study of animal carcinogenesis to evaluate both a positive as well as a null or negative effect, must be clearly defined and stated when the results of the experiments are reported. To simply state that exposure of these animals to an electromagnetic field of a given time and intensity produced no effect upon cancer incidence, tumor number, latency, tumorigenicity etc. is not a scientifically accurate or sufficient statement. What must be stated clearly is the statistical power of that given animal experiment to detect or measure a change and that no change was detected that was greater than this number[†].

5.3.2   Current animal cancer studies

The bulk of scientific evidence to date indicates that it is extremely unlikely that electromagnetic or RF fields are serving as classical initiators of carcinogenesis in a manner analogous to ionizing radiation. The studies done indicate that it is highly unlikely that these low-energy electromagnetic fields are capable of causing direct damage to DNA, resulting in a mutation in a gene which is inheritable from one generation to the next. It is more likely mechanistically that if these fields are capable of influencing the cancer incidence in the human

---

* An extremely large animal study was performed once by the National Institute of Health, termed 'The Mega Mouse Study' in order to establish that a linear relationship actually existed during a high dose to low dose extrapolation for a chemical initiating agent (National Institute of Health, 1993).

† As stated previously, the average animal experiment does not have the power to detect an increase in cancer incidence or tumorigenicity greater than between 1 in 10 and 1 in 20, i.e. 5–10%.

population in a positive manner that the most likely effect would be upon the promotional or co-promotional aspects of carcinogenesis (Reiners *et al.*, 1990; Takigawa *et al.*, 1983; Stuchly *et al.*, 1991; McLean *et al.*, 1991). Promotional or co-promotional chemicals are incapable of causing any increase in animal cancer rates, even in large doses when given alone. However, when given in addition to classical chemical agents which cause low-level mutations in DNA, are capable of markedly increasing the overall tumor incidence and numbers of tumors.

A number of animal studies have been designed to assess both the promotional and co-promotional effects of fields (Stuchly *et al.*, 1991; McLean *et al.*, 1991). We are in the process of performing a complex series of animal experiments in which rats are exposed to either simulated digital or FM cellular phone emissions. The animals have been administered a carcinogen, ethylnitrosourea (ENU), transplacentally during fetal development. These are lifetime studies where the animals are exposed both to a digital or FM cellular phone fields for several days prior to birth following ENU administration and throughout their lifetime of two years. It is our belief that if these cellular phone fields are capable of altering or affecting the cancer outcome, it is most likely to be at a promotional or co-promotional level in which we would expect to see some alteration in the numbers or types of tumors in the animals receiving the low doses of carcinogen. Our studies have been designed to assess the ability of the cellular phone fields to increase cancer incidence rather than decrease it. Thus, the level of carcinogen which is administered is very low and it has been designed to produce a very low increase in cancer incidence in primary brain tumors (in the order of 10–15%).

5.4   SUMMARY

Several conclusions can be made in relation to the series of experiments performed assessing the ability of cultured cells to respond to RF amplitude-modulated fields. It appears that cells in culture have the ability to sense or respond to RF fields provided they are amplitude-modulated at low frequency. The increases in ODC activity which were seen in the low-frequency amplitude-modulated fields were not observed in the absence of amplitude modulation or at higher amplitude modulation frequencies. Further studies in this regard, particularly being performed by Litovitz and his colleagues, who are studying the coherent and time-dependent application of fields in relation to noise, appear to be proceeding rapidly and should provide further insight into the mechanisms involved in field tissue or field cell interaction. It does appear that cells are capable of responding or sensing low-energy RF fields if they have a certain low frequency modulation component. Thus the question concerning the potential health risk of exposure to low-energy electromagnetic fields in general and RF fields in particular cannot be dismissed out of hand because the cells are not able to respond to these fields. However, whether such a biological response (such as elevated ODC activity) leads to a negative health effect (such as increased cancer), remains an open and unanswered question. Further investigations into the potential health effects of electromagnetic fields, particularly in relation to cancer, should be pursued in conjunction with studies designed to more fully understand the basic mechanistic parameters involved. It is not clear that animal cancer models have sufficient statistical power to be able to rule out the potential deleterious health effects of field exposure of the human population. None of the animal studies which are currently being performed have sufficient power to eliminate the concerns of an environmental risk of exposure to electromagnetic fields. No animal experiment to date has the ability to state with certainty that the given EMF field applied did not cause for example a 1–5%, increase in a cancer endpoint – an enormously significant number in relation to environmental human exposure. The inherent power of animal cancer experiments, however, could be highly significant if they show a stimulatory or inhibitory effect of field exposure.

REFERENCES

Adey, W.R. (1981) *Physiological Reviews*, **61**, 435–514.

Byus, C.V., Pieper, S.E. and Adey, W.R. (1987) *Carcinogenesis*, **8**, 1385–1389.

Byus, C.V., Kartun, K., Peiper, S. *et al.* (1988) *Cancer Res.*, **48**, 4222–4226.

Byus, C.V. (1990) *Acute Myelogenous Leukemia: Progress and Controversies*, Wiley-Liss, Inc., pp. 51–60.

Byus, C.V. and Wu, V.S. (1991) *J. Cell. Physiol.*, **149**, 9.

Cain, C.D., Donato, N.J., Byus, C.V. *et al.* (1986) *International Conference on Electric and Magnetic Fields in Medicine and Biology*, pp. 9–13.

Cain, C., Thomas, D.L. and Adey, W.R. (1993) *Carcinogenesis*, **14**, 955–960.

Cain, C.D., Thomas, D.L., Ghaffari, M. *et al.* (1995) *OrnitHine Decarboxylase Activity, Exported Polyamines and Magnetic Field Strength Dependency in C3H10T^1/2.* Proceedings of the 17th Annual Bioelectromagnetic Society, pp. 19–20.

Chomzcynski, P. and Sacchi, N. (1987) *Analytical Biochem.*, **162**, 156–159.

Cranor, C.J. (1993) *Regulating Toxic Substances: A Philosophy of Science and Law*, Oxford University Press, New York, pp. 1–252.

van Daalen Wetters, T., Macrae, M., Brabant, M. *et al.* (1989) *Mol. Cell. Biol.*, **9**, 5484–5490.

Goodman, R. Weisbrot, D., Uluc, A. *et al.* (1992) *Bioelectromagnetics*, **13**, 111–118.

Hannan, C., Jr. and Liang, Y. (1995) *Magnetic Field Effects on Multidrug Resistant Human Tumor Cells.* Proceedings of the 17th Annual Bioelectromagnetic Society, p. 10.

Hawel, L., III, Tjandrawinata, R.R. and Byus, C.V. (1994a) *Biochim. Biophys. Acta*, **1222**, 15–26.

Hawel, L., III, Tjandrawinata, R.R., Fukumoto, G.H. *et al.* (1994b) *J. Biol. Chem.*, **269**, 7412–7418.

Heby, I. and Persson, L. (1990) *TIBS*, **15**, 153–158.

Litovitz, T.A., Krause, D. and Mullins, J.M. (1991) *Biochem. Biophys. Res. Commun.*, **178**, 862–865.

Litovitz, T.A., Krause D., Montrose, C.J. *et al.* (1994) *Bioelectromagnetics*, **15**, 399–409.

Mattsson, M.-O., Mild, K.H. and Rehnholm, U. (1992) Proceedings of the First World Congress for Electricity and Magnetism in Biology and Medicine, p. 44.

McCormick, F. (1978) *Biochem. J.*, **174**, 427–432.

McLean, J.R., Stuchly, M.A., Mitchel, R.E. *et al.* (1991) *Bioelectromagnetics*, **12**, 273–287.

Mevissen, M., Löscher, W., Lerchl, A. *et al.* (1995) *Possible Mechanisms of the Tumor Copromoting Effect of Magnetic Field Exposure in a Rat Breast Cancer Model.* Proceedings of the 17th Annual Bioelectromagnetic Society, p. 50.

National Institute of Health (1993) *Risk Assessment in the Federal Government: Managing the Process.* National Academy Press, Washington, D.C., pp. 1–191.

Pegg, A.E. (1986) *Biochem. J.*, **234**, 249–262.

Phillips, J.L., Haggren, W., Thomas, W.J. *et al.* (1990) *Biochim. Biophys. Acta*, **1222**, 15–26.

Porter, C.W., Pegg, A.E, Granis, B.M. *et al.* (1990) *Biochem. J.*, **268**, 07–212.

Reiners, J.J. Pavone, A., Rupp, T. *et al.* (1990) *Carcinogenesis*, **11**, 128–137.

Somjen, D., Yariv, M., Kaye, A.M. *et al.* (1983) *Adv. Polyamine Res.*, **4**, 713–718.

Stuchly, M.A., Lecuyer, D.W. and McLean, J. (1991) *Bioelectromagnetics*, **12**, 261–271.

Tabor, C.W. and Tabor, H. (1984) *Ann. Rev. Biochem.*, **53**, 749–790.

Takigawa, M., Verma, A.K., Simsiman, R.C. *et al.* (1983) *Cancer Res.*, **43**, 3732–3738.

Tjandrawinata, R.R. and Byus, C.V. (1995) *Biochem. J.*, **305**, 291–299.

U. S. Congress, Office of Technology Assessment (1987) *Identifying and Regulating Carcinogens.* OTA-BP-H-42 (Washington, D.C.), U. S. Government Printing Office, November, 1987, pp. 1–249.

Valtersson, U., Mild, K.H., Mattsson, M. O. (1995) *Ornithine Decarboxylase Activity in Humanlymphoblastoid Cell Line in the Presence of 50 Hz Magnetic Fields.* Proceedings of the 17th Annual Bioelectromagnetic Society, p. 20.

Wallace, H.M. and Keir, H.M. (1981) *Biochim. Biophys. Acta*, **676**, 25–29.

Wei, L.X., Goodman, R. and Henderson A. (1990) *Bioelectromagnetics*, **11**, 269–272.

Wu, V.S., Donato, N.J. and Byus, C.V. (1981) *Cancer Res.*, **42**, 3384–3391.

Wu, V.S. and Byus, C.V. (1984) *Biochem. Biophys. Acta*, **804**, 89–99.

6
Review of epidemiological studies

Ulf Bergqvist

6.1 INTRODUCTION

The increasingly widespread use of cellular phones, and the general proliferation of radiofrequency (RF) or microwave equipment in modern telecommunications, have generated an increasing interest in possible adverse health consequences of the ensuing exposure to RF fields. Epidemiological studies offer – in principle – powerful tools for evaluating the impact on humans of occupational or environmental exposures. In a recent 'opinion piece', Goldsmith (1995) summarized that he 'presents evidence that sufficient microwave exposures are associated with all four of these outcomes ...', one outcome being cancer. A WHO report (1993), on the other hand, concluded that 'epidemiological ...studies do not provide clear evidence of detrimental health effects in humans from exposure to RF fields'. It thus appears prudent to review epidemiological studies of RF exposures, with particular emphasis on studies relevant to mobile telecommunication situations.

6.2 SELECTION OF REPORTS FOR THE REVIEW

Studies related to radiofrequency fields and/or microwaves and various adverse health effects were obtained using MEDLINE resources – supplemented by checking reference lists of thus available reports. With a few exceptions, reports were limited to those appearing in peer-review publications. It was quickly found that none of these studies had specifically looked at RF exposures due to mobile telecommunication systems. Any study including exposure or assumed exposure to RF or microwaves was considered relevant for the purpose of the review – the results are then discussed below in terms of possible relevance to telecommunication use situations. After screening available studies, the review concentrated on those concerning cancer, ocular or neurasthenic effects.

Mobile Communications Safety
Edited by N. Kuster, Q. Balzano and J.C. Lin
Published in 1997 by Chapman & Hall, London. ISBN 0 412 75000 7.

Some studies on possible effects of RF exposure on reproductive or pregnancy outcomes exist, both after maternal (Källén *et al.*, 1982; Kolmodin-Hedman *et al.*, 1988; Larsen *et al.*, 1991; Ouellet-Hellstrom *et al.*, 1993) and after paternal exposure (Sigler *et al.*, 1965; Lancranjan *et al.*, 1975). It was observed, however, that these studies were based on occupations with substantial exposures to fairly high RF fields to other parts of the body than the head (Allen *et al.*, 1994; Skotte, 1986; Lancranjan *et al.*, 1975; Kolmodin-Hedman *et al.*, 1988). Although further studies of e.g. female physiotherapists being exposed to microwave or short-wave diathermy appear warranted (WHO, 1993; Goldsmith, 1995), these studies were not considered relevant for the purpose of this review.

6.3   EVALUATION AND CAUSAL INFERENCE

Epidemiology can be defined as the study of the occurrence of illness. It is a powerful tool for evaluating statistical associations between disease and exposure. Within that framework, careful evaluations are needed to ascertain whether a noted association could be due to random variations (chance?), to other factors (confounders?) or to the selection of the population under study.

The shift from a discussion of a statistical association to a causal one is not trivial, however. Hill (1965) suggested that several items such as the strength of the association, the consistency across studies, the plausibility, the presence of experimental evidence and of a biological gradient should all be considered when attempting to evaluate the causality of a finding. He did, however, caution that 'none of my nine viewpoints can bring indisputable evidence for or against the cause-and-effect hypothesis and none can be required as a *sine qua non*' (see also comments made by Rothman, 1986). The International Agency for Research on Cancer (IARC), which evaluates relationships between cancer and various agents, normally considers both epidemiological and experimental evidence.

In this review, epidemiological support for the hypotheses linking radiofrequency radiation and fields with adverse health effects is evaluated. The reader should take note of the fact that a total evaluation of such a hypothesis normally require also other data. This is briefly reiterated in terms of the noted epidemiological findings in the summary.

A further consideration is the methodological quality of the reviewed epidemiological papers. IARC has also published some quality criteria (IARC, 1991) for use when evaluating epidemiological studies:

• The study population, disease and exposure should be well defined by the authors. Cases should be identified independently of exposure, and likewise, exposure should be assessed independently of disease. This normally precludes using studies with self-selected participants, as well as studies with low response rates.

- Design and analysis should take into account other factors (confounders) that could influence the risk of disease.
- The authors should report the basic data on which conclusions are founded, also when sophisticated statistical analyses are performed, at least as to numbers of exposed or nonexposed cases and controls or observed and expected cases.
- The statistical methods used for estimation of risks and control of confounding should be clearly stated, and considered appropriate.

Basically, these items are useful in ensuring that adequate control of bias and confounding exist in a study. In addition, the size of the study is an important consideration in the weighting of any information derived thereof. Case reports and correlation studies (ecological studies) are rarely used in evaluation, as major uncertainties in their causal interpretations exist.

In principle, these criteria are used in the evaluation below. The long time span of these studies (1965–1995) should, however, be kept in mind – epidemiology has developed considerably in these years, with increasing attention both as to new statistical tools and to problems of confounding and bias.

Studies with insufficient distinction between exposure to extremely low frequency (ELF) fields and RF fields do present a specific problem in the context of this review, see further discussion below.

6.4   REVIEW OF STUDIES RELEVANT TO CANCER

A number of studies have presented data on the possibility of an association between cancer and RF exposure. Of these, the studies by Lin *et al.* (1985) and Milham (1985) compared cancer mortality between various job categories with presumed high or low exposure to electromagnetic fields. There were, however, no distinctions made between exposure to low frequency fields and RF exposure groups. A similar situation exists concerning reports of neuroblastoma in children of fathers with 'electromagnetic occupations' (Spitz *et al.*, 1985; Johnson *et al.*, 1985). Therefore, these studies were not included in the following review. The ecological study by Lester and Moore (1982) was likewise not included. The remaining seven studies are reviewed below.

6.4.1   Methodological descriptions of the cancer studies

Lilienfeld and co-workers (1978) examined the mortality and morbidity of a cohort of employees at the U. S. embassy in Moscow, and compared them with employees from other U. S. embassies in East European countries. Between 1963 and 1975, microwave radiation of maximum 0.05 W/m² lasting 9 hours/day at frequencies between 0.5 and 10 GHz were detected at certain locations in the

Moscow embassy. (Prior to 1963, routine checks also suggested the existence of these signals.) Checks at the other embassies did not reveal RF irradiation except for background levels. All 4388 individuals who worked or lived at any of these embassies at any time between January 1953 and June 1976 were included in the study – 42% of which were from the Moscow embassy. Health data were obtained from medical records as well as health-oriented questionnaires. Medical records were traced and reviewed for 71%, and questionnaires returned from 42% of the study population – these percentages were similar for individuals from Moscow and from the other embassies.

Robinette et al. (1980) examined the health records of 41 000 U. S. naval personnel enlisted during the Korean war. Selection of these men were based on six occupational groups, three classified as 'high' and three classified as 'low' RF exposure based on earlier measurements. Data on morbidity were ascertained for 1952–1976 with exception of some years (record unavailability), while mortality data were obtained up to 1974. More detailed exposure related data were obtained from other military records for all dead (435) and 5% randomly chosen living men (960). Based on these data, individuals in the high exposure groups were also given a 'hazard number' depending on their opportunity for exposure.

Milham (1988) examined the mortality of 67 000 male amateur radio operators in California and Washington State, by record linkage between licence information and death records, and compared the results with the general (U. S. national) population.

Selvin et al. (1992) examined childhood cancers among 50 000 children (<21 years of age) around a microwave tower in San Francisco. Exposure was approximated by distance from the tower, with those living within 3.5 km of the tower defined as 'exposed'.

In another study, Maskarinec and Cooper (1993) performed a case-control study of 70 children living in the vicinity of a radio tower in Hawaii, again with distance to the tower as a surrogate for exposure – the dividing line between 'exposed' and 'unexposed' was here 4.2 km. This latter study was developed around a cluster specified both in space (Waianae Coast, Hawaii) and time (1977–1984), which provided (at least) 7 of the 14 cases.

Armstrong et al. (1994) performed a nested case-control study of electric utility workers in France and Québec, Canada. All 2700 cancer cases occurring in 1970–1988 (Québec) or in 1978–1989 (France) were included, as were 4000 matched controls from the same utilities. Job-exposure matrices were determined for these utility workers, and measurements of job-specific exposures were made by individuals carrying a meter sensible to 10–15 MHz transient field exposures, and expressed as the proportion of time in which the electric field exposure exceeded 200 V/m. Later added information suggested that the meters also exhibited sensitivity to fields of higher frequencies (e.g. 150–300 MHz), and were sensitive to transmissions from walkie-talkies as well as car and truck radios (Armstrong et al., 1994), but this remains – at present – a suggestion only, since a proper calibration in the higher frequency range was not performed.

Szmigielski (in press) examined the cancer morbidity in the Polish career military personnel between 1971 and 1985, with cancer incidences obtained from military hospital records. The size of the cohort varied between 118 500 and 142 200 (mean 127 800), the majority being between 30–49 years of age. Classification of personnel posts as exposed or not was performed by safety personnel, where posts with exposures of less than $2\,W/m^2$ were considered non-exposed. At 'exposed' posts, pulse-modulated field levels at frequencies of 0.15–3.5 GHz were generally found to vary between 2–6 W/m^2. Apart from this, there were no individual assessments of exposure levels or duration. Between 3400 and 4600 individuals were considered exposed at any one year. Information on 'EM exposure' was also obtained from the medical records.

Hematologic and lymphatic cancers were investigated in all studies, with varying degree of specificity as to e.g. specific leukaemias, Hodgkin's disease, other lymphomas, etc. Brain or CNS cancers were studied by Lilienfield and co-workers (1978), Milham (1988), Selvin et al. (1992), Armstrong et al. (1994) and Szmigielski (in press). Cancers in the digestive tract as well as lung or other respiratory tract cancers were investigated by Lilienfield and co-workers (1978), Robinette et al. (1980), Milham (1988), Armstrong et al. (1994) and Szmigielski (in press). Melanoma and other skin cancers were investigated by Armstrong et al. (1994) and Szmigielski (in press). Some other cancer sites were investigated in a few studies – see further below.

Essentially all studies included measures to eliminate confounding by age or gender. The study by Armstrong and co-workers (1994) also adjusted for a number of other factors (ionizing radiation, chemicals, smoking and socioeconomic status).

6.4.2   Results and discussion – cancer and RF

These seven studies are shown in Table 6.1, and their main results are discussed in the text below, separated into a discussion on adult and childhood cancers.

Adult cancers and RF – five studies

Lilienfield and co-workers (1978) did not observe an excess of cancer in the Moscow cohort, neither compared to the (U.S.) national average nor compared to other U.S. embassies in Eastern Europe. The standard mortality ratio (SMR) for the former comparison was 0.9 (0.5–1.4), based on 19 cases (values in parenthesis give the 95% confidence interval). For specific cancer sites, only 4 sites yielded more than one case; lung (n=5, SMR 0.9; 0.3–2.0), digestive organ (n=3, SMR 0.6; 0.1–1.9), leukaemia (n=2, SMR 2.5; 0.3–9.0) and breast cancer (n=2, SMR 4.0; 0.5–14.4). For the comparison embassies, the SMR's

Table 6.1 Summary of seven studies relevant to RF and cancer.

Study	Population base	Final study size	Overall results according to the author(s)
Studies on adults			
Lilienfield (1978)	U.S. embassy personnel	1209 in Moscow vs 1883 other countries	No deleterious effects noted
Robinette (1980)	Radar personnel	20 109 with 'high' vs 20 781 'low' exposure	Effects on mortality not clearly perceptible
Milham (1988)	Amateur radio operators	67 829 operators	Significant excess mortality of some hematologic cancers
Armstrong (1994)	Electric utility workers	2679 cases 3476 controls	Lung cancers associated with exposure to transient fields
Szmigielski (in press)	Military personnel	3720 exposed among 127 800 personnel	Higher morbidities were found for several neoplasms
Studies on children			
Selvin (1992)	Children around microwave tower	22 700 'close' 28 000 'further away'	No distance-dependent relation between cancer and microwave tower
Mascarinec (1993)	Children around radio tower	14 cases, 56 controls (based on a cluster)	Chance remains a possibility, but pattern reduces this

were slightly higher than in Moscow for all cancers, lung cancer and digestive organ cancers (all with SMR $\approx$ 1), and slightly lower than in Moscow for leukaemia and breast cancer (SMR 1.8; 0.4–5.3 and 2.4; 0.5–7.0, respectively). These results are clearly insufficient to indicate a cancer effect of working at the irradiated Moscow embassy. It should be emphasized, however, that the limited number of cancer cases makes this study rather non-informative in comparison with the other studies.

Robinette *et al.* (1980) did not find excess mortality ratios for the 'high' vs the 'low' exposed group for cancers in digestive organ, respiratory tract, nervous system, lymphatic/hematopoietic system or in other cancer sites (as a group). The hazard number, however, yielded one significant finding; those with high hazard numbers (i.e. high potential for RF exposure) had a mortality ratio of 2.2 from respiratory tract malignancies, which was significantly higher than those with lesser hazard numbers ($p < 0.05$). Adjustments were made for year of birth.

Milham (1988) found increased SMR's for radio amateurs for certain cancer sites; brain cancer 1.4 (0.9–2.0), Hodgkin's disease 1.2 (0.4–2.9), leukaemia 1.2 (0.9–1.7) and cancer in other lymphatic tissue 1.6 (1.2–2.2). For leukaemias, the excess was essentially restricted to acute myeloid leukaemia (1.8; 1.0–2.8). For other cancer sites (stomach, intestines, liver, pancreas, the respiratory system, prostate, urinary bladder and kidney), the SMR's were not elevated (≤ 1.1). There were no adjustments for confounders apart from those inherent in the SMR calculations, but the author indicated that these amateur radio operators were over-represented in occupations with presumed exposure to electric and magnetic fields, in addition to being exposed to e.g. soldering fumes etc. within their hobby activity. It is thus difficult to separate these results indicative of their hobby activity (with RF exposure) from their occupational activity (with presumed exposure also to extremely low frequency fields).

Armstrong et al. (1994) examined certain cancer sites that were selected a priori; hematologic cancers (including leukaemias), brain cancer and melanoma. No associations with exposure to transient fields were found. Investigations of other cancer types (not a priori selected) did, however, yield some indications of an effect. For stomach cancers, the odds ratio (OR) and its 95% confidence interval was 2.01 (0.96–4.18), but the excess odds were essentially confined to one of the utilities (in France), and did not show a clear dose-response relationship.

The suggested relationship with lung cancer (OR=1.27; 0.96–1.68) was more indicative, in that a clear dose-response relationship existed. The overall association was stronger if exposure was evaluated (retrospectively) for at least 20 years prior to the hypothesis. On the other hand, the association was again essentially limited to one of the utilities (Québec). Adjustments for coal tar, ionizing radiation, cadmium and asbestos reduced the odds ratio to 1.14 (0.82–1.58), but retained a high odds ratio of 3.41 (1.63–7.12) for those in the highest exposure group (≥ 90 percentile exposure). The authors caution, however, that the facts of 1) measurements used not being precisely understood and limited by job heterogeneity, 2) findings of an association made at only one utility, 3) an absence of a lung cancer mortality increase in Québec utility workers as a whole compared to the general population, and 4) an absence of a priori hypothesis, all limit a causal interpretation of the lung cancer findings (Armstrong et al., 1994).

Szmigielski (in press) observed excess occurrence of cancers among exposed personnel at several cancer sites; esophageal and stomach 3.2 (1.8–5.1), colorectal 3.2 (1.5–6.2), liver and pancreas 1.5 (0.8–3.0), skin (including melanoma) 1.7 (0.9–4.1), nervous system (including brain) 1.9 (1.1–3.5) and thyroid 1.5 (0.8–2.6). For hemopoietic/lymphatic malignancies, excess risk ratios were found for Hodgkin's disease 3.0 (1.3–4.4), lymphoma (non-Hodgkin) and lymphosarcoma 5.8 (2.1–9.7), chronic lymphocytic leukaemia 3.7 (1.4–5.2), acute lymphoblastic leukaemia 5.7 (1.2–18.2), chronic myelocytic leukaemia 13.9 (6.7–22.1) and acute myeloblastic leukaemia 8.6 (3.5–13.7). Incidence ratios for oral cavity, pharynx, laryngeal and lung, bone or kidney and prostate cancers did not deviate substantially from 1, suggesting an absence of an excess risk. There was a slight decrease in the incidence ratios with age for both all cancers and for hemopoietic/lymphatic malignancies. The author concluded that these results did not prove a causal link, but showed an urgent need for further studies.

This study presents some problems for a reviewer. On the one hand, the observed excess risk ratios are large with – for some – rather convincing confidence intervals. On the other hand, the large odds ratios for a variety of different cancer sites do offer some grounds for methodological considerations, which are not fully answered by the report. For one thing, it is not clear how the exposure information was obtained. Such information was apparently available both from annual data for all personnel, and from reports of cancer cases. Was the designation of 'exposed' vs 'unexposed' derived from only the first source or from both, and – especially if the latter was the case – could the exposure information have been influenced by the case status? Furthermore, the retrospectivity of the exposure data was not described – was the exposure status relevant to the year of diagnosis, or to service years prior to diagnosis? It appears that person-years at risk were not computed, which would have been preferably for a dynamic population. Finally, some information on certain possible confounders was apparently available, but apart from age, adjustments for other factors – e.g. possible carcinogen exposures other than RF exposure – appear not to have been made. In the absence of information on these points, it is not feasible to evaluate the possible bias – if any – due to these considerations. The decision made in this review is to accept these findings as suggestive when they are supported by findings of at least one other of the studies reviewed here.

Adult cancers and RF – summary

These five studies of adult cancers vary considerably in exposure assessments, where e.g. only one study is based on (job-specific) actual measurements (Armstrong *et al.*, 1994). Likewise, it appears that only that study has included adjustments for possible confounders other than age and gender. These and other disparities between studies make any attempt at drawing overall conclusions from them rather difficult. Nevertheless, cancer at four sites warrant further discussion (see below) – for other cancer sites, results are either non-positive, or appear only in single studies.

Two studies suggested an association between lung or respiratory system cancer and RF exposure; that of Robinette *et al.* (1980) and that of Armstrong and co-workers (1994). It can be noted that both studies did find stable or indicative results in the highest exposure groups only. On the other hand, most of the counterarguments that were raised by Armstrong *et al.* (1994) still apply. In addition, the study by Robinette and co-workers (1980) did not adjust for the possible influence of smoking. The reviewer can only agree with Armstrong *et al.* that a causal association between RF exposure and lung cancer is suggested, but cannot be considered to be established by these results alone. It should be noted that none of the other studies (Lilienfield *et al.*, 1978; Milham, 1988; Szmigielski, in press) indicated any excess lung cancers among the 'exposed'.

For stomach cancers, two studies (Armstrong *et al.*, 1994; Szmigielski, in press) suggested excess cancer among the 'exposed', while the other did not (Lilienfield *et al.*, 1978; Robinette *et al.*, 1980; Milham, 1988). It should be noted that Szmigielski reported combined result for stomach and esophagus cancers, whereas Armstrong *et al.* reported results for stomach cancers, with variations in specificity also in the other studies. This, together with the uncertainty expressed by Armstrong *et al.*, and detailed above also for the study by Szmigielski, do further detract somewhat from the credibility of these findings.

For brain or nervous system cancers, for acute myeloid leukaemia and for non-Hodgkin's lymphoma (except lymphosarcoma), support for excess incidence or mortality was found in the studies by Milham (1988) and Szmigielski (in press), but not in the other studies. Neither of the positive studies appear to have adjusted the results for other confounders except for age, and Milham noted a possible covariation of the exposure with (presumably) extremely low frequency (ELF) field exposure during occupational activity. Since these cancer sites are currently candidates for associations with ELF fields, the noted findings are difficult to evaluate in terms of RF exposure*.

The summary evaluation of adult cancer studies are – as should be clear from the above – influenced by certain methodological aspects of the reviewed studies; low numbers (Lilienfield *et al.*, 1978), presumed confusion with ELF exposures (Milham, 1988), as well as unclear documentation of methodology (Szmigielski, in press). In conclusion, the findings of respiratory tract or lung cancer are suggestive but do require further studies. Indications of associations between other cancers and RF exposure appear rather uncertain for leukaemia, lymphoma, brain and stomach cancer, and limited to non-existent for other sites.

Childhood cancers and RF

Selvin *et al.* (1992) estimated risk ratios of children closer to, compared to further away than 3.5 km from, a microwave tower, and found that these risk ratios did not deviate from chance findings; the p-values were 0.82, 0.27, 0.24 and 0.36 for leukaemias, brain cancer, Hodgkin's disease and non-Hodgkin's lymphoma, respectively. Investigations based on other measures related to distance yielded a similar lack of indication of an effect.

Maskarinec and Cooper (1993) found that the odds ratio for a childhood leukaemia case living less than 4.2 km from a broadcasting tower (vs further away) was 2.1 (0.7–16.4). They suggested that the 'unusual age, sex and type of

---

* Note also the decision not to include certain job title studies with major ELF influence above.

leukaemia pattern' reduced the likelihood of a chance explanation of the cluster. They also suggested that 'closeness to the radio station may be confounded by socioeconomic status or exposure to hazardous chemicals' – but no data were offered on this suggestion in the rather brief report.

The fact that this latter study was based on a cluster effectively precludes making generally applicable conclusions from it. The study by Selvin and co-workers (1992) suggests that distance from the microwave tower was not a risk indicator. Taken together, these two studies fail to establish or strongly indicate an effect of living close to microwave or radio towers on childhood cancers. On the other hand, their limited size, the paucity of reported details in one of them and the lack of any data on the individual or group exposure to RF radiation makes it impossible to verify a lack of effect of such exposures on childhood cancers.

6.5   REVIEW OF STUDIES RELEVANT TO OCULAR EFFECTS

Eight studies have included endpoints related to ocular effects such as lens opacities and cataracts or eye irritation. After an examination of methodological aspects of these studies, six studies dealing with lens opacities or cataracts were included in the review, while two studies were not (Majewska, 1968; Hollows *et al.*, 1984), because the published reports did not include sufficient information about selection procedures and response rates, and the latter did not include adjustment for important confounders such as age. Further elaborations of the six selected studies are reported below.

Two studies investigated eye irritation among workers with plastic sealers or welders (Bini *et al.*, 1986; Kolmodin-Hedman *et al.*, 1988); both found an excess reporting of eye irritation among the exposed workers – but with limited details reported. In the study by Kolmodin-Hedman and co-workers (1988), it was noted that the work situations also included handling materials known to be eye irritants – but no confounder analysis was performed. The paucity of reported details about the effects and the analysis makes these results clearly insufficient for any conclusions to be made. Thus, for the purpose of this review, these ocular effects will not be further considered.

6.5.1   Methodological descriptions of lens opacity studies

Cleary and co-workers (1965) performed a case-control study of U. S. military veterans from World War II and the Korean War, based on military records (to determine job tasks) and hospital records (to determine case status). 5110 white male veterans of the army and the air force who were born after 1910 were admitted to the study. Cases were individuals with cataracts, while control individuals were those admitted to the same hospital, but for different (random) diagnoses. For about 10% of the individuals, data were considered insufficient for analysis.

Cleary and Pasternack (1966), also performed a cross-sectional study of 1295 individuals working at 16 microwave installations. Non-exposed individuals were selected 'from the same locations and occupational environment', presumably implying that they worked at the same installations. There is no information as to whether any workers declined participation in or were omitted from the study; the numbers given refer to the final number of individuals, on which the analysis was made.

Siekierzynski and co-workers (Czerski et al., 1974; Siekierzynski et al., 1974a; 1974b) performed a cross-sectional study of 841 male microwave workers, age 20–45 years. Exposed individuals were those 507 exposed at levels between 2 and 60 W/m^2 while the 334 non-exposed individuals were those exposed below 2 W/m^2, based on individual spot measurements. The exposed individuals were somewhat younger (56% being $\leq$30 years of age) than the non-exposed group (42% being $\leq$30 years of age), motivating the authors to perform age-specific analyses.

Odland and co-workers (1973) examined a group of 697 individuals at eight U.S. air force bases. The selection procedure was performed at each base according to certain criteria – primarily geared to the presumed exposure. There is no information as to possible refusals to participate. A similar procedure was utilized by Shacklett et al. (1975), where 817 U.S. air force individuals at eight U.S. air force bases were examined. Medical examinations in both of these studies were performed by the same medical officers, at partly overlapping time periods (1970–1972 and 1971–1974, respectively). The degree of overlap in individuals examined, if any, has not been reported.

Appleton and co-workers (1975) examined 2343 individuals at 5 U.S. army bases. Again, selection of individuals were done at each base in accordance with general criteria. All personnel with histories of exposure (ever having worked with microwave equipment) were requested to attend.

The most common exposure assessment method used in these studies was to assign an individual to one of two distinct groups, e.g. radar vs non-radar or 'microwave' worker or not (Cleary et al., 1965; Odland et al., 1973; Shacklett et al., 1975; Appleton et al., 1975). In one study, questionnaire data were used to develop an exposure score, taking details of operating power, distances etc. into account (Cleary et al., 1966). In another study, microwave workers were separated according to measured exposure levels (Czerski et al., 1974).

In general, lens opacities refer to the finding of increased optical density regions in the eye's lens, while the clinical entity cataract also includes the observation that these optical densities are sufficient to cause a decrease in visual acuity. In a study by Cleary and co-workers (1965), the endpoint was a diagnosed cataract according to hospital records, except that cataracts with certain known causes such as wound trauma, diabetic etc. were excluded. In other studies by Cleary and Pasternack (1966), Odland *et al.* (1973), Siekierzynski and co-workers (1974a), Shacklett *et al.* (1975) and Appleton and co-workers (1975), the occurrence of specified lens opacities as noted by e.g. slit-lamp examination was studied. These observed changes were normally insufficient for cataracts to be clinically manifested. In some studies, other related changes such as the presence of vacuoles and posterior subcapsular iridescence (PSCI) were also investigated (Odland *et al.*, 1973; Shacklett *et al.*, 1975; Appleton *et al.*, 1975).

All studies included here made adjustments for age or at least reported age-specific strata of associations between exposure and effects. In addition, adjustments for other factors were reported in a few studies; for ionizing radiation (Cleary *et al.*, 1966), military branch (Cleary *et al.*, 1965), employment duration (Cleary *et al.*, 1966; Siekierzynski *et al.*, 1974a) and family history of cataract-relevant disorders (Odland *et al.*, 1973). Analytical procedures were seldom performed in accordance with current epidemiological procedures, often the reporting consisted of percentage of findings in different groups. In two studies, though, linear regression analyses were performed (Cleary *et al.*, 1966; Siekierzynski *et al.*, 1974a). Detailed reporting of basic age-specific data have sometimes enabled subsequent analyses to be performed, see further comments and e.g. calculations of odds ratios by the reviewer below.

6.5.2   Results and discussion – RF and ocular effects

A summary of the studies and the authors' own evaluation of the study results are given in Table 6.2.

In the study by Cleary *et al.* (1965) on cataracts, the results were reported as a risk of 0.67 for radar vs non-radar workers, with a χ^2 of 1.26. Adjusting for military branch (army or air force) and age did not materially change this estimate. Based on reported data, the odds ratio with 95% confidence interval was calculated as 0.67 (0.36–1.24).

Cleary and Pasternack (1966) related – by a linear regression analysis – the occurrence and/or intensity of some lens changes with an exposure score. Although age was the dominant factor, also duration of microwave work and exposure score contributed significantly to the lens opacity. In a figure showing linear regressions between lens changes and age, the one for the exposed group increased faster with increasing age than the one for the non-exposed group, making the authors suggest that the microwave associated effect could be seen as an increased lens 'aging'. The exposure score in this study was composed of various descriptives of microwave employment; average power output, mode of power termination, frequency of viewing open microwave waveguides, frequency of experiencing cutaneous heating due to exposure and distances to power generating equipment. Certain information was not available, such as operating frequency, pulse duration etc. For these reasons, the exposure score could not be interpreted in terms of energy absorption or power density (Cleary *et al.*, 1966).

Siekierzynski and co-workers (1974a) reported age and employment duration-specific associations with lens opacities of different grades – no significance was found according to the authors. Based on presented data, odds ratios with 95% confidence intervals have been calculated, and concur with the authors' evaluation. Comparing grades 3–5 (many opacities, increasing and/or causing visual impairment) with grade 1 (no opacities), the odds ratio for exposed vs non-exposed was 1.1 (0.7–1.7). It may bear comment, that the age-specific odds ratios were 1.9 (0.9–3.8) ($\leq$30 years old) and 1.2 (0.7–2.2) (>30 years old). There were no such age variations when comparing grade 2 (single opacities) with grade 1 (no opacities), the overall (crude) odds ratio was 1.1 (0.8–1.5).

In the study by Odland *et al.* (1973), no significant associations were noted between exposure and lens changes. Recalculated odds ratios were 1.0 (0.5–1.7) for exposed vs non-exposed individuals regarding the presence of either opacity, vacuoles and/or PSCI. No change in these results after age adjustments or adjustments for family history was found, apart from a non-significant increase (1.7; 0.9–3.4) of opacities, vacuoles and PSCI with exposure in individuals with a family history of diabetes mellitus, non-traumatic cataract, glaucoma, and grossly defective visions. In a possibly related study by Shacklett and co-workers (1975), the same general absence of positive findings were noted. Recalculated odds ratios for exposed vs unexposed were 0.9 (0.6–1.2), 1.0 (0.8–1.3) and 0.9 (0.7–1.2) for opacities, vacuoles and PSCI, respectively. Age-stratified odds ratios were similar.

Finally, the study by Appleton *et al.* (1975) again failed to show evidence of an association, with recalculated odds ratios of 0.8 (0.6–1.0), 0.9 (0.7–1.0) and 0.8 (0.7–0.9) for opacities, vacuoles and PSCI, respectively. Again, age-stratified odds ratios were similar to these crude odds ratios. In 1972, Appleton and co-workers reported on the results of one part of this study (Appleton *et al.*, 1972), with a similar non-positive conclusion by the authors. This preliminary study was later commented on by Frey (1985), who suggested that that study was indeed positive, and by Wike and Martin (1985), who responded by asserting that both studies by Appleton and co-workers were indeed non-positive when properly analyzed (e.g. by log-linear analysis).

Overall, these studies are clearly not demonstrating an effect of RF radiation exposure on cataracts or their precursors, lens opacities. The positive finding in one study has not been supported by findings in other studies, as seen in Table 6.2. It is, however, appropriate to insert a cautionary note here, since the positive study by Cleary and Pasternack (1966) is one of two studies that has exposure data beyond that of occupational categories only – and where the second study by Siekierzynski *et al.* (1974a) includes one suggestive although nonsignificant age-specific finding. The age-specific associations in these two studies were, however, opposite (larger differences for older age groups by Cleary and Pasternack, larger differences for younger age groups for Siekierzynski *et*

Table 6.2 Summary of six studies on lens opacities/cataracts and RF.

Study	Population base	Final study size	Overall results according to the author(s)
Case-control study of cataracts			
Cleary (1965)	Military personnel	2946 cases 2164 controls	No evidence in support of microwave work causing increased cataracts
Cross-sectional studies of lens opacities			
Cleary and Pasternack (1966)	Microwave workers	736 exposed 559 nonexp	A significant increase in certain specific lens defects with exposure score
Siekierzynski (1974a)	Microwave workers	507 exposed 334 nonexp	No dependence of lens changes on exposure or on duration
Odland (1973)	Military personnel	377 exposed 320 nonexp	The study failed to show any differences due to exposure
Shacklett (1975)	Military personnel	477 exposed 340 nonexp	No significant difference was found
Appleton (1975)	Military personnel	1542 exposed 801 nonexp	No difference between groups were demonstrated

al.). A conceivable explanation of the difference between the positive study by Cleary and Pasternack and the others could be differences due to varying degree of exposure misclassification – with the positive study perhaps having a somewhat more accurate exposure assessment. On the other hand, essentially all studies have shortcomings especially as to the accuracy of the selection procedures, and few studies have included data permitting the assessment of participation rates among those originally selected.

On balance, the opinion of this reviewer is that these studies fail to demonstrate an association between microwave or radar work and lens opacities, but that they fall short in fully asserting the non-existence of such an effect. Apart from methodological shortcomings in some studies, the major problem is the limited exposure assessment in these studies. Inclusion of the item 'experiencing heating' in the exposure score in the one positive study (Cleary *et al.*, 1966) is interesting in that it could suggest that an effect – if there indeed is one – would be consistent with exposure capable of producing heat sensation. Unfortunately, the report does not describe the contribution of the item 'cutaneous heating' – nor whether the noted association is still present in the absence of heating.

6.6   REVIEW OF STUDIES RELEVANT TO NEURASTHENIC AND OTHER SYMPTOMS

Some early Soviet reports of neurasthenic symptoms (including fatigue, head-aches, lack of concentration, sleep disturbances, weakness, decreased libido etc.) suggested that these were associated with work with RF-emitting equipments. Various methodological aspects preclude, however, the drawing of definite con-clusions from these studies. For reviews, see e.g. Albert and Sherif (1982), Michaelson (1982), Roberts and Michaelson (1985) or WHO (1993). The pos-sibility of neurasthenic or similar symptoms being related to RF exposures has been investigated in six more recent studies with (generally) improved method-ology.

6.6.1   Methodological descriptions of neurasthenic studies

Hamburger and co-workers (1983) performed a cross-sectional study of 5187 male physiotherapist workers, 3004 of whom (58%) responded to a mailed questionnaire on personal data, symptoms and work history of diathermy use. Questionnaire data on years of experience and treatments administered per week were used to classify the respondents as highly exposed or not in terms of microwaves or shortwaves.

Bini *et al.* (1986) reported on a detailed survey of plastic sealers, and briefly also reported a health survey of 63 female workers, some of whom were using these sealers, and who were compared with 'unexposed' workers. Measured electric field head exposures varied between 120 V/m and more than 1000 V/m (median 400 V/m) at frequencies about 27 MHz. Few details about selection of participants were given, though.

Kolmodin-Hedman and co-workers (1988) studied a group of 113 plastic weld-ing operators (51 men and 62 women) and compared them to 23 female sewing machine operators[†]. Also in this study, measurements of exposures at the plas-tic welding machines were made – at 50% of the exposed group's workplaces, the equivalent power density exceed $50 \, W/m^2$ at least in one measuring point. The majority of the exposed workers also reported light burns at least yearly due to touching metallic objects in the RF fields.

In a study by Nilsson *et al.* (1989), 17 radar mechanics and 12 referents were examined. Measurements of RF exposures (at 1.3–10 GHz, pulsed) were made – these were generally very low unless the covers were removed, which actually was often done by the engineers. At such times, exposure could exceed $10 \, W/m^2$.

For details of the studies by Siekierzynski *et al.* (1974b) and Robinette *et al.* (1980) see above.

[†] The authors commented on the lack of a suitable male comparison group.

Symptoms related to neurasthenic syndrome or psychological or neurological disorders were examined by Siekierzynski *et al.* (1974b), Robinette *et al.*
(1980), Kolmodin-Hedman and co-workers (1988) and Nilsson *et al.* (1989).
Upper-limb paresthesias (numbness) were examined by Bini *et al.* (1986) and
Kolmodin-Hedman and co-workers (1988). Heart related disorders or symptoms were ascertained by hospital records (Robinette *et al.*, 1980), examination (Siekierzynski *et al.*, 1974) or by questionnaires (Hamburger *et al.*, 1983).
Cerebrospinal fluid samples were taken in one study (Nilsson *et al.*, 1989) for
cytological analysis.

Matching or adjustments for the possible influence of other variables were
performed in several studies for age (Hamburger *et al.*, 1983; Siekierzynski *et
al.*, 1974b; Robinette *et al.*, 1980; Bini *et al.*, 1986; Nilsson *et al.*, 1989), for
ionizing radiation (Hamburger *et al.*, 1983) and for life style (Bini *et al.*, 1986).

6.6.2   Results and discussion of neurasthenic effects of RF

These six studies are summarized in Table 6.3.

In the study by Siekierzynski *et al.* (1974b), no association was found between neurotic syndrome and RF exposures, the recalculated odds ratio was
0.9 (0.6–1.2), with no age variation. Likewise, there was no association between
'abnormal ECG' and RF exposure; the crude odds ratio was 0.9 (0.5–1.5).

Hamburger and co-workers (1983) found an association between use of short-
wave or microwave diathermy equipment and heart disease, as reported in a
questionnaire. The reported odds ratios for frequent use of shortwave and microwave equipment was 3.4 (1.6–7.4) and 2.5 (1.1–5.8), respectively.

Admission rates due to mental, psychoneurotic or personality disorders or due
to diseases of the circulatory system to navy or to veteran hospitals were not
higher for the high exposure groups compared to the low exposure groups, as
shown by Robinette and co-workers (1980). In some cases, e.g. mental disorders,
the navy hospital admission rates were significantly higher for the low exposure
groups (6.4/1000 per year, vs 5.2/1000 per year, p<0.001). The authors caution
that limited data on non-veteran hospitalization, variations in age etc. limit the
conclusions that can be made.

Nilsson *et al.* (1989) found no clinical neurological differences between exposed
and referents, nor was any found regarding psychometric tests, although a non-
significant increase in subjective psychiatric symptoms were noted. Analysis
of cerebrospinal fluids revealed no major differences, but specific differences in
some detailed analyses were noted – in one iso-electric focusing related protein
band.

Bini and co-workers (1986) found a statistically significant association between exposure and upper-limb paresthesia. There was, on the other hand, no
significant association between central nervous system findings and exposure.
No numerical data were given.

Table 6.3 Summary of six studies on neurasthenic symptoms, heart problems and paresthesias.

Study	Population base	Final study size	Overall results according to the author(s)
Studies of neurasthenic or related symptoms			
Siekierzynski (1974b)	Microwave workers	507 exposed 334 nonexp	No dependence of functional disturbances on exposure or on work duration
Robinette (1980)	Military personnel	20 109 'high' 20 781 'low' exp	No health effects were associated with exposure
Kolmodin-Hedman (1988)	Welders vs sewers	62 vs 23 women	Some difference between exposed and non-exposed women as to neurasthenia
Nilsson (1989)	Military personnel	17 exposed 12 non-exp	No significant differences for subjective or clinical endpoints
Studies of upper limb paresthesias			
Bini (1986)	Plastic sealers	63 workers 30 'exposed'	Statistical significant association between exposure and upper-limb paresthesia
Kolmodin-Hedman (1988)	Welders vs sewers	62 vs 23 women	Significant difference between exposed and non-exposed women as to paresthesia
Studies of heart related disorders			
Siekierzynski (1974)	Microwave workers	507 exposed 334 nonexp	No dependence of functional disturbances on exposure or on work duration
Robinette (1980)	Military personnel	20 109 'high' 20 781 'low' exp	No health effects were associated with exposure
Hamburger (1983)	Physiotherapists	3004 men (58% response rate)	A significant association between frequent diathermy use and heart disease

Kolmodin-Hedman *et al.* (1988) found a higher percentage of neurasthenic symptoms among exposed (20%) than among referent women (9%) – the difference was not, however, statistically significant, the calculated odds ratio being 2.7 (0.6–13.3). Headaches or tiredness were not more common among exposed than non-exposed. It should be noted that 53% of the exposed women, but only 26% of the referents, reported 'psychologically stressing work' in the interviews. Paresthesia of the hands were found among 53% of the exposed and 22% of the referent women (calculated odds ratio of 4.1; 1.4–12.4). The authors report a significant correlation also with measured exposure levels (no further data given). Exposed and non-exposed groups of women were fairly matched for age, but no analysis of confounding was reported. (The limited size of the study presumably made this unfeasible.).

In summary, this limited number of studies have not revealed any solid or consistent evidence for a neurasthenic effect of RF exposure. The increased occurrence of neurasthenic symptoms found in one study among exposed individuals (Kolmodin-Hedman *et al.*, 1988) must be evaluated with some reserve, since a) the difference does not appear to be significant (according to recalculated odds ratios), and b) no analysis was reported as to whether the excess occurrence of stressful work that was reported could explain the difference.

In some contrast to this, an effect on upper-limb numbness (paresthesia) was found in both studies that included that endpoint (Kolmodin-Hedman *et al.*, 1988; Bini *et al.*, 1986), although a firm evaluation of these data are somewhat difficult due to the paucity of reported details, and the absence of any confounder analysis. It should be noted that both studies reported very high exposure levels; median exposure at $50 \, W/m^2$ (Kolmodin-Hedman *et al.*, 1988) and $400 \, V/m$ (Bini *et al.*, 1986), respectively, at frequencies about $27 \, MHz$ (specified by Bini *et al.*).

Results pertaining to heart disorders or related outcomes are difficult to evaluate because of the lack of reported details on the specific endpoints. Nevertheless, only one of the studies does include an indication of an effect on subjectively reported heart disorders (Hamburger *et al.*, 1983). The self-reporting of both effect and exposure and the low response rate (58%) do, however, detract from the credibility of the finding – the authors caution that bias could have been introduced.

6.7   EXPOSURE TO RF FIELDS AND SUMMARY OF SOME RESULTS

In the review above, positive indications were noted in the studies by Robinette *et al.* (1980) and Armstrong and co-workers (1994) as to (primarily) respiratory cancer, Cleary and Pasternack (1966) as to lens opacities, and Bini *et al.* (1986) and Kolmodin-Hedman *et al.* (1988) as to paresthesia. Some additional findings were made, but were questioned on methodological grounds (see above), these are therefore not included in the following discussion.

A summary of the populations under study as well as assumed exposure levels is given in Table 6.4. The evaluation is made with reference to IRPA/INIRC limits of exposure for RF fields (Duchéne *et al.*, 1990).

As can be seen in Table 6.4, studies with positive indications of an effect of the presumed or measured RF exposure are all based on populations where the exposure appear to be above current IRPA/INIRC occupational limits of

Table 6.4 Probable exposure levels in studies with some positive indications of effects.

Study	Endpoint indicated as exposure related	Exposed population	Reported exposure frequencies and levels	Evaluation of exposure levels[*]
Robinette (1980)	Respiratory cancer	Military radar operators	Potentially high exposure, no levels reported	Above?[†]
Armstrong (1994)	Stomach(?) & lung cancers	Electric utility workers	>200 V/m at 10-15MHz, measured for job categories	Above
Cleary and Pasternack (1966)	Lens opacities	Microwave workers (radar)	Exposure score used	Above?[‡]
Bini (1986)	Paresthesia	Plastic sealers	400 V/m at 27 MHz	Above
Kolmodin-Hedman (1988)	Paresthesia	Plastic welders	>50 W/m² for 50%, at 27 MHz(?)	Above

[*] Above = above the relevant IRPA/INIRC occupational guideline levels (Duchéne, et al., 1990) for relevant frequencies.

[†] Possibility of high exposures as suggested by the authors and also evaluated using data from Allen et al. (1994).

[‡] Evaluated based on inclusion of heating sensation in exposure score.

exposure. Although this observation is weakened by the paucity of adequate exposure measurements, it is still apparent that these reviewed studies have failed to suggest adverse health effects of RF exposures below the occupational (or public) exposure limits.

As remarked initially, various points need to be discussed when evaluating the possible causal inference of those statistical associations, with information drawn both from epidemiological and experimental studies. In the reviewers viewpoint, the findings cited above for cancer do not strongly support a causal association, due to the lack of consistency across the epidemiological studies, and the lack of support from experimental studies (WHO, 1993). Positive findings on lens opacities are limited both regarding epidemiological studies (see above) and experimental studies (WHO, 1993), and those experimental indications that do exist appear to be associated with very high exposure levels (WHO, 1993; Duchéne et al., 1990). The findings of excess occurrence of paresthesia appear more consistent in that both studies investigating this effect did find indications of excess occurrence in relation to high exposures.

In terms of common or public mobile telecommunication situations, exposure levels of the same order of magnitude as the current basic limits may conceivably occur after local head exposure to some cellular phones when assuming a worst possible exposure situation – although realistic exposure situations do appear to result in substantially lower levels. In this respect, it should be noted that – except for lens opacities – none of the indicated effects (see Table 6.4) appear relevant to local head exposure. Public whole body exposure levels in mobile telecommunication situations should to be considerably below current basic limits. It should also be noted that three of the six studies cited in Table 6.4 involve frequencies well below those primarily relevant to mobile telecommunications.

A conclusion from this is that the only finding in Table 6.4 with a possible relevance – in terms of exposure localization and frequency – to mobile telecommunications is that of Cleary and Pasternack (1966) on lens opacities – and that single finding was not supported by results of other studies (see further discussion above). Furthermore, the inclusion of the heating sensation item in the exposure score used indicates that substantially higher exposure levels are required than could conceivably appear in mobile telecommunication situations. This is also in line with the experimental evidence of cataractogenesis and RF exposures (WHO, 1993). In essence, this review was therefore unable to find information suggesting an adverse health effect of RF exposures similar to those due to common or public use of mobile telecommunication systems.

6.8   FURTHER EXPOSURE ASSESSMENT IN MOBILE PHONE SITUATIONS

It is equally clear that well-conducted epidemiological studies of mobile telecommunication systems would be a valuable asset in further discussions. The experience gathered from the studies reviewed above, suggest that one of the important improvements that needs to be made is in exposure assessment techniques. As should be clear from other parts of this publication, precise exposure assessments in cellular phone situations require detailed information from individuals that may be difficult to obtain in a large scale epidemiological study.

One course of action could conceivably be a nested case-control, where the study base would consist of a large number of individuals using mobile phones, and where ongoing registrations of their extent of mobile phone usage would be made. After an appropriate time – allowing for a sufficient long latency period for e.g. cancer induction – cases in this study base would be identified, and appropriate controls selected. Registry information on mobile phone use may then, together with questionnaire or interview-derived information on type(s) of phones used/owned, way of usage and other factors of interest, form the basis for a reasonable exposure assessment. Obviously, checks need to be built in to guard against or at least detect differential misclassification due to the possibility of case-specific recall[‡]. Likewise, information about a variety of confounders need to be ascertained.

6.9   SUMMARY

In summary, the review presented here has suggested a few indications of effects of RF exposure on paresthesia, and possibly also on lung cancer and ocular lens changes. These indications were found in groups which were probably exposed above current occupational exposure limits. Due to this, and also in light of the varied methodology of the studies involved, the paucity of good exposure measurements, and the lack of experimental studies supporting the lung cancer finding, none of these findings appear to motivate further restrictions of exposure. Thus, this review essentially concurs with that of the WHO report (1993).

The present review was unable to find any firm results suggesting an effect at RF exposure situations comparable to those encountered by common use of mobile telecommunication systems. This was partly due to the overall paucity of positive indications in generally applicable RF studies, and partly due to the limited relevance of these studies to the use of mobile telecommunication systems.

Nevertheless, further epidemiological investigations of possible RF-related effects are warranted – again in concurrence with the view of the WHO report (1993). Such research should include efforts to investigate specifically situations involving common or public use of mobile telecommunications.

REFERENCES

Albert, E. N. and Sherif, M. F. (1982) Interactions of nonionizing radiation with the nervous system, in *Biomedical Thermology*, Alan R Liss, New York, pp. 219–225.

Allen, S. G., Blackwell, R. P., Chadwick, P. J. *et al.* (1994) Review of Occupational Exposure to Optical Radiation and Electric and Magnetic Fields with Regard to the Proposed CEC Physical Agents Directive. *NRPB R265*. National Radiological Protection Board, Didcot, UK.

Appleton, B., Hirsch, S., Kinion, R. O. *et al.* (1975) Microwave lens effects in humans. *Archives of Ophthalmology*, **93**, 257–258.

[‡] The registration of phone usage could presumably provide a basis for such checks.

Armstrong, B., Thériault, G., Guénel, P. et al. (1994) Association between Exposure to Pulsed Electromagnetic Fields and Cancer in Electric Utility Workers in Quebec, Canada, and France. American Journal of Epidemiology, 140, 805–820.

Bini, M., Checcucci, A., Ignesti, A. et al. (1986) Exposure of workers to intense RF electric fields that leak from plastic sealers. Journal of Microwave Power, 33–40.

Cleary, S. F., Pasternack, B., and Beebe, G. W. (1965) Cataract incidence in radar workers. Archives of Environmental Health, 11, 179–182.

Cleary, S. F. and Pasternack, B. S. (1966) Lenticular changes in microwave workers. Archives of Environmental Health, 12, 23–29.

Czerski, P., Siekierzynski, M., and Gidynski, A. (1974) Health surveillance of personnel occupationally exposed to microwaves. I. Theoretical considerations and practical aspects. Aerospace Medicine, 45, 1137–1142.

Duchéne, A. S., Lakey, J. R. A., and Repacholi, M. H. (1990) IRPA Guidelines on Protection Against Non-Ionizing Radiation, Pergamon Press, New York.

Frey, A. H. (1985) Data analysis reveals significant microwave-induced eye damage in humans. Journal of Microwave Power, 20, 53–55.

Goldsmith, J. R. (1995) Epidemiologic evidence of radio frequency radiation (microwave) effects on health in military, broadcasting, and occupational studies. International Journal of Occupational and Environmental Health, 1, 47–57.

Hamburger, S., Logue, J. N., and Silverman, P. M. (1983) Occupational exposure to non-ionizing radiation and an association with heart disease: an exploratory study. Journal of Chronic Diseases, 36, 791–802.

Hill, A. B. (1965) The environment and disease: Association or causation? Proceedings of the Royal Society of Medicine, 58, 295–300.

Hollows, F. C. and Douglas, J. B. (1984) Microwave cataracts in radiolinemen and controls. Lancet, Aug 18, 406.

IARC (1991) IARC monograph programme on the evaluation of carcinogenic risks to humans, in IARC Monographs on the evaluation of carcinogenic risks to humans. Volume 52. Chlorinated drinking-water; chlorination by-products; some other halogenated compounds; cobalt and cobalt compounds, International Agency for Research on Cancer, Lyon, pp 15–36.

Johnson, C. C. and Spitz, M. R. (1985) Neuroblastoma: case-control analysis of birth characteristics. Journal of the National Cancer Institute, 74, 789–792.

Kolmodin-Hedman, B., Mild, K. H. et al. (1988) Health problems among operators of plastic welding machines and exposure to radiofrequency electromagnetic fields. International Archives of Occupational and Environmental Health, 60, 243–247.

Källén, B., Malmquist, G., and Moritz, U. (1982) Delivery outcome among physiotherapists in Sweden: Is non-ionizing radiation a fetal hazard? Archives of Environmental Health, 37, 81–84.

Lancranjan, I., Maicanescu, M., Rafaila, E. et al. (1975) Gonadic function in workmen with long-term exposure to microwaves. Health Physics, 29, 381–383.

Larsen, A. I., Olsen, J., and Svane, O. (1991) Gender-specific reproductive outcome and exposure to high-frequency electromagnetic radiation among physiotherapists. Scandinavian Journal of Work, Environment and Health, 17, 324–329.

Lester, J. R. and Moore, D. F. (1982) Cancer mortality and air force bases. Journal of Bioelectricity, 1, 77–82.

Lilienfeld, A. M., Tonascia, J., Tonascia, S. et al. (1978) Foreign service health status study – evaluation of health status of foreign service and other employees from selected eastern European posts. Final report. *NTIS PB-288 163.* Department of State, Washington DC.

Lin, R. S., Dischinger, P. C., Conde, J. *et al.* (1985) Occupational exposure to electromagnetic fields and the occurrence of brain tumours. *Journal of Occupational Medicine,* **27,** 413–419.

Majewska, K. (1968) Investigations on the effect of microwaves on the eye. *Polish Medical Journal,* **7,** 989–994.

Maskarinec, G. and Cooper, J. (1993) Investigation of a childhood leukaemia cluster near low-frequency radio towers in Hawaii. *American Journal of Epidemiology,* **138,** 666.

Michaelson, S. M. (1982) Health implications of exposure to radiofrequency/microwave energies. *British Journal of Industrial Medicine,* **39,** 105–119.

Milham, S. (1985) Mortality in workers exposed to electromagnetic fields. *Environmental Health Perspective,* **62,** 297–300.

Milham, S. (1988) Increased mortality in amateur radio operators due to lymphatic and hematopoietic malignancies. *American Journal of Epidemiology,* **127,** 50–54.

Nilsson, R., Hamnerius, Y., Mild, K. H. *et al.* (1989) Microwave effects on the central nervous system – a study of radar mechanics. *Health Physics,* **56,** 777–779.

Odland, L. T., Penikas, V. T., and Graham, R. B. (1973) Radio-frequency energy: a hazard to workers? *Industrial Medicine & Surgery,* **July/August,** 23–26.

Ouellet-Hellstrom, R. and Stewart, W. F. (1993) Miscarriages among female physical therapists who report using radio- and microwave-frequency electromagnetic radiation. *American Journal of Epidemiology,* **138,** 775–786.

Roberts, N. J. and Michaelson, S. M. (1985) Epidemiological studies of human exposures to radiofrequency radiation. *International Archives of Occupational and Environmental Health,* **56,** 169–178.

Robinette, C. D., Silverman, C., and Jablon, S. (1980) Effects upon health of occupational exposure to microwave radiation (radar) *American Journal of Epidemiology,* **112,** 39–53.

Rothman, K. (1986) *Modern Epidemiology,* Little, Brown and Company, Boston.

Selvin, S., Schulman, J., and Merrill, D. W. (1992) Distance and risk measures for the analysis of spatial data: a study of childhood cancers. *Social Science in Medicine,* **34,** 769–777.

Shacklett, D. E., Tredici, T. J., and Epstein, D. L. (1975) Evaluation of possible microwave-induced lens changes in the United States air force. *Aviation, Space and Environmental Medicine,* **46,** 1403–1406.

Siekierzynski, M., Czerski, P., Gidynski, A. *et al.* (1974a) Health surveillance of personnel occupationally exposed to microwaves. III. Lens translucency. *Aerospace Medicine,* **45,** 1146–1148.

Siekierzynski, M., Czerski, P., Milczarek, H. *et al.* (1974b) Health surveillance of personnel occupationally exposed to microwaves. II. Functional disturbances. *Aerospace Medicine,* **45,** 1143–1145.

Sigler, A. T., Lilienfield, A. M., Cohen, B. H., and Westlake, J. E. (1965) Radiation exposure in parents of children with mongolism (Down's Syndrome). *Bulletin, Johns Hopkins Hospital,* **117,** 374–399.

Skotte, J. (1986) Reduction of radiofrequency exposure to the operator during shortwave diathermy treatments. *Journal of Medical Engineering & Technology*, **10**, 7–10.

Spitz, M. R. and Johnson, C. C. (1985) Neuroblastoma and paternal occupation. A case-control analysis. *American Journal of Epidemiology*, **121**, 924–929.

Szmigielski, S. Cancer morbidity in subjects occupationally exposed to high frequency (radiofrequency and microwave) electromagnetic radiation. *Science of the Total Environment* (in press).

WHO (1993) *Electromagnetic Fields (300 Hz to 300 GHz)*. Environmental Health Criteria 137. World Health Organization, Geneva.

Wike, E. L. and Martin, E. J. (1985) Comments on Frey's 'Data analysis reveals significant microwave-induced eye damage in humans'. *Journal of Microwave Power*, **20**, 181–184.

PART III

Biological Research Activities

7

Biological research in North America

Asher R. Sheppard

7.1 INTRODUCTION

Biological effects of radiofrequency (RF) electromagnetic fields have been a subject of investigation in many North American laboratories over the past fifty years. A rising level of interest was evident over the decades of the nineteen hundred sixties, seventies and early eighties but, as noted by others (Michaelson *et al.*, 1995), research activities declined from the mid-1980s until the mid-1990s.

Now, there is renewed interest in the biological effects of electromagnetic fields, spurred by the need for gathering information for new uses of RF energy in wireless comunications, the need for refinements in the standards for radiofrequency electromagnetic exposure, and by the need to resolve issues left unsettled by past research. As a result, there are now many new opportunities for laboratory research in which new laboratory techniques and protocols can be applied to questions about the potential for stimulation or enhancement of tumor-related processes, effects on the central and peripheral nervous systems, and several topics in cell biology that can be related to a general interest in possible health effects.

The vitality of the new investigations is a result of the ability of researchers to take advantage of the astounding growth in instrumentation and knowledge that support the profusion of knowledge in genetics, neuroscience, and cell biology. Motivated by the technologies of the wireless communications industry, modulation-dependent effects and the responses of animals exposed under near-field conditions figure prominently in current research. In contrast, much of the research done in prior years was concerned with continuous wave (CW) waveforms and the narrow pulses used for radar systems. Of the non-radar modulation possibilities, only sinusoidal amplitude modulation had been tested at any depth in research conducted before the mid 1990s.

Mobile Communications Safety
Edited by N. Kuster, Q. Balzano and J.C. Lin
Published in 1997 by Chapman & Hall, London. ISBN 0 412 75000 7.

In order to provide the most up-to-date information, this chapter rests heavily on experimental ideas that are either newly in progress or still in the final planning stages. For this reason neither experimental details nor results can be fully given. The author can only satisfy the reader's curiosity about several current projects with suggestions on how such research might progress, based on the current stage of planning. Hopefully, the reader will soon be able to match the research ideas given in this chapter with data appearing in publications.

The sources of funding for research on biological effects of RF fields reflects changes in society, particularly in the USA where private corporations of the wireless communications industry rather than the United States government are expected to be the major sponsors of research over the next several years. In contrast, earlier cycles of RF fields biological research were sponsored by branches of the US military services, government agencies in the environmental and health-protective spheres, and manufacturers of home, commercial and military RF equipment (especially microwave ovens, industrial equipment, and radar).

7.2   PAST RESEARCH

Three questions from earlier research help motivate new research: (1) Do modulated or unmodulated RF fields enhance any of the processes related to cancer? (2) Do modulation-dependent effects such as those related to altered 'calcium efflux' play a role in biological responses and pathogenesis? (3) Are there robust phenomena involving non-thermal mechanisms of interaction (such as compromise of the blood-brain barrier and altered calcium metabolism) and do such mechanisms lead to harmful effects? Of these, the question of cancer has loomed largest. Likely, this is not only because of biological issues but because of a burst of publicity concerning brain cancer and the use of cellular telephones.

7.2.1   Cancer studies in the past

Past studies of cancer in laboratory animals have involved whole body exposures and a variety of waveforms, often at energy levels sufficient to raise body temperature. The research studies are few in number and do not give conclusive evidence addressing questions about the appearance of cancer after prolonged whole body exposures. Although cancer figures importantly in public health assessments for genotoxic chemicals and ionizing radiation, historically there has been scant attention to the possibility of a RF association with cancer. Indeed, very little of past laboratory research in North American countries was specifically designed to detect cancer effects. Until recently there was no research giving direct evidence about exposures to the RF fields typical of wireless communications, particularly with regard to brain cancer. Therefore the studies discussed below in section 7.3 have only indirect precedents and these are relatively few in number.

Mice were chronically exposed by Prausnitz and Susskind (1962) to a pulsed 9200 MHz signal at 100 mW/cm^2 for 4.5 minutes per day, 5 days per week, over a period of 59 weeks. For this high level of exposure the specific absorption rate (SAR) was estimated to be 40 W/kg (Kirk, 1984), but the relatively short exposure duration limited the body temperature rise to an average of 3.3°C. Among the effects reported by the authors were 'leukosis', a term indicating an abnormal number of white blood cells and used by the authors to group several forms of cancer of the white blood cells, although histopathological details are missing. A statistical reanalysis of the data by Kirk (1984) indicated that the rate of leucosis among the exposed mice was *not* statistically significant by the usual criterion (P < 0.05).

Preskorn *et al.* (1978) exposed fetal mice *in utero* to 2450 MHz fields, 35 W/kg, for 20 min/day over a 4 day period. After birth, at age 16 days, the young mice were injected with sarcoma (cancer) cells. Subsequent evaluation of the tumors showed a significant delay in tumor formation among the exposed mice, but final tumor numbers were not significantly different.

Spalding *et al.* (1971) exposed mice to an 800 MHz RF field over a period of almost six months for 2 hours per day at a power density of 4.3 W/m^2, corresponding to an estimated SAR of 12.9 W/kg. The level, frequency and CW nature of this exposure resemble the circumstances for some types of wireless communications signals, but the SAR is considerably greater. The authors reported no adverse health effects (apart from heat effects) and no deleterious effects, although lifespan was slightly increased.

A signal with fast rise time and narrow pulses of high peak intensity (447 kV/m) was used during exposures of rats over a period of 658 days, 23 hours per day by Baum *et al.* (1976) who reported no adverse effects of exposure.

Chou *et al.* (1992) reported a lifetime study of 100 rats exposed to circularly polarized fields producing SARs which ranged from 0.4 to 0.15 W/kg as the animals grew in size. Compared to controls, there were no robust physiological effects of exposure after more than two years of exposure to 2450 MHz fields pulsed at 800 Hz with square-wave modulation at 8 Hz. No significant effects were found on survival time, growth and development, immune responses and blood chemistry as examples from a battery of 155 measured parameters. However, the incidence of primary malignant tumors summed over all target sites was nearly fourfold higher among the exposed rats. Benign tumors of the adrenal gland were also increased, but not the total of all benign tumors. These equivocal findings on tumor incidence have been a stimulus for further research aimed at discovering if there is an effect of RF fields on the cancer process.

7.2.2   Athermal, non-thermal and thermal effects

A number of terms have been used to describe the relative exposure levels in laboratory studies although their meaning is not fixed: athermal, non-thermal, and thermal. Although definitions vary, these terms can be distinguished and ranked according to the potential degree of temperature rise (Sheppard, 1996). If exposures are so low that a significant temperature rise would not occur even in the absence of special cooling devices, exposures can be called 'non-thermal', but if temperature is held constant by removal of heat that would otherwise cause significant temperature increase, exposures can be called 'athermal', and if the RF energy is sufficiently strong and allowed to elevate temperature, exposures are 'thermal'. For *in vitro* studies, heat affects cellular and biochemical responses through a change in chemical reaction rates which can be sensitive to changes in temperature of less than one degree Celsius. In animal studies, temperature changes not only influence biochemical events and cellular physiology, but can bring about adaptive physiological responses in animal behavior (panting, perspiration, lowered activity, etc.). In general, *in vitro* research concerns exposures in the athermal and non-thermal regimes because, even at high levels, exposure systems usually are designed to maintain constant temperature. Effects under non-thermal conditions are controversial because some observers believe the only manner of interaction is by the heating effect of absorbed microwave energy. For this reason, heating is suspected in any situation where biological effects seem to occur.

7.2.3   Prior studies on biological effects of CW RF fields

A large body of research, much of it conducted in the USA and Canada, concerns potential effects on animal physiology, cellular functions, and biochemical functions in cells and tissues. There has been a concentration of research on the effects of RF fields on chromosomes, DNA and DNA repair, and cell reproduction. Several recent reviews provide an encyclopedic approach to this body of research worldwide (e.g. Hitchcock *et al.*, 1995; Michaelson *et al.*, 1995; Scientific Advisory Group on Cellular Telephone Research, 1994; World Health Organization, 1993). An older review conducted by the United States Environmental Protection Agency is still valuable for its detail, depth of critical analysis, and completeness (Elder *et al.*, 1984).

Many studies on chromosomes, DNA, and related areas concerning the genome have been conducted with CW and pulsed RF fields. Uniformly negative results were found over a large number of standardized tests using rodents and rodent cells, insects, bacteria and yeast, such as in tests for the genotoxicity of chemicals, drugs and ionizing radiation. In particular, barring changes in temperature, the literature is generally consistent in showing no RF-related effects on chromosome aberrations, mitosis, mutation rates, bacterial cell survival, and

DNA repair (for review, Michaelson *et al.*, 1995). There are examples of studies reporting effects on chromosome aberrations (Heller, 1970; Yao, 1978; Chen *et al.*, 1974) and germ cells (Manikowska-Czerska *et al.*, 1985), but these stand out as the exceptions among many other tests of genetic processes with negative results. The exceptional nature of these positive findings does not, of course, confer judgment on their accuracy, but instead is an expression of the fact that even if there are circumstances where RF energy affects the genetic apparatus, such circumstances are uncommon. The general conclusion remains that under most conditions, and especially when there is no possibility of temperature increase, RF is not genotoxic in the manner of certain chemicals and ionizing energy.

Cell biologists and biochemists have probed many features of cell physiology and biochemistry. Effects on cell proliferation and the kinetics of the cell cycle have been studied with particular interest because of a possible connection to the abnormal growth of tumor cells. Most evidence indicates that RF energy is not capable of initiating damage in DNA, consistent with the low energy of microwave photons and the low strength of the electric and magnetic fields of microwave electromagnetic fields. However, studies of cell transformation in C3H/10T$\frac{1}{2}$ cells by Balcer-Kubiczek and Harrison (1985; 1989; 1991) showed that 120 Hz pulse-modulated microwaves (2450 MHz) acted like a tumor initiator when microwave exposures were combined with a tumor promoting agent (the phorbol ester, TPA). The microwave exposure had no independent effect on transformation. The cell transformation assay identifies colonies of cells which grow densely as a result of the loss of the normal inhibitions against overgrowth. The appearance of dense plaques of cells amongst a background of cells growing in a normal monolayer is an *in vitro* model for the uncontrolled growth of tumor cells *in vivo*. The provocative results from these experiments were obtained in various experiments covering SARs from 0.1 to 4.4 W/kg. Exposures were made in the aperture of a waveguide and exposure was controlled by the depth in water of the samples. Modulation at 120 Hz was produced by the full-wave rectification of the magnetron power supply (Balcer-Kubiczek *et al.*, 1991).

Cleary *et al.* (1990) reported on the influence of a 2 hour exposure to 27 and 2450 MHz RF fields in the range 5 to 200 W/kg on cultured brain tumor (glioma) cells. One, three, or five days after RF exposure, thymidine and uridine uptake studies were conducted to measure DNA and RNA synthesis, respectively. There were both increases and decreases in uptake ('biphasic' responses). Because of strong cooling, temperature change was not believed to be a factor and the authors characterized the effects as 'isothermal'. Because uptake changes were greater three days after exposure than either one or five days after exposure, the results were interpreted as 'a kinetic cellular response to RF radiation', suggesting the possibility of long-term disruption of the regulation of cell-cycling. The relevance of this study to wireless communications exposures is uncertain because of the relatively high SARs, the unknown relation between the nucleotide measurements and any actual increase in cell numbers, and the occurrence of biphasic results. Despite these and other questions, this study has been a stimulus to renewed interest in studies of cell cycle kinetics and cell proliferation. Other researchers have also found changes in DNA synthesis, such as the inhibition reported by Chang *et al.* (1980), who worked with leukemia cells, or the increased DNA synthesis in *Neurospora* cells reported by Dutta and Verma (1993) who exposed at SARs so low that heating is not a question (≥ 0.001 W/kg, 915 MHz, CW) with a peak effect at 0.1 W/kg. Verma and Dutta (1992) and Dutta and Verma (1992) reported changes for a variety of genes (c-myc, c-ras, enolase, U6, and rRNA) up to 8 hr after exposure. Earlier studies in immune system cells (Hamrick *et al.*, 1977; Lin *et al.*, 1977; Blackman *et al.*, 1979) provided evidence that the cells were uninfluenced by RF exposures. Byus *et al.* (1988) found no effects of 450 MHz fields (1 mW/cm^2, amplitude modulated) on DNA synthesis in hepatoma cells. Meltz and Walker (1987) found no changes in DNA synthesis after exposures to several frequencies (35, 850 and 1200 MHz) at SARs in the range 0.39 to 2.7 W/kg.

The interest in the genetic apparatus also includes evaluations of damage to DNA. When uncoiled, as occurs during transcription and replication for cell division, DNA is most subject to damage that can be detected by several tests. Damage can occur through random errors and damage from toxic chemicals (for example, by natural products such as the free radicals produced by metabolism or toxic chemicals taken in from foods, water, air or skin contact). Damage to DNA by ionizing radiation has been studied extensively and this body of research establishes a paradigm, perhaps inappropriate, for testing of RF fields. Several tests of DNA and chromosomes are used to evaluate genetic damage *in vitro*. These include studies of mutation in bacterial cultures, chromosomal aberrations, DNA fragmentation, and rates of DNA repair following intentional DNA damage. Many such tests have been done with RF fields (e.g. for reviews, McCann *et al.*, 1993; Scientific Advisory Group on Cellular Telephone Research, 1994) and the results lead to the general conclusion that RF energy is not genotoxic. In addition to research in bacterial systems, Meltz and colleagues conducted a series of studies with multiple carrier frequencies in the range 350 to 2450 MHz using both CW and pulsed waveforms, and SARs in the range from 0.04 to 40 W/kg over the various studies (Meltz *et al.*, 1989; 1990; Ciaravino *et al.*, 1991). Their tests included chromosome aberrations studies, tests for DNA damage and DNA repair following damage by either ultraviolet light or the mutagens proflavin, adriamycin or mitomycin C. The findings were consistently negative. The few instances of apparent weak positive effects could not be repeated.

A number of physiological and behavioral studies have been conducted at non-heating levels. Lary *et al.* (1983) found no effects on rat embryos exposed *in utero* at a level that produced a whole body average of 0.4 W/kg (100 MHz) to the mother. D'Andrea *et al.* (1986a; 1986b) observed behavioral differences in a shuttle box test – but not physiological effects – for rats chronically exposed at levels as low as 0.1 W/kg, 2450 MHz. On the other hand, Lebovitz (1983) reported on behavioral changes which were the same for both CW and pulse-modulated RF under athermal conditions for which no temperature rise was measured (3.6 W/kg, 1300 MHz). Lebovitz drew the conclusion that even though temperature was not elevated, a thermal mechanism caused the observed effects. For additional information, see Postow and Swicord (1996) who tabulate 34 studies in which the effects of pulsed and CW fields were studied.

7.2.4   Prior studies on biological effects of modulated RF fields

The origin of many questions still current in bioelectromagnetics research is a behavioral study of electroencephalographic patterns in cats exposed to sinus-oidally-modulated 147 MHz RF fields that was conducted more than twenty years ago at UCLA by Suzanne Bawin, Ross Adey and colleagues. Bawin *et al.* (1973) found that cats could be behaviorally trained if the RF carrier was modulated at frequencies corresponding to frequencies dominant in certain brain wave patterns. Subsequently, Bawin investigated brain calcium levels in chick brain (Bawin *et al.*, 1975) in an effort to follow-up on the behavioral phenomena and Adey *et al.* (1982) reported on calcium responses in cat brain during exposure to modulated RF. In her original studies, Bawin used a 147 MHz RF field (flux density of $1 \, mW/cm^2$) sinusoidally-modulated at several extremely low frequencies and under conditions where exposure could not significantly change temperature (Tenforde, 1980). The peak response was for 16 Hz modulation. Unmodulated signals and modulation frequencies much above and below 16 Hz had no influence, leading to the concept of frequency windows. Blackman *et al.* (1979) and Sheppard *et al.* (1979) reported power windows, a concept later expanded upon by Blackman and his colleagues.

Many subsequent studies of 'calcium efflux' have been conducted, including extensive work on ELF-modulated RF and direct ELF fields by Blackman and colleagues, but there is no unanimity on the significance and reproducibility of the calcium efflux phenomena. Specific results and the window concepts of calcium efflux have been fully or partially replicated in work by Blackman (1989 for review), Byus *et al.* (1984), a number of *in vitro* studies with neuroblastoma cells (Dutta *et al.*, 1994; 1992; 1989). Blackman's body of work extended the range of phenomena (especially for ELF fields). Other extensions are represented by *in vitro* studies in a heart muscle preparation (Schwartz *et al.*, 1993; 1990; Wood *et al.*, 1992). However, the reported phenomena are not large (typically a change of about 20% or less) and several groups have been unable to replicate the original reports (Albert *et al.*, 1987). Others have found no effects on tissue-associated calcium ion levels using similar techniques but different waveforms. Pulse-modulated 147 MHz fields did not influence chick brain calcium (Shelton *et al.*, 1981; Merritt *et al.*, 1982).

Although calcium efflux phenomena have been an undoubted stimulus to bioelectromagnetics research, they remain controversial because the phenomena have not been directly linked to specific physiological responses nor has a detailed biophysical mechanism been developed to explain the modulation dependence, that is, to identify nonlinear response elements that would serve as detectors of the modulation envelope. Adey developed a conceptual model in which transduction occurs along the cell plasma membrane surface by an interaction of the RF field with extracellular charged moieties of integral cell membrane proteins (Bawin et al., 1975; 1978; Adey, 1981). Pickard and co-workers made theoretical (Pickard et al., 1978) and experimental studies of demodulation in plant cells (Pickard et al., 1981; Gokhale et al., 1985; Brunkard et al., 1984) and invertebrate neurons (Sheppard et al., 1984). Their results were consistent with biophysical models for transmembrane demodulation which show that nonlinear ion dynamics can contribute a small ELF signal if the carrier frequency is below about 1 to 10 MHz. But for higher frequencies, transmembrane demodulation does not occur because ions cannot cross the membrane within one cycle of the applied field.

Pulse modulation is necessary for the microwave hearing effect whereby pulses (approximately 1 to 100 μs in duration) are detected as audible clicks if the exposure is high enough (above approximately 0.4 J/m^2 during pulses shorter than 30 μs). The thermo-elastic model is accepted as the mechanistic explanation for microwave hearing. In this model, the heating which occurs during a microwave pulse causes expansion of the tissues within the head (brain, fluids and other matter) with a resulting stimulation of the auditory sense via the cochlea. Because the threshold for microwave hearing is relatively high, thermoelastic expansion has not figured in studies of the potential health effects of RF exposure to wireless technologies. However, the possibility that hearing of pulsed waveforms influences animal studies should not be overlooked (Lai et al., 1987a; 1987b).

Many of the studies discussed above are notable because they involve tests under non-thermal conditions. In addition, tests where biological responses depend on modulation characteristics can, in principle, provide compelling demonstrations of effects that are independent of heating. Non-thermal effects also can be shown convincingly when the power level is so low that significant heating could not occur. Such experiments have been reported but not universally accepted. The in vitro calcium efflux studies discussed above were conducted under just such non-thermal conditions where amplitude-modulated radiofrequency fields at certain frequencies – but not the unmodulated carrier – produced positive effects.

Animal studies with positive findings with modulated fields are few in number. Adey and coworkers reported modulation effects on calcium levels in vivo in experiments on cat brain (Adey et al., 1982) and Kues et al. (1985) found that pulsed RF caused more damage to corneal endothelium than CW signals of the same power density. Pulse-modulated, but not CW RF fields at both thermal and athermal levels affected the development of lymphoblastoid cells in culture (Czerska *et al.*, 1992).

7.3 NEW RESEARCH IN LABORATORY ANIMALS

7.3.1 Cancer studies

Laboratory animal research studies are now planned or under way to address questions about the possible influence of exposures to wireless communications fields on tumor growth. Because the head is exposed when using portable cellular transceivers, the focus of current projects is brain cancer. None of the research in North America is expected to address the issues of spontaneous tumor growth raised by whole-body exposures in previous research. The possibilities for experimental studies of spontaneous brain cancer in laboratory animals are limited. The natural incidence of central nervous cancer in common rat strains is typically 3% over the animal's lifespan. With such low natural incidence, very large numbers of rats are needed to get a population with statistically useful numbers of tumors. If the study size is inadequate, it would not be possible to make strong conclusions about any RF effect or its absence. One approach is to expose rats throughout life as a model for chronic use of RF telecommunications devices. If, as has been considered, exposures are restricted to one side of the animal head, tumor laterality could indicate a RF-specific effect on brain tumors.

As an alternative to the large number of rats needed for a study of spontaneous tumors, fetal rats can be exposed to a carcinogenic chemical which produces tumors of the central and peripheral nervous systems. When N-ethyl-N-nitrosourea (ENU) is administered to a mother rat late in pregnancy, it passes across the placenta and preferentially affects cells of the developing nervous system. The incidence of nervous system tumors depends upon the amount of ENU administered, the species of rat, and the time during the gestational period at which it is given. It is possible to obtain a population of rat offspring that will have a predictable incidence of glial cell tumors, tumors of the cranial nerves, meninges, spinal nerves, and certain ependymal sites. The details of tumor numbers and sites vary from strain to strain. The Fischer 244 rat, widely used for lifetime testing of chemicals, and the Sprague-Dawley rat are both used in studies of ENU-initiated tumors.

A principal outcome of such studies is a comparison of the numbers of tumors in rats exposed to radio frequency fields and those sham exposed. The time of tumor appearance is a key indication of whether tumor growth may have been promoted by RF exposure and the size. The number of tumors per rat provides another index of the relative growth of tumors in both groups. Careful examination of the brain is needed to detect tumors of microscopic size which may be a substantial part of the total number of tumors. The histological features of the tumors (degree of anaplasia and metastatic properties) also are valuable data. Other data of interest include comparisons of tumor location which might show some relation to SAR. SAR is highly non-uniform throughout the brain and spinal cord of exposed animals.

The ENU dose (for example 5, 10 or 20 mg/kg body weight of the mother) must be chosen so that tumors appear with a time course suitable for the duration of the study. The experimenter faces additional choices, such as whether a study should last most of the rat lifespan (two years or more) or be terminated in mid-life. These choices influence both the biological and statistical sensitivity of a study. Insight into the possible mechanisms for RF effects on tumorigenesis is useful in evaluating alternative experimental designs, but, as the following discussion indicates, it is not always possible to avoid trade-offs of one valuable feature for another.

The timing and manner of RF exposure require consideration of a number of factors that bear on the ENU tumor model. Because ENU is administered but once to the fetus and is quickly eliminated from the rats' bodies (mothers and fetuses), the damage to cellular DNA occurs but once. If RF energy is presumed to have a synergetic effect at the time of this original DNA lesion, it is necessary to irradiate the animals at the time of ENU administration. However, the rapid development of the rat brain continues through the final days of gestation and for weeks after birth. On this basis it can be argued that RF exposure to newborn and juvenile rats is most significant. Depending on ENU dosage and characteristics of individual animals, the development of tumors can take most of the natural lifespan. In view of these mechanistic factors, it appears that lifetime exposure is advisable during exploratory studies. The rapid growth of rats and the difficulties of maintaining relatively constant SARs add to the complexity of such experiments.

In studies of animals exposed to RF, the choice of frequency bears significantly on the degree to which animal exposure can resemble the pattern of energy deposition in the much larger body of exposed humans. However, relevance to the frequencies and waveforms of wireless technology push experimenters to use actual communication frequencies such as 835 and 915 MHz, although this can present severe difficulties if the laboratory is close to an active communications site and must therefore avoid interference with commercial activities.

The statistical design of large animal studies of tumor growth requires optimization of many factors so that the study has the greatest practical power to provide conclusive evidence on the chosen hypothesis. One rat tumor study undertaken in North America utilized relatively low doses of ENU so that macroscopic and microscopic tumors would develop in a minor fraction of the population, approximately 15% over the rat lifetime. In this way the experimenters hoped to maximize the power to observe a doubling in tumor incidence, but gave up the ability to have similar power to observe a decline in tumor incidence among the exposed animals. Another study will use a higher ENU dose and will terminate the experiment after about one year, thereby achieving considerable cost savings while forgoing the possibility of observing the tumor process in aged rats.

Transplantation of tumor cells into adult animals provides an alternative model for the study of tumor processes. Rat glioma cells may be grown in culture and injected in carefully controlled numbers into specific brain sites. Later, upon sacrifice, the extent of tumor growth can be evaluated with precision. This model is often used to test the efficacy of antineoplastic agents. It also can show whether RF energy influences growth processes of the implanted cells. Of course, since the injected cells were already transformed to a tumorigenic state at the time of injection, this model cannot provide evidence on possible RF influences on the transformation process.

7.4   NEW RESEARCH CONDUCTED *IN VITRO*

7.4.1   Cell proliferation

Regulation of the cell cycle is an important feature of normal cell growth. Disruption of normal cell cycling is strong evidence of a cell gone awry as is the case for the rapid and uncontrolled growth of cancer cells. Studies of the rate at which cells grow provide partial evidence about growth regulation which is governed by the genome. Commonly, cells are cultured for several generations under carefully controlled conditions and their numbers evaluated after several doubling times, that is, after several days for typical mammalian cells. Cell counts can be made visually under the microscope or with electronic instruments. Cell proliferation can also be estimated indirectly from measurements of the uptake of thymidine and uridine which are utilized, respectively, for synthesis of new DNA and RNA of the daughter cells.

Stagg made direct tests of proliferation in the widely-studied C6 glioma cell. Cells were exposed to a TDMA signal (0.1, 1.0 and $10\,\text{mW/cm}^2$; 0.21, 2.1 and $21\,\text{mW/kg}$). The preliminary report (Stagg *et al.*, 1995) indicates no reliable effects on cell numbers as directly determined from cell counts as well as the thymidine uptake technique. However, because the cell type and exposure conditions of Stagg's experiment do not replicate those of Cleary *et al.* (1990), it will be interesting to learn the results from replication studies in which exposure conditions will closely match those of Cleary, both at $27\,\text{MHz}$ and at $2450\,\text{MHz}$. Because the LN71 glioma cell line used by Cleary *et al.* (1990) is uncommon, if similar results are not found with a cell line such as C6, additional cell lines may have to be tested. In any event it will be useful to know if changes in cell growth occur with other cells, especially so if this *in vitro* observation is to weigh importantly in public health considerations. S. Motzkin (Polytechnic

University, New York) has begun a replication of the Cleary *et al.* study at both 27 and 2450 MHz.

The growing interest in bioeffects of wireless technology promises to yield new research approaches to questions about possible alterations in cell growth regulation. Researchers such as those mentioned above will, no doubt, continue their investigations to include additional waveforms of interest to wireless technology. Special interest attends modulation patterns that have low frequency patterns resembling in some characteristics (for example, pulse repetition rate or low frequency Fourier components) the character of the sinusoidal amplitude modulation frequencies effective in the calcium efflux studies.

One promising approach found in North American laboratories is a study of growth curves and cell cycling. Modern laboratory machines such as the FACS (fluorescence-activated cell sorter) permit screening and sorting of cells. In a typical RF study using flow cytometry, the investigator exposes cells to CW and modulated RF fields (such as 835 MHz over a SAR range surrounding 1 W/kg) for periods that bracket the typical mammalian cell cycle, for example, 4, 8, 16 and 24 hours. Exposures can be done in standard petri dishes or, where larger volumes are needed, vessels as large as the T-75 flask. Cells such as mouse fibroblasts (C3H/10T$\frac{1}{2}$), or human-derived tumor cells (glioma, HeLa) can be grown in monolayer in a medium supplemented by fetal calf serum and held in an incubator at constant temperature (37°C). The numbers of cells in the growth (G1, G2), synthesis (S) or mitotic (M) phases of the cell cycle are automatically scored and comparisons made between sham-exposed samples and cells given various exposures.

7.4.2   Cell transformation

Studies of cell transformation using wireless technology signals are of strong interest. Studies of transformation in C3H/10T$\frac{1}{2}$ cells exposed can answer the question of whether microwave fields in general – or the particular signals used for communications – cause cell transformation in combination with TPA, as reported in the studies by Balcer-Kubiczek and Harrison (1985; 1989; 1991) discussed above. Variations on the standard transformation assay may also prove useful in evaluating the possible effects of microwaves on cell growth. In one variant, already used to test extremely low frequency fields (Cain *et al.*, 1993), two types of C3H/10T$\frac{1}{2}$ cells are grown together. Because of growth control signals emanating from the parental cell type, the uncontrolled growth pattern of the second cell type is suppressed. However, should RF energy disrupt communication of these suppressive signals or otherwise interfere with the cell growth of both cell types, abnormal growth patterns could emerge. Once again, TPA plays a central role in the conduct of these experiments and, should positive results occur, it may be possible to better understand the mechanism for any microwave effects on cell transformation.

7.4.3 Gene expression

A flow cytometry study, while providing useful data in itself, can be coupled to other probes of the cellular apparatus. In that event, the cell cycle data become useful as a form of quality control to assure that cell cycle-dependent changes do not influence additional tests. One such test is an evaluation of the expression of the pattern of messenger RNAs (mRNAs) produced by cells from the DNA gene template according to a regulated program of gene transcription. Following RF exposure, cells are biochemically treated to extract the mRNAs which are then examined by electrophoresis, a means to display the mRNAs according to their relative molecular masses. The array of RNAs on the electrophoretic gel produces a characteristic pattern of bands. The change in band strength (or appearance and disappearance of a particular band) indicates an alteration of the cellular apparatus that regulates gene expression. Such changes are easily produced by exposure of cells to hormones and other biochemicals and by changes in temperature of several degrees. As indicated above, previous research on the ODC enzyme and related studies suggest that sinusoidally modulated fields might alter gene expression. However in the case of ODC, there were no changes in DNA synthesis accompanying the changes in ODC activity. The simple occurrence of a change in gene expression does not, of course, immediately point to a deleterious effect, but studies underway or soon to be begun will help answer the question, 'Do RF fields cause changes in gene expression in the absence of temperature change?'

An interesting variant of the study of gene expression is to examine structural elements of the nuclear biochemical machinery themselves rather than the products of gene transcription as just described. To do so, following exposure, the investigator separates the proteins associated with the cell nucleus ('nuclear matrix proteins') using electrophoresis and stains specific for the nuclear proteins. As in all such studies, confirmation of any effects that may appear require careful analysis for experimental artifacts such as might happen from differences in handling which affect temperature or cell growth factors. Additional detailed investigations would be needed to identify the particular proteins affected by RF exposure and the aspects of RF exposure (such as modulation, intensity, or duration) which influence nuclear proteins.

Genes such as c-fos, c-myc, and c-jun are activated by many cell signals and play an early role in a sequence of events that can lead to expression of other genes and gene products related to cell proliferation. Typically, activity of these genes increases with a characteristic time course following application of a stimulus to the cell. These genes are known as proto-oncogenes for their role in the proliferation of cancer cells but play a role in many normal cell activities. Tests for the activity levels and time course of gene activity can be useful markers of the biological activity of RF fields. Suitable experiments may use C3H/10T$^1/_2$ fibroblasts, lymphocytes and lymphoblastoid cells, PC-12 cells, and others. Exposure and assay protocols need to take into account the normal time course of gene activation. C-fos, for example, can reach a peak in about thirty minutes whereas c-jun takes about forty-five minutes and each may return to baseline levels thereafter. On the other hand, baseline levels could be changed after several hours or days of exposure and stand as evidence for long-lasting changes in gene activity. Significant changes in cell genetic function should be reflected in protein synthesis and cell growth. The techniques of molecular biology have matured in recent years and there is now widespread recognition of the importance of internal controls so that any changes can be referred to an invariant gene, for example, a 'housekeeping gene' such as GAPD. Observation of a change in gene expression is not of itself a strong clue to any specific biological effects and there may not be disease-related consequences from a change in gene expression. However, changed gene expression would point to the occurrence of a biological interaction that might be linked to others having greater physiological specificity. Cell protein synthesis is the end result of the expression of mRNAs and it is important to supplement investigations of gene expression with investigations of protein expression that can establish that the proteins encoded by the genes are in fact synthesized.

7.4.4   DNA damage

Although the existing *in vitro* evidence quite strongly indicates that RF energy is non-genotoxic, there is no evidence specific to the modulated signals used in wireless communications and there are two recent studies of cells from animals exposed *in vivo* that stand in contradiction to the overall conclusions from *in vitro* research on genotoxicity. The recent evidence is found in reports of DNA damage following chronic low level exposures to mice in work conducted by researchers in India (Sarkar *et al.*, 1994) and acutely-exposed rats in a study done in the U. S. A. (Lai and Singh, 1995; 1996).

As a result, researchers in North America are conducting additional *in vitro* research on DNA integrity following RF exposures. One such study involves DNA fragments from the nuclei of cells exposed *in vitro* or in a living animal and then treated in a strongly alkaline environment that cleaves the two strands of DNA. The extent of DNA migration under a strong electric field (electrophoresis) is proportional to the size and shape of the DNA fragments. When seen under a fluorescence microscope, the DNA fragments create a comet-like cloud whose tail contains those fragments that move furthest from the original site in the nucleus because they are smallest and most mobile (Singh *et al.*, 1988; Tice *et al.*, 1990; and for review, Fairbairn *et al.*, 1995). They represent the fraction of total DNA that has suffered single-strand breaks. Double-strand breaks, of greater relevance to the heritable mutations that might relate to cancer and reproductive hazards, can also be measured by working at neutral pH. A valuable feature of the comet assay is that DNA effects are observed in single cells. The primary outcomes of a comet assay are the amount of DNA that migrated and the extent of migration. These are often presented as distributions of 'tail length' and 'tail moment'. Comet assays of cells exposed *in vitro* complement those from *in vivo* studies but do not substitute for experiments in which tissues come from exposed animals. Scientists are at work studying DNA exposed to wireless communications signals under both conditions.

7.4.5   Studies in cell physiology

Radio frequency bioeffects can be studied *in vitro* by many means that do not directly concern DNA but take a more physiological approach. Among these are studies of cell differentiation, cell-to-cell communication, and the protein fibers that make up the cellular cytoskeleton. For studies of differentiation, models exist to follow pluripotent stem cells as they mature to become fully differentiated somatic cells. D3 embryonic mouse cells can be followed in culture for several days as they mature into differentiated cell lines with the properties of nerve cells, heart muscle cells, and white blood cells of the myeloid series. The numbers of differentiated cells can be evaluated by flow cytometry and immunostaining can be used to identify the appearance and quantity of blood cells whereas heart muscle cells become apparent by their rhythmic beating. Cell-cell communication is important in many epithelial tissues and of interest because of the aberrant cell-cell communication that marks cancer cells. Intercellular proteins bridge the gap between cells and permit cell-to-cell transfer of ions, small molecules, and electrical signals. The integrity of such cell-cell communication or its alteration by RF exposure provides opportunity for another test. The fibers that make up the cytoskeleton are important structural elements used for communication of chemical messages to and from the cell nucleus. Fluorescent dyes that bind to the cytoskeletal proteins allow its direct visualization and observations of any changes that might occur after exposure. Excitable cells such as cardiac muscle or nerve cells from the peripheral nervous system are useful for physiological studies because their temporal properties permit analysis of subtle changes in membrane function that would affect either cell-cell communication (as in heart muscle) or the flux of ions that underlies electrical activity of nerve and muscle. Thus, tests of cell firing rate, strength/duration curves, and tests of compound action potentials in nerves can provide evidence of physiological effects but with no direct bearing on questions focused on cancer.

In cells, a balance between free radicals and free radical scavengers is required for normal physiologic functioning and an imbalance constitutes 'oxidative stress'. Oxidative stress may be a causative factor in observations of DNA damage because the elevated levels of DNA damage that occur when antioxidants are in relative short supply may overcome the mechanisms of DNA repair. To conduct such experiments, cells are exposed to RF fields and tested for the levels of oxidative metabolic products such as hydrogen peroxide and superoxide radical, levels of antioxidants such as superoxide dismutase, and levels of DNA damage and repair. Positive controls may include agents such as heat shock and ultraviolet light which it is known affect oxidative stress.

7.5   CONCLUSIONS

A number of North American laboratories are actively studying animal and cell systems using a wide range of biological models. Most studies address the possibility that RF energy or specific RF waveforms may be tumorigenic in animals or cause cancer-related changes in cell systems. Many *in vitro* studies raise hypotheses involving possible effects on nuclear DNA. Both *in vivo* and *in vitro* investigations are reactions to a specific concern about brain cancer and therefore many utilize brain cancer cells or exposures to the brain. Many other experiments are mechanistic in nature and use diverse cell systems chosen for the specific needs of a biological model. At the time of writing, results were not available from the new generation of studies specific to wireless technology. The acquisition of data has already begun in many laboratories and the reader can look forward to a large number of research reports in the next few years. Although scientific research rarely if ever provides conclusive evidence with the initial round of study, it is possible that many of the first round studies will be fruitful. This follows from the fact that there is prior research with modulated, unmodulated, and pulse-modulated RF fields which can aid in interpretation of the new data.

Despite the appearance that there are a great number of studies ongoing or planned, some areas for investigation remain to be explored using fields relevant to wireless technology. Whole-body exposures have been given little emphasis because of the attention gained by the stronger exposures to the head of a cellular telephone user. Exposures from cellular base stations and exposures from other uses of modulated signals have figured in public concerns but received little research attention. Should research at levels used for the current generation of research validate health concerns specific to modulation characteristics, additional studies with chronic whole-body exposure will be needed.

The proliferation of modulation schemes underscores the need to develop a comprehensive biophysical model for the interactions of modulated RF fields with biological tissues. A successful model would reduce the need to conduct a new biological experiment for every novel modulation scheme. Some observers believe that such a model already is at hand because, it can be argued, there are no known biophysical mechanisms for electrobiological detection of either frequency or amplitude modulation at microwave frequencies and no biological effects unless a significant temperature change occurs. If this view is correct, support would come in the form of uniformly negative results from the new research spawned by the interest in cellular telephone bioeffects.

This chapter is being written as a new wave of investigations begins into the potential biological and health effects of exposures to RF energy modulated for communications purposes. The outcome of the research program will be valuable not only for the public and wireless technology companies, but for a deeper understanding about the interaction of electromagnetic energy with biological systems.

REFERENCES

Adey, W.R. (1981) Tissue interactions with nonionizing electromagnetic fields. *Physiol Rev*, **61**, 435–514.

Adey, W.R., Bawin, S.M. and Lawrence, A.F. (1982) Effects of weak amplitude-modulated microwave fields on calcium efflux from cat cerebral cortex. *Bioelectromagnetics*, **3**(3), 295–307.

Albert, E.N., Slaby, F., Roche, J. *et al.* (1987) Effect of amplitude-modulated 147 MHz radio frequency radiation on calcium ion efflux from avian brain tissue. *Radiat Res*, **109**(1), 19–27.

Balcer-Kubiczek, E.K. and Harrison, G.H. (1985) Evidence for microwave carcinogenesis *in vitro*. *Carcinogenesis*, **6**(6), 859–864.

Balcer-Kubiczek, E.K. and Harrison, G.H. (1989) Induction of neoplastic transformation in C3H/10T^1/$_2$ cells by 2.45 GHz microwaves and phorbol ester. *Radiat Res*, **117**(3), 531–537.

Balcer-Kubiczek, E.K. and Harrison, G.H. (1991) Neoplastic transformation of C3H/10T^1/$_2$ cells following exposure to 120 Hz modulated 2.45 GHz microwaves and phorbol ester tumor promoter. *Radiat Res*, **126**(1), 65–72.

Baum, S.J., Ekstrom, M.E., Skidmore, W.D. *et al.* (1976) Biological measurements in rodents exposed continuously throughout their adult life to pulsed electromagnetic radiation. *Health Phys*, **30**(2), 161–166.

Bawin, S.M., Gavalas, R.J. and Adey, W.R. (1973) Effects of modulated very high frequency fields on specific brain rhythms in cats. *Br Res*, **58**, 365–384

Bawin, S.M., Kaczmarek, L.K. and Adey, W.R. (1975) Effects of modulated VHF fields on the central nervous system. *Ann NY Acad Sci*, **247**, 74–80.

Bawin, S.M., Sheppard, A. and Adey, W.R. (1978) Possible mechanisms of weak electromagnetic field coupling in brain tissue. *Bioelectrochemistry and Bioenergetics*, **5**, 67–76.

Blackman, C.F., Elder, J.A., Weil, C.M. *et al.* (1979) Induction of calcium-ion efflux from brain tissue by radio-frequency radiation: effects of modulation frequency and field strength. *Radio Science*, **14**, 93–98.

Blackman, C.F., Kinney, L.S., House, D.E. *et al.* (1989) Multiple power-density windows and their possible origin. *Bioelectromagnetics*, **10**(2), 115–128.

Brunkard, K.M. and Pickard, W.F. (1984) The membrane potential of characean cells exposed to amplitude-modulated, low-power 147 MHz radiation. *Bioelectromagnetics*, **5**(3), 353–356.

Byus, C.V., Kartun, K., Pieper, S. *et al.* (1988) Increased ornithine decarboxylase activity in cultured cells exposed to low energy modulated microwave fields and phorbol ester tumor products. *Cancer Research*, **48**, 4222–4226.

Byus, C.V., Lundak, R.L., Fletcher, R.M. *et al.* (1984) Alterations in protein kinase activity following exposure to cultured human lymphocytes to modulated microwave fields. *Bioelectromagnetics*, **5**, 341–351.

Cain, C.D., Thomas, D.L., and Adey, W.R. (1993) 60 Hz magnetic field acts as co-promoter in focus formation of C3H/10T$^1\!/_2$ cells. *Carcinogenesis*, **14**(5), 955–960.

Chang, B.K., Huang, A.T. and Joines, W.T. (1980) Inhibition of DNA synthesis and enhancement of the uptake and action of methotrexate by low-power-density microwave radiation in L1210 leukemia cells. *Cancer Res*, **40**(4), 1002–1005.

Chen, K.M., Samuel, A. and Hoopingavner, R. (1974) Chromosomal aberrations of living cells induced by microwave radiation. *Environ Lett*, **6**, 37.

Chou, C.-K., Guy, A.W., Kunz, L.L. *et al.* (1992) Long-term, low-level microwave irradiation of rats. *Bioelectromagnetics*, **13**(6), 469–496.

Ciaravino, V., Meltz, M.L. and Erwin D.N. (1991) Absence of a synergistic effect between moderate-power radio-frequency electromagnetic radiation and adriamycin on cell-cycle progression and sister-chromatid exchange. *Bioelectromagnetics*, **12**, 289–298.

Cleary, S.F., Liu, L.M. and Merchant, R.E. (1990) Glioma proliferation modulated *in vitro* by isothermal radiofrequency radiation exposure. *Radiat Res*, **121**(1), 38–45.

Czerska, E.M., Elson, E.C., Davis, C.C. *et al.* (1992) Effects of continuous and pulsed 2450 MHz radiation on spontaneous lymphoblastoid transformation of human lymphocytes *in vitro*. *Bioelectromagnetics*, **13**(4), 247–259.

D'Andrea, J.A., DeWitt, J.R., Emmerson, R.Y. *et al.* (1986a) Intermittent exposure of rats to 2450 MHz microwaves at 2.5 mW/cm^2: behavioral and physiological effects. *Bioelectromagnetics*, **7**(3), 315–328.

D'Andrea, J.A., DeWitt, J.R., Emmerson, R.Y. *et al.* (1986b) Behavioral and physiological effects of chronic 2450 MHz microwave irradiation of the rat at 0.5 mW/cm^2. *Bioelectromagnetics*, **7**(1), 45–56.

Dutta, S.K. and Verma, M. (1992) *In vivo* DNA synthesis of specific genes enhanced by low-dose-rate 915 MHz, CW microwave radiation (Abstract). First World Congress for Electricity and Magnetism in Biology and Medicine, Lake Buena Vista, p. 111.

Dutta, S.K. and Verma, M. (1993) *In vivo* DNA synthesis of specific genes enhanced by low-dose-rate 915 MHz, CW microwave radiation, in *Electricity and Magnetism in Biology and Medicine* (ed M. Blank), San Francisco Press, San Francisco, 525–527.

Dutta, S.K., Das, K., Ghosh, B. *et al.* (1992) Dose dependence of acetylcholinesterase activity in neuroblastoma cells exposed to modulated radio-frequency electromagnetic radiation. *Bioelectromagnetics*, **13**(4), 317–322.

Dutta, S.K., Gosh, B. and Blackman, C.F. (1989) Radio frequency radiation-induced calcium ion efflux enhancement from human and other neuroblastoma cells in culture. *Bioelectromagnetics*, **10**(2), 197–202.

Dutta, S.K., Verma, M. and Blackman, C.F. (1994) Frequency-dependent alterations in enolase activity in escherichia coli caused by exposure to electric and magnetic fields. *Bioelectromagnetics*, **15**(5), 377–383.

Elder, J.A. and Cahill, D.F. (eds) (1984) *Biological Effects of Radiofrequency*

Radiation, Research Triangle Park, United States Environmental Protection Agency.

Fairbairn, D.W., Olive, P.L. and O'Neill, K.L. (1995) The comet assay: a comprehensive review. *Mut Res,* **339,** 37–59.

Gokhale, A.V. and Pickard, W.F. (1985) Evidence that Characean membrane transport is not significantly altered by incident electromagnetic radiation. *Radiat Res,* **102**(3), 300–306.

Hamrick, P.E. and Fox, S.S. (1977) Rat lymphocytes in cell culture exposed to 2450 MHz (CW) microwave radiation. *J Microw Power,* **12**(2), 125–132.

Heller, H.J. (1970) Cellular effects of microwave radiation, in *Biological Effects and Health Implications of Microwave Radiation* (ed S. F. Cleary), HEW Publication, Rockville, Bureau of Radiological Health, 116–121.

Hitchcock, R.T. and Patterson, R.M. (eds) (1995) *Radio-frequency and elf electromagnetic energies: A handbook for health professionals,* Van Nostrand, Reinhold, New York, 551 pp.

Kirk, W.P. (1984) Life span and carcinogenesis, in *Biological Effects of Radiofrequency Radiation* (eds J. A. Elder and D. F. Cahill), Research Triangle Park, U.S. Environmental Protection Agency, 5-106 to 5-111.

Kues, H.A., Hirst, L.W., Lutty, G.A. *et al.* (1985) Effects of 2.45 GHz microwaves on primate corneal endothelium. *Bioelectromagnetics,* **6,** 177–188.

Lai, H., Horita, A., Chou, C.-K. *et al.* (1987a) Low-level microwave irradiations affect central cholinergic activity in the rat. *J Neurochem,* **48**(1), 40–45.

Lai, H., Horita, A., Chou, C-K. *et al.* (1987b) A review of microwave irradiation and actions of psychoactive drugs. *IEEE Trans Eng Med Biol,* **6,** 31–36.

Lai, H. and Singh, N.P. (1995) Acute low-intensity microwave exposure increases DNA single-strand breaks in rat brain cells. *Bioelectromagnetics,* **16**(3), 207–210.

Lai, H. and Singh, N.P. (1996) Single- and double-strand DNA breaks in rat brain cells after acute exposure to radio frequency electromagnetic radiation. *Int J Radiat Biol,* **69,** 513–521.

Lary, J.M., Conover, D.L. and Johnson, P.H. (1983) Absence of embryotoxic effects from low-level (nonthermal) exposure of rats to 100 MHz radio frequency radiation. *Scand J Work Environ Health,* **9**(2), 120–127.

Lebovitz, R.M. (1983) Pulse-modulated and continuous-wave microwave radiation yield equivalent changes in operant behavior of rodents. *Physiol Behav,* **30**(6), 891–898.

Lin, J.C. and Peterson, W.D. (1977) Cytological effects of 2450 MHz CW microwave radiation. *J Bioeng,* **1**(5/6), 471–478.

Manikowska-Czerska, E., Czerski, P. and Leach, W.M. (1985) Effects of 2.45 GHz microwaves on meiotic chromosomes of male CBA/CAY mice. *J. Hered.,* **76**(1), 71-73.

McCann, J., Dietrich, F., Rafferty, C. *et al.* (1993) A critical review of the genotoxic potential of electric and magnetic fields. *Mut Res,* **297,** 61–95.

Meltz, M.L., Eagan, P. and Erwin, D.N. (1990) Proflavin and microwave radiation: absence of a mutagenic interaction. *Bioelectromagnetics,* **11,** 149–157.

Meltz, M.L., Eagan P. and Erwin, D.N. (1989) Absence of mutagenic interaction between microwaves and mitomycin C in mammalian cells. *Environ Mol Mutagen,* **13**(4), 294–303.

Meltz, M.L., Walker, K.A. and Erwin, D.N. (1987) Radiofrequency (microwave) radiation exposure of mammalian cells during UV-induced DNA repair synthesis. *Radiat Res*, **110**, 255–266.

Merritt, J.H., Shelton, W.W. and Chamness, A.F. (1982) Attempts to alter $^{45}Ca^{2+}$ binding to brain tissue with pulse-modulated microwave energy. *Bioelectromagnetics*, **3**(4), 475–478.

Michaelson, S.M. and Elson, E.C. (1996) Interaction of nonmodulated and pulse modulated radio frequency fields with living matter: experimental results, in *Handbook of Biological Effects of Electromagnetic Fields* (eds C. Polk and E. Postow), CRC Press, Boca Raton, 435–533.

Pickard, W.F. and Barsoum, Y.H. (1981) Radio-frequency bioeffects at the membrane level: separation of thermal and athermal contributions in the characeae. *J Membr Biol*, **61**, 39–54.

Pickard, W.F. and Rosenbaum, F.J. (1978) Biological effects of microwaves at the membrane level: Two possible athermal electrophysiological mechanisms and a proposed experimental test. *Math Biosci*, **39**, 235–253.

Postow, E. and Swicord, M.L. (1996) Modulated fields and 'window' effects, in *Handbook of Biological Effects of Electromagnetic Fields* (eds C. Polk and E. Postow), CRC Press, Boca Raton, 535–580.

Preskorn, S.H., Edwards, W.D. and Justesen, D.R. (1978) Retarded tumor growth and greater longevity in mice after fetal irradiation by 2450 MHz microwaves. *J Surg Oncol*, **10**(6), 483–492.

Sarkar, S., Ali, S. and Behari, J. (1994) Effect of low power microwave on the mouse genome: a direct DNA analysis. *Mut Res*, **320**, 141–147.

Schwartz, J-L., House, D.E. and Mealing, G.A.R. (1990) Exposure of frog hearts to CW or amplitude-modulated VHF fields: Selective efflux of calcium ions at 16 Hz. *Bioelectromagnetics*, **11**(4), 349–358.

Schwartz, J-L. and Mealing, G.A.R. (1993) Calcium-ion movement and contractility in trial strips of frog-heart are not affected by low-frequency-modulated, 1 GHz electromagnetic radiation. *Bioelectromagnetics*, **14**(6), 521–533.

Scientific Advisory Group on Cellular Telephone Research (1994) *Potential public health risks from Wireless technology: Research agenda for the development of data for science-based decision making*. Scientific Advisory Group on Cellular Telephone Research, Washington, DC.

Shelton, W.W. and Merritt, J.H. (1981) *In vitro* study of microwave effects on calcium efflux in rat brain tissue. *Bioelectromagnetics*, **2**(2), 161–167.

Sheppard, A.R., Bawin, S.M. and Adey, W.R. (1979) Models of long-range order in cerebral macromolecules: Effects of sub-ELF and of modulated VHF and UHF fields. *Radio Sci*, **14**(6S), 141–145.

Sheppard, A.R. (1996) Where does the energy go? Microwave energy absorption in biological objects on the microscopic and molecular scales, in *State of the Science Symposium*, Washington, Wireless Technology Research, LLC (in press).

Sheppard, A.R., Pickard, W.F. and Bawin, S.M. (1984) Measurements in aplasia neurons detect no transmembrane demodulation of extremely-low-frequency amplitude-modulated 450 MHz fields. *Bioelectromagnetics Society, 6th Annual Meeting*, p. 50.

Singh, N.P., McCoy, M.T., Tice, R.R. *et al.* (1988) A simple technique for quantitation of low levels of DNA damage in individual cells. *Exp Cell Res*, **175**, 184–191.

Spalding, J.F., Freyman, R.W. and Holland, L.M. (1971) Effects of 800 MHz electromagnetic radiation on body weight, activity, hematopoiesis and life span in mice. *Health Physics*, **20**, 421–424.

Stagg, R.B., Thomas, W.J, Jones, R.A. *et al.* (1995) Cell Proliferation in C6 Glioma Cells Exposed to a 836.55 MHz Frequency Modulated Radiofrequency Field (Abstract). Bioelectromagnetics Society, 17th Annual Meeting, June, Boston, MA, 45–46.

Tenforde, T.S. (1980) Thermal aspects of electromagnetic field interactions with bound calcium at the nerve cell surface. *J Theor Biol*, **83**, 517.

Tice, R.R., Andrews, P.W., Hirai, O. *et al.* (1990) The single cell gel (SCG) assay: an electrophoretic technique for the detection of DNA damage in individual cells. *Adv Exp Med Biol*, **283**, 157–164.

Verma, M. and Dutta, S.K. (1992) *Enhanced transcription of specific genes coded by various RNA polymerases induced by 915-MHz, CW microwave radiation. (Abstract).* First World Congress for Electricity and Magnetism in Biology and Medicine, Lake Buena Vista, p. 43.

Wood, A.W., Lubinas, V., Joyner, K.H. *et al.* (1992) Calcium efflux from toad heart: a replication study, in *Electricity and Magnetism in Biology and Medicine* (ed M. Blank), San Francisco Press Inc., San Francisco, 482–484.

World Health Organization (1993) *Electromagnetic fields (300 Hz to 300 GHz). Environmental Health Criteria*, Vol. 137, Geneva, World Health Organization, 290 pp.

Yao, K.T. (1978) Microwave radiation-induced chromosomal aberrations in corneal epithelium of Chinese hamsters. *J Hered*, **69**(6), 409–412.

8

European research on the effects of RF fields on biological systems

Bernard Veyret and Peter Semm

8.1 INTRODUCTION

In this chapter, we shall focus on European research related to health aspects of mobile communications. We made sure that this review was as comprehensive as possible.

At the present time, European research is not sponsored by any governmental research councils and foundations, nor by the European Commission. In France and Germany, for example, Telecom agencies are working with university partners. Such academic research activity is sometimes criticized in the media for a lack of independence.

The various research topics are reviewed in alphabetical order: behaviour, cancer, development, EEG and sleep, genetics, immune system, literature survey, melatonin, neuronal responses, and proliferation *in vitro*. The European programme COST 244 on 'biomedical effects of electromagnetic fields' is described briefly.

8.2 BEHAVIOR

Deutsche Telekom is sponsoring a study by M. Bornhausen at Neuherberg (München, Germany) on the learning behaviour of young rats. The mothers of these rats will be exposed to the GSM signal throughout their pregnancy. Behaviour will be assessed using Skinner boxes: this method has been successfully used to monitor the influence of chemicals, such as mercury, on learning behaviour.

There is preliminary evidence that a reflex behaviour of crickets (kicking reflex) is influenced by pulse-modulated 900 MHz radiation at power densities of

Mobile Communications Safety
Edited by N. Kuster, Q. Balzano and J.C. Lin
Published in 1997 by Chapman & Hall, London. ISBN 0 412 75000 7.

$0.1 \, \text{mW/cm}^2$ (group of P. Semm, University of Frankfurt, sponsored by Deutsche Telekom). This reflex activity, which can be excited by applying air puffs or touching sensory hairs, decreased by about 30% upon microwave exposure which suggests an alteration of the electric activity of the neurones involved.

8.3   CANCER MODELS

Tumour growth under exposure to low-level microwaves was investigated at the University of Bordeaux, France (Chagnaud *et al.*, 1995). Rats were injected on day 0 with benzo(a)pyrene and tumours appeared in 100% of the animals, approximately 100 days post-injection. The sensitivity of this model had been tested previously using antibodies (anti benzo(a)pyrene-like molecules, etc.). The date of appearance of tumours and the survival time of the animals were affected. Exposure to pulse-modulated microwaves (900 MHz, GSM signal, far-field, $200 \, \mu\text{mW/cm}^2$, SAR of 0.27 W/kg) started on days 20, 40 or 75 and lasted 10 days (2 h/day, 5 days/wk). There were 10 animals in each of the exposed or sham-exposed groups. Levels of autoantibody against phosphatidylinositol (tumour marker) and tumour size were also assayed regularly. Results of these studies showed no differences between groups in any of the parameters (to be published).

At the University of Kuopio, Finland (J. Juutilainen), a study is in progress on possible cancer-promoting effects of continuous or pulsed (GSM) 900 MHz microwaves in CBA/s mice. Ionizing radiation is used as the initiating agent. Animals are exposed for 1.5 h/day, 5 days/wk (average SAR of 1.5 W/kg for CW microwaves and 0.35 W/kg for GSM modulation).

A study on brain cancer, using the rat brain glioma model, was performed by Salford and co-workers (1993c; 1993d) in Lund, Sweden. The animals were exposed to 915 MHz microwaves (CW or 4, 8, 16, 200 Hz modulation, 7 h/day, 5 days/wk for 2–3 wk). There was no statistically significant difference in tumour growth between exposed and sham-exposed groups under any exposure conditions.

At ENEA in Rome, Italy, the non-thermal effects of 900 MHz exposure on the proliferation of neoplastic cells, and in particular as regards tumoral activation, are being studied (Marino *et al.*, 1995). A TEM cell, designed at ENEA and at the University La Sapienza, was used to expose groups of 12 mice (SAR of 0.4 W/kg). Three-month-old hybrid mice are used. Adenocarcinoma cells were injected in the mice's hind feet. In a first experiment, animals were exposed for 60 h over 10 days, starting 3 days after injection, and tumour volume was monitored between days 10 and 30. In a second experiment, mice were exposed when tumour size was $200 \, \text{mm}^3$ until it reached $1000 \, \text{mm}^3$. No statistically significant differences in tumour sizes were found between exposed and sham-exposed groups in either experiments.

A group from the University Clinic of Tübingen, Germany (H. Bartsch and C. Bartsch, sponsored by Deutsche Telekom) is looking at the co-promoting role of GSM-modulated microwaves in the development of DMBA-induced tumours in rats. Special chambers have been designed to expose each animal under optimal controlled conditions. The melatonin level of the urine will also be assayed during the experiment.

In some earlier work done in Budapest, Hungary, Somosy et al. (1991) showed that amplitude-modulated microwaves (2.45 GHz, square-wave 16 Hz modulation, 0.0024–2.4 W/kg) yielded more morphological cell changes than did CW microwaves. The amount of free negative charges on cell surface decreased following irradiation with AM microwaves, but remained unaffected under CW exposure.

8.4 DEVELOPMENT

It had been reported that chicken embryos did not survive EM field exposure at 1.2 GHz, at power densities below those of the safety standards (Varga, 1989). Similar experiments with chicken and pigeons are being conducted at the University of Frankfurt (P. Thalau, Group of P. Semm). Special chambers have been designed for optimal computer-controlled egg rolling, temperature, and exposure. Additionally, the melatonin level will be measured in those animals which ultimately survive exposure, and a histopathological examination will be performed on the disabled and non-surviving subjects. A comparison is planned between effects on chicken and pigeons.

In Budapest, Hungary, Thuroczy et al. (1995) showed that mortality increased among the progenies of CFLP mice exposed during gestation (19 days) for 100 min/day to microwaves (2.45 GHz, square-wave modulation at 50 Hz and GSM modulation: 217 Hz, 1/8 duty factor, SAR 0.63–4.23 W/kg). Whereas litter number was reduced by 7.4% in the sham group by day 20, it was reduced by 13.8% in the three groups combined that were exposed to CW or 50 Hz AM or 217 Hz AM microwaves (3 mW/cm² average incident power). Results were thus independent of the modulation. Postnatal increase in body and organ weight was not affected by prenatal exposure.

8.5 EEG AND SLEEP

The research group of M. Hietanen at the Institute of Occupational Health in Helsinki, Finland, is investigating the effects of exposure to RF fields on the functional state of the human brain. The EEGs of human volunteers are recorded with and without exposure.

The effect of exposure of rats to GSM modulated microwaves has been investigated by Thuroczy and co-workers (1995), at the National Research Institute for Radiobiology and Radiohygiene in Budapest, Hungary. Following 30 min exposure at $3 \, \text{mW/cm}^2$ (2.45 GHz, 2.5 W/kg SAR), the response of the central nervous system was observed by quantitative electroencephalography (EEG) and visual evoked potential (VEP) recording. No changes were observed in the early (PO, N1) or late (P2, N3) latency times of VEP. However, the delta bands of the EEG power spectrum were increased, while the alpha and beta bands amplitudes decreased in the first 5 minutes following exposure.

A group in Giessen, Germany (sponsored by Deutsche Telekom) recently observed EEG changes in volunteers exposed to the GSM signal (Reiser et al., 1995). These alterations were comparable to the pharmacological changes that are induced by small doses of diazepam (Lai et al., 1991) or by a minor analgesic activation of the endogenous opioid system.

At the department of psychiatry of the University of Mainz in Germany, the group of J. Röschke, sponsored by Deutsche Telekom, has recently published their results on the influence of GSM telephone on sleep (Mann et al., 1996). This study on human volunteers showed a hypnotic effect, a shortening of sleep onset latency, and REM suppressive effect. Moreover, the EEG signal was altered during REM sleep.

8.6   GENETICS

Under the sponsorship of Belgacom, and in collaboration with L. Martens and C. de Wagter at the University of Gent, Belgium, the group of L. Verschaeve (VITO, Mol, Belgium) is studying the cytogenetic effects of microwaves emitted by mobile communication systems (GSM). Various in vitro endpoints are checked: chromosome aberrations, sister chromatid exchanges, micronuclei and DNA fragmentation (comet assay). Ongoing studies include investigation of the dose-effect relationship and the possible synergetic effects with other agents (H_2O_2, mitomycin-C and X-rays). Biomonitoring of exposed workers is also in progress. Additionally, the VITO group (Maes et al., 1995) recently described the effects on whole blood samples placed next to a base station antenna (5 cm away, 49 V/m, 2 h exposure). Although some genetic damage was observed (chromosome aberrations), these authors concluded that microwaves emitted by a base station are not sufficient to induce genetic effects in the general population. In the same paper, a pilot study on 6 workers was also described. These workers had been exposed for a minimum of 1 h/day for at least a year to microwaves at various frequencies including 900 MHz. There was no statistically significant difference in genotoxicity parameters between exposed and control groups.

The Croatian National Research Action Programme recently sponsored investigations on subcellular and cellular mutagenic effects of RF radiations: in a follow-up study on workers exposed to various RF radiations, genotoxicity tests were performed and, in a pilot study, animals were exposed to 7.7 GHz microwaves. Experiments were also performed *in vitro* on the mutagenic effects of 27 and 100 MHz RF radiations on human lymphocytes (Croatian report to COST 244, 1994).

Deutsche Telekom are planning a study at the Neuropathological Institute of the University of Bonn (O.D. Wiestler) on genetic changes that are known to correlate with induced tumour growth in the rat brain.

S. Diener and P. Eberle, in Braunschweig, Germany, have studied the effects of 450, 900 and 1800 MHz electromagnetic fields on mutations in genes and chromosomes and on cell growth (Diener *et al.*, 1996). Human lymphocytes were exposed for 29–70 hours in TEM or GEM cells. There were no change in chromosome aberration rate, sister chromatide exchange, micronucleus number and in cell proliferation (work sponsored by the Forschungsgemeinschaft Funk FGF).

8.7   IMMUNE SYSTEM

The effects of CW or AM microwave exposures on the immune system of mice were studied in Budapest by Elekes and Thuroczy (1995). Mice were immunized with sheep red blood cells on the second day of exposure (2.45 GHz, 50 Hz modulation, SAR of 0.14 W/kg). CW microwave exposure increased the number of antibody-producing cells in the spleen of male mice. AM microwave exposure induced significant elevations of spleen weight, spleen index and antibody-producing cell counts in the spleen of male mice. It must be noted that immune parameters were not affected at all in female mice.

8.8   LITERATURE SURVEY

A recent literature review by the group of P. Semm (University of Frankfurt, Germany, sponsored by Deutsche Telekom) sorted out reports leading to new developments from fact-findings papers. The criteria applied in this selection were the comprehensive description of the experimental conditions, the independent replication of the experimental results, and the publication in peer-reviewed journals. A few results were thus considered as well documented: blood brain barrier permeability changes, neuronal responses, modifications of the growth rate of yeast cells and of chemically-induced tumors.

Two additional literature reviews concerning melatonin and cancer are in progress (J. Olcese, Hamburg, European Pineal Research Group, and C. Bartsch, Tübingen, sponsored by Deutsche Telekom).

In Poland, S. Szmigielski (1993) published a comprehensive review of results obtained *in vitro* on the carcinogenicity of microwaves associated with mobile communication.

8.9   MELATONIN

Since the hormone melatonin is linked to the occurrence of certain kinds of hormone-related cancer, a study on melatonin synthesis in rats was initiated by L. Vollrath (University of Mainz, Germany, sponsored by Deutsche Telekom). So far effects have not been found on melatonin level nor on rat behavior. However, as data were pooled for day- and night-time, a shift was not easily detectable by this method. In addition, behavioural tests were not quantitative since they depended upon observations of anatomists. All experiments were conducted at field intensities below the levels given in the safety standards.

In birds, there is preliminary evidence that the nocturnal peak of melatonin synthesis is shifted following exposure (Group of P. Semm, University of Frankfurt, sponsored by Deutsche Telekom). Special chambers have been designed for controlled light, temperature and exposure conditions. Experiments were done at low field intensities and melatonin level was measured every hour throughout day and night. However, this study warrants further investigation and replication as the control group showed an untypical melatonin time-course.

The effects of (pulsed) EM fields on melatonin synthesis in healthy human volunteers are being investigated by Röschke (Department of Psychiatry, University Clinic of Mainz, Germany, sponsored by Deutsche Telekom). Additionally, several other hormones (ACTH, Thyroxin, etc.) will be assayed under the same exposure conditions.

The effects of pulsed EM fields on saliva melatonin content in human volunteers will be investigated by L. Vollrath at the Anatomical Institute in Mainz, Germany (sponsored by Deutsche Telekom). Special mobile exposure chambers have been designed to allow for control of all experimental conditions.

8.10   NEURONAL RESPONSES

8.10.1   Nervous system

The objective of the Semm group (University of Frankfurt, sponsored by Deutsche Telekom) was to investigate the specific effects of GSM-modulated microwaves on the central nervous system of birds. Data were collected in Frankfurt by Dr. Beason (State University of New York at Geneseo), who was asked to replicate the previous Semm experiment. Thirty-eight spontaneously active units were recorded, and 20 of them showed some response to the stimulation: 13 responded with excitation and 7 responded with inhibition. The remaining 18 cells showed no discernible response. Three cells that responded to the modulated carrier were also tested using a CW signal at the same carrier frequency, and with either the same peak power or the same average power. All of these cells exhibited a response only to the amplitude-modulated carrier and not to the unmodulated one. All responses were recorded at intensities of 0.1–0.5 mW/cm^2. There are still some doubts left about the fact that the electrode itself may cause changes in cell activity by producing 'hot spots'. The results of this study and that of the previous one will soon be submitted for publication (Semm *et al.*, 1995b).

Very similar results were obtained by the same group using Russian Gun oscillators. These devices produce an EM field at 53 GHz, modulated at 16.6 Hz and with a power density of 0.1 mW/cm^2. These applicators have been frequently used for therapeutic purposes and, according to Russian scientists, with large reproducible effects. In future experiments, recordings will be performed using various insects. Additionally, the dependence of neuronal responses on endogenous opioids (Lai *et al.*, 1991) and/or on melatonin will be assessed in mice.

In collaboration with the Frankfurt University, a neuropathology group at the University Clinic of Mainz (J. Bohl, sponsored by Deutsche Telekom) will assess the animals (mice) in which single neurones responded to EM fields, for changes in different transmitters (acetylcholine, noradrenaline, endorphins and enkephalins, etc.) using immuno-histochemical and other staining methods.

A biologist at the University of Braunschweig, Germany, had used the PASP-method (Peripheral Autonomous Surface Potential) to study the possible effects of EM fields. In contrast to earlier publications where he stated otherwise, this scientist now agrees that these potentials are not changed significantly in volunteers exposed to microwaves (Damboldt *et al.*, manuscript in preparation). At the University Clinic of Freiburg, Breisgau, Germany (M. Braune, sponsored by Deutsche Telekom), the human autonomic nervous system will be investigated under microwave exposure, using different methods (reflexes, Doppler measurements, cognition tests, blood pressure).

The group of Persson in Lund, Sweden, has worked for many years on the possible effect of RF radiations on the permeability of the blood-brain barrier (BBB). At first, these studies were addressing the health problems related to exposure of patients to the EMFs produced by magnetic resonance imaging (MRI) devices. Further studies were directed to mobile communications EMFs (Salford *et al.*, 1993a, 1993b, 1994): exposure of Fischer 344 rats in a TEM transmission line chamber to 915 MHz microwaves at SARs between 0.016 and 5 W/kg showed significantly more albumin leakage than in control animals (8%), with pulse-modulated (30%) or with CW fields (40%).

In Nîmes, France (R. de Seze and L. Miro), the level of cerebral neurotransmitters was assayed on slices of brains of rats exposed *in vivo* (GSM signal, 200 μW/cm^2, far-field, 6 h/day; 5 days/wk, 4 wk). Analysis of the slices by immuno-histology is in progress.

A study is being conducted as a joint project by the Max-Plank Institutes for Neurological Research in Köln and the Swiss Federal Institute of Technology in Zürich under Motorola Sponsorship. This study investigates whether electromagnetic fields cause an acute reaction and injury to the CNS. The brain of the rats will be exposed to the varying strength levels which would be produced by mobile phones. The effects on the activation of specific genes and the histology of brain tissue will be examined at various times after exposure.

8.10.2   Neuroendocrine responses

At the University Hospital in Nîmes, (R. de Seze and L. Miro, in collaboration with French Telecom), the level of the hypothalamo-pituitary hormones (FSH, TSH, GH, LH, ACTH, PRL) was assayed before, during and after exposure of human volunteers to 'real-life' GSM telephone signals (2 h/day; 5 days/wk, 4 wk). The results are being analyzed and, so far, no influence of the signals on hormone levels has been noticed (de Seze *et al.*, 1996). Further studies will be performed, in collaboration with Motorola, to assess the possible effects of exposure on the circadian level of 5 hormones, including melatonin.

In Rome, Italy, experiments are planned at ENEA (Marino and co-workers) on the detection of effects of 900 MHz exposure on the hypothalamus and the pituitary. These involve quantitative analysis of FSH and LSH in mice using radio-immuno assays.

8.11   PROLIFERATION OF CELLS *IN VITRO*

Following their earlier ELF experiments, P. Raskmark and S. Kwee (Aalborg, Denmark) are continuing with experiments on cultured cells exposed in a TEM cell to 960 MHz fields modulated at 217 Hz. These authors have found preliminary evidence of effects under certain exposure conditions.

Effects on proliferation of cells exposed to microwaves is being studied in Bordeaux, France (J.-L. Chagnaud and B. Veyret). Various cells lines (Molt4: human lymphocytes, GH3: rat pituitary cells and C6: glioma cells) are exposed or sham-exposed for 4 hours to 900 MHz microwaves (GSM signal, 200 μW/cm^2) in thermostat-controlled containers placed in anechoic rooms. Control samples are kept in regular incubators. Proliferation is assayed 24 and 48 h after plating using a colorimetric assay. The effects of changes in exposure or temperature conditions are being investigated.

Recent results of the Brinkmann group in Braunschweig, Germany (sponsored by FGF), have shown no influence of exposure to GSM-modulated 900 and 1800 MHz fields on human leukemic cell cultures placed in GTEM cells (Fitzner *et al.*, 1996).

Among the well-documented effects of microwaves in the literature are Grundler's findings as regards to both increases and decreases in yeast cell growth rate, depending on frequency (at around 40 GHz). A follow-up study is planned together with a genetic approach by Prof. Kohli (University of Bern, Switzerland, sponsored by Deutsche Telekom and Swiss PTT). Current results have not yet confirmed Grundler's results. The same group is going to extend this investigation on yeast cells to mobile phone frequencies.

8.12   COST 244

In 1990 a new COST programme was proposed by the Faculty of Bioelectrical Engineering, University of Zagreb, Croatia. This proposal, COST 244, concerning the 'biomedical effects of electromagnetic fields' was adopted in October 1992 and has since helped foster research efforts in Europe. The main emphasis has been on mobile communications since COST 244 was placed under the umbrella of the Technical Committee for Telecommunications of the European Commission. This programme now includes 21 countries (Austria, Belgium, Bulgaria, Croatia, Czech Republic, Denmark, Finland, France, Germany, Greece, Hungary, Italy, Latvia, Netherlands, Poland, Slovakia, Slovenia, Spain, Sweden, Switzerland, United Kingdom). There are now 135 institutions, involving more than 500 scientists, working on 160 projects. The programme, which is headed by L. Koren (chairman, Zagreb) and P. Bernardi (vice chairman, Rome), is divided into three working groups:

  (i) Epidemiology and human health effects
      (chairman: A. Wennberg, Stockholm)
 (ii) Basic research
      (chairman: N. Leitgeb, Graz)
(iii) System applications and engineering
      (chairman: G. D'Inzeo, Rome).

In parallel to these three 'horizontal' working groups a 'vertical' coordination group has been set up to deal with all aspects of mobile communications research: this committee, MCCC (mobile communications coordination committee), is composed of four scientists and headed by P. Bernardi, Rome. The primary function of this committee is to coordinate the organization of workshops on mobile communications and to make sure that an executive summary is prepared after each workshop and circulated widely. The MCCC will also monitor the progress of all collaborative activities related to mobile communication research within COST 244. The following workshops have already been held: 'Mobile communications and ELF fields' (Bled, Slovenia, December 1993); 'Instrumentation and measurements in bioelectromagnetics research' (Plzen, Czech Republic, April 1994); 'Electromagnetic hypersensitivity' (Graz, Austria,

September 1994); 'Physical phantoms and numerical methods' (Rome, Italy, November 1994); 'Exposure assessment and quality control' (Athens, Greece, March 1995); 'Biological effects relevant to amplitude-modulated RF fields' (Kuopio, Finland, September 1995). A congress to conclude round I of the programme, was held in March 1996 in Nancy, France. This congress was common to both COST 244 and the EBEA (European Bioelectromagnetics Association). A second 4-year round will start in the Fall of 1996. Information about workshops, publications and other activities can be obtained from the COST 244 secretariat or through Internet (gopher carnet.hr).

8.13   CONCLUSION

In conclusion, European research on health aspects of mobile communications has already produced new data on biological effects of modulated microwave exposure. In particular, the different parts of the nervous system appear to be responding to these stimuli, and modulated waves seem to be more effective than continuous waves. It is likely that animal behavior will reflect some of these neuronal responses. However, there is still a lack of reliable biological studies of long-term exposure to RF fields. Extrapolation of the few known biological effects to human health is so far totally impossible.

It is clear that coordination on the national and international level – with the exception of COST 244 -- is almost completely absent at the present time. A report to the European commission was recently written by J. Bach Andersen (1995) describing the status and the needs of European research in this area. Further progress in European research on health aspects of mobile communications will certainly benefit from the European initiative to be launched as coordinated programme in 1997.

REFERENCES

Bach Andersen, J., Johansen, C., Frolund Pedersen, G. *et al.* (1995) On the possible health effects related to GSM and DECT transmissions. *Report of a contract with the European Commission.*

Chanaud, J.-L., Veyret, B. and Després, B. (1995) *Effects of pulsed microwaves on chemically-induced tumors.* 17th annual meeting of the Bioelectromagnetics Society, Boston, p. 28.

Damboldt, T., Dombeck, P., Droste, H. *et al.* (1994) *Research on biological effects of microwave electromagnetic fields carried out by Deutsche Telekom.* 16th annual meeting of the Bioelectromagnetics Society, Copenhagen, p. 71.

Damboldt, T., Dombeck, P., Hollmann, H. *et al.* (1995) Is a measurement of the evoked skin potential useful for detecting influences of electromagnetic fields on the human nervous system. *Bioelectromagnetics* (in press).

Damboldt, T., Dombeck, P., Hollmann, H. *et al.* (1995) *The PASP is not suitable as an indicator for influences of EM fields on the human nervous system.* 8th COST 244 Workshop on Biomedical Effects Relevant to Amplitude-Modulated RF Fields, Kuopio.

Diener, S. and Eberle, P. (1996) Cytogenic studies on the effects of mobile telephone radio waves. *Newsletter Edition Wissenschaft*, **4**, p. 15.

Elekes, E., and Thuroczy, G. (1995) Sexual differences in the immune response of mice exposed to continuous or amplitude modulated microwaves. *Bioelectromagnetics* (in press).

Fitzner, R., Langer, E., Zemann, E. *et al.* (1996) *Growth behaviour of human leukemic cells (promyelocytes) influenced by high frequency electromagnetic fields (1.8 GHz pulsed and 900 MHz pulsed) for the investigation of cancer promoting effects.* 18th annual meeting of the Bioelectromagnetics Society, Victoria.

Lai, H., Carino, M.A., Wen, Y.F. *et al.* (1991) Naltrexone pretreatment blocks micro-wave-induced changes in central cholinergic receptors. *Bioelectromagnetics*, **12**, pp. 27–33.

Maes, A., Collier, M., Slaets, D. *et al.* (1995) Cytogenetic effects of microwaves from mobile communication frequencies (GSM). *Electromagnetobiology* (in press).

Mann, K. and Röschke, J. (1996) Effects of pulsed high-frequency electromagnetic fields on human sleep. *Neuropsychobiol*, **33**, pp. 41–47.

Marino, C. (1994) *Preliminary studies on biological effects of microwaves: in vivo experimental models.* 16th annual meeting of the Bioelectromagnetics Society, Copenhagen, p. 70.

Marino, C., Antonini, F., Avella, B. *et al.* (1995) *900-MHz effects on tumoral growth in in vivo systems.* 17th annual meeting of the Bioelectromagnetics Society, Boston, pp. 191–193.

Reiser, H.-P., Dimpfel, W. and Schober, F. (1995) The influence of electromagnetic fields on human brain activity. *Eur. J. Med. Res.*, **1**, pp. 27–32.

Salford, L.G., Brun, A., Eberhardt, J.L. *et al.* (1993a) Permeability of the blood brain barrier induced by 915 MHz electromagnetic radiation; continuous wave and modulated at 8, 16, 50 and 200 Hz. *Bioelectrochem. Bioenerg.*, **30**, pp. 293–301.

Salford, L.G., Brun, A., Eberhardt, J.L. *et al.* (1993b) *Permeability of the blood brain barrier induced by 915 MHz EM radiation, [CW and Modulated] at various SARs.* 1st World Congr for Elec & Magn in Biol & Med, Blank, M. (ed), San Franscisco Press, pp. 599–602.

Salford, L.G., Brun, A., Eberhardt, J.L. *et al.* (1993c) *Experimental studies of brain tumor development during exposure to continuous and pulsed 915 MHz radio frequency radiation.* 1st World Congr for Elec & Magn in Biol & Med, Blank, M. (ed), San Franscisco Press, pp. 379–381.

Salford, L.G., Brun, A., Eberhardt, J.L. *et al.* (1993d) Experimental studies of brain tumour development during exposure to continuous and pulsed 915 MHz radiofrequency radiation. *Bioelectrochem. Bioenerg.*, **30**, pp. 313–318.

Salford, L.G., Brun, A., Eberhardt, J.L. *et al.* (1994) Permeability of the blood brain barrier induced by 915 MHz electromagnetic radiation, continuous wave and modulated at 8, 16, 50 and 200 Hz. *Micros. Res. Tech.*, **27**, pp. 535–542.

Semm, P. (1995a) *Neuronal responses to high frequency electromagnetic fields in the central nervous system of birds.* 17th annual meeting of the Bioelectromagnetics

Society, Boston, p. 38.

Semm, P., Dombek, P., Hollmann, H. *et al.* (1995b) Neuronal responses to high frequency low intensity electromagnetic fields in the avian brain. *Bioelectromagnetics* (in press).

de Seze, R., Després, B., Miro, L. *et al.* (1994) *Experimental studies on the possible effects of cellular telephones.* 16th annual meeting of the Bioelectromagnetics Society, Copenhagen, p. 71

de Seze, R., Miro, L., Privat, A. *et al.* (1995) *Effects of pulsed microwaves on rat neurotransmitters.* 17th annual meeting of the Bioelectromagnetics Society, Boston, p. 189.

de Seze, R. Albertin, V., Rouzier-Panis, R. *et al.* (1996) *Effects on human of microwaves emitted by GSM-type mobile Telephones: chronobiological rhythm of ACTH.* 18th annual meeting of the Bioelectromagnetics Society, Victoria.

Somosy, Z., Thuroczy, G., Kubasova, T. *et al.* (1991) Effects of modulated and continuous microwave irradiation on the morpology and Coll surface negative charge of 3T3 fibroblasts. *Scanning Microscopy,* **5**, pp. 1145–1155.

Szmigielski, S. (1993) *In vitro assays for carcinogenicity of microwave fields associated with mobile communication.* Proceedings of the COST 244 meeting on Mobile Communications and Extremely Low Frequency Fields, Simunic, D. (ed), Bled, Slovenia, pp. 56–63.

Thuroczy, G., Elekes, E., Kubinyi, G. *et al.* (1993) *Biological effects of modulated and CW microwave exposure: in vivo experiments in immunology and neurophysiology.* Proceedings of COST 244 Mobile communications an ELF, Simunic, D. (ed), pp. 64–74.

Thuroczy, G., Kubinyi, G., Nagy, N. *et al.* (1995) Measurements of visual evoked potentials (VEP) and brain electrical activity (EEG) after GSM-type modulated microwave exposure on rats, in *Advanced Computational Applied Electromagnetics,* Honma,T. (ed), Elsevier Press, pp. 384–395.

Varga, A. (1989) Physical Environment and Human Health. Springer.

9

Biological research in the Asia-Pacific area

Michael H. Repacholi and Masao Taki

9.1 INTRODUCTION

This chapter provides an overview of past and current research conducted in laboratories and on exposed populations in the Asia-Pacific region. Countries in this region actively conducting some research include Australia, China and Japan. Other countries in the region may be conducting research but have either published locally in journals not available outside the country and are not abstracted by journals such as Current Contents, or are unknown to the author. In many cases there are only abstracts of conferences conducted in English, but no paper is subsequently published in an English journal. Only a small amount of research is being conducted in any country in the Asia-Pacific region. Thus this review concentrates on a few key results.

The World Health Organization noted in its most recent review (WHO, 1993), that, while current studies do not indicate that exposure to radio frequency fields (RF) at environment levels cause any known detriment to health, there should be more studies to make better health risk assessment from exposure to low-level RF fields. Because of the rapid technological advances made in telecommunications, particularly in the use of devices such as mobile telephones, and the potential for exposure of large segments of the population to RF fields, increasing pressure has been placed on governments and standards setting organizations to ensure that exposure to low-level RF fields has no associated adverse health consequences.

Mobile Communications Safety
Edited by N. Kuster, Q. Balzano and J.C. Lin
Published in 1997 by Chapman & Hall, London. ISBN 0 412 75000 7.

9.2   PAST RESEARCH

9.2.1   Australia

The only research into biological effects of RF fields conducted in Australia has been by Dr. Andrew Wood and co-workers at the Swinburn University of Technology in Melbourne, Victoria, and by Dr. Michael Repacholi and co-workers at Royal Adelaide Hospital in South Australia. The latter research is being completed and will be described under current research.

Wood *et al.* (1993) have recently published a replication study on calcium efflux from toad heart. This was a replication of the Schwartz *et al.* (1990) study that reported an increase in the movement of calcium ions in frog hearts exposed to RF (240 MHz) fields amplitude modulated at 16 Hz. Other studies have reported enhanced movement of calcium ions from avian brain hemispheres (Adey, 1981; Blackman *et al.*, 1982) and Graham *et al.* (1991) had produced evidence to suggest that ELF fields modify the heart rate in human volunteers. It was important that any effect of exposure to RF fields modulated at ELF frequencies on calcium be confirmed since these ions play a critical role in the normal physiology of the heart and are responsible for excitation-contraction coupling.

Groups of 80 toad hearts were sham exposed or exposed in a TEM cell to 240 MHz fields modulated at 16 Hz, and SARs of 0.15, 0.18, 0.24, 0.30 or 0.36 mW/kg for 30 minutes. Determinations were made on the movement of calcium ions using ^{45}Ca as a tracer. Wood and co-workers concluded that there was no effect at the SARs and frequency chosen.

9.2.2   China

A large number of abstracts have been published for meetings of the Bioelectromagnetics Society. It is apparent that there are a few research groups investigating biological effects of RF fields, but rarely are the papers published in an English language journal. This makes assessment and follow-up of the results virtually impossible. Some of the investigators and institutions involved in RF research include: Liu and co-workers at the Shanxi Medical College and Beijing Air Force Hospital; Jixi and colleagues at the Northwest Telecommunications Engineering Institute, and Zhong-gi and co-workers at the Military Medical College in Xi'an; Chiang and co-workers at the Zhejiang Medical University in Hangzhou; and Zhao and co-workers at the Beijing Medical University.

In a paper providing the highlights of mm-wave bioeffects research conducted in China since 1984, Li (1988a) reported that the combined effect of haematoporphyrin derivative (HPD) and 39 GHz field-exposure (3 mW/cm^2, 30 min/day for 3 days) on MGC-80-3 gastric carcinoma cells significantly reduced cell viability compared to HPD alone. Exposure of mice to 36 GHz fields (1 mW/cm^2, 15 or 30 min/day for 5 days) was reported to increase white-blood-cell count in peripheral blood, increase glycogen deposits in the liver, and increase pyknosis of the nuclei of megakaryocytes in the bone marrow. When the left middle fingers of 90 healthy human volunteers was exposed to 38 GHz fields at 6 mW/cm^2 for 15 minutes, extension and dilation of capillary loops, blood velocity changes and white blood cell rolling were observed.

A few researchers have been involved in determining if microwaves can cause any changes in cells in culture. Li *et al.* (1988a) report that in human hepatoma (SMMC-7721) cell cultures in monolayer, when exposed to 36 GHz fields at 1 or 2 mW/cm^2 for 15 or 30 min, morphological changes were observed using scanning electron microscopy. When the cells were exposed *in vitro* to 1, 2 or 3 mW/cm^2 for 30 min/day for 1, 2 or 3 days there was a significant reduction in cloning ability without any increase in cell mortality, and there was a loss of DNA content. The same research team reports that pre-exposure of female mice to 304 rads of ^{60}Co γ-rays and 24 hours later, exposure to 36 GHz fields at 3 mW/cm^2 for 30 min/day for 5 days, increased the formation of the colony forming unit – culture (CFU-C) in the bone marrow compared to the sham exposed group (Li *et al.*, 1988b). This result had previously been found *in vitro*. Given the shallow depth that 36 GHz fields penetrate tissue, it seems likely that the results given above would have a bearing on human exposure only if heating was the predominant mechanism.

In a pilot study to determine if 2450 MHz fields could promote colon cancer in mice initiated with dimethylhydrazine, Shao *et al.* (1988) reported that exposure to 10 mW/cm^2 (but not when tested at lower power densities of 1 or 5 mW/cm^2) significantly accelerated its development in infant mice, suggesting a thermal mechanism. In this study Balb/c mice were exposed to CW fields in an anechoic chamber in the E-orientation at 0, 1, 5 or 10 mW/cm^2, 3 h daily, 6 sessions per week for over 5 months. A tumour promoter (TPA) was administered once per week for 10 weeks, commencing on the third week. In their peer reviewed publication on this study, the authors reported that they could not find any promoting effect of microwave exposure (Wu *et al.*, 1994). The SARs in the study were estimated to be 10–12 W/kg.

Liu and co-workers report various effects from *in vivo* studies on rodents exposed to 2450 MHz fields (Liu *et al.*, 1988; Liu *et al.*, 1991a; 1991b). Groups of 20 mice were exposed to CW fields at 20, 30 or 40 mW/cm^2 (no exposure duration given) and compared to a sham exposed group and a positive control group exposed to 150 R of ionizing radiation. The authors report that the microwave exposure increased the micronucleus rate in polychromatic erythrocytes of femur bone marrow. Microwave fields also caused deformation of sperm shape, affected germs cells more than somatic cells. There was a higher sperm teratogeny rate with a tendency of increasing effect with exposure to higher power density. In a later report, Liu and Liu (1991a) conducted the same experiment using pulsed 250 MHz fields (pulsing regime not given) and again reported changes in sperm morphology in the groups exposed to 30 and $40\,mW/cm^2$ but not at $20\,mW/cm^2$. It seems apparent that microwave heating played a major role in producing these results since the exposure levels were relatively high.

In order to determine causes of lessened libido and menstruation disorders in workers exposed to microwaves, Liu and Liu (1991b) studied the effects of 2450 MHz fields on American SD rats. Groups of 10 (half males and half females) were exposed to 20, 40, 60, or $80\,mW/cm^2$ for 30 min/day for 3 days. Statistically significant differences in blood testosterone and progesterone levels were found in the highest exposed group. Increases in menstruation disorders appeared. In a similar type of study, Liu et al. (1992a) reported increases in the blood enzyme, lipid peroxidase (LPO), with increasing dose up to $60\,mW/cm^2$. Exposures to $80\,mW/cm^2$ caused the LPO to decrease with increasing dose. The authors note that LPO is an important factor for gene mutation, chromosomal aberration and carcinogenesis and that if the LPO is high this could increase the risk of carcinogenesis. Nie and Yuan (1992) reported an increase in the activity of choline acetyltransferase (ChAT) in the brains of mice exposed to 2450 MHz microwaves at $10\,mW/cm^2$ (SAR 11.4 W/kg). Follow-up studies were underway; however, it should be noted that the relatively high levels of exposure would result in elevated temperatures in the mice.

Investigations of the effects of microwave exposure on humans have been reported from Chinese laboratories. In a study of 121 workers exposed to RF fields (<30 MHz), the high exposure group ($\geq 100\,V/m$), Liu et al. (1992b) reported changes in their electrocardiograms (ECG) compared to the low exposure group (<100 V/m). The investigators suggested that 100 V/m should be the limit in an RF standard. When the level of the -SH groups was observed in the serum of these high frequency workers, no difference was observed (Liu et al., 1992).

9.2.3   Japan

Biological effects research commenced in Japan in the seventies. The primary objective was to determine if there were health effects resulting from RF exposure that required limits to be established in standards (Amemiya, 1994). Some of the earlier research included a study indicating reduced growth in the thymus following long-term, low-level irradiation of mice to 400 MHz and 900 MHz fields (Saito et al., 1988).

In studies on anaesthetized frog, Miura and Okada (1991) provided evidence for a mechanism of vasodilation that may depend on an increase in Ca^{2+} outflow through the plasma membrane of the smooth muscle and/or an increase in Ca^{2+} influx through the sarcoplasmic reticulum. The exposure parameters leading to the effect on vasodilation were: 10 MHz fields, 1 V (peak to peak), 7.3 mG, 2.19 V/cm field applied 50% of the time at 10 kHz burst rates. Since Ca^{2+} ATPase is activated by cyclic GMP which is produced by the enzymic action of guanylate cyclase, the authors suggested the electromagnetic field exposure may activate guanylate cyclase to facilitate cyclic GMP production.

Exposure of fertile eggs to 428 MHz fields at 5.5 mW/cm^2 for more than 20 days caused increased embryo death and teratogenic effects as well as delayed hatching (Saito et al., 1991). The authors claimed that the effects were not due to any temperature increase. In a follow-up study, Saito et al. (1993) produced further evidence that chronic exposure to 428 MHz fields at 4 mW/cm^2 prolonged the incubation period. In a companion study on mice, Saito et al. (1993) reported that 1 mW/cm^2 exposure altered the immune system by suppressing cell-mediated immune competence by local delayed hypersensitivity.

In Japan there is increasing concern among the population about possible adverse health effects from exposure to chronic levels of RF fields from wireless communications. Those involved with the technology recognise the necessity for evaluation of safety through further research. Thus the level of funding for fundamental research is now increasing to answer questions related to the health problems expressed by the population. A major animal study to provide further information on the safety of cellular telephones commenced towards the end of 1995.

9.3   CURRENT RESEARCH

9.3.1   Australia

The rapid rise in the use of mobile telephones in Australia, and the associated concerns voiced by the general public about possible health effects from exposure to the RF fields from the telephone antennas and base stations, has resulted in an increased amount of research to address these concerns. This has included both *in vitro* and *in vivo* studies.

RF fields have been reported in a few animal studies to increase incidence of various cancers. However, these studies are insufficient to establish that RF field exposure can lead to an increased incidence of cancer. As a result, Repacholi and co-workers have been conducting a study to determine whether long-term exposure of female, Eμ-pim1 transgenic mice (van Lohuizen et al., 1989) to 900 MHz fields can increase the normal incidence of cancer in these cancer-prone mice, especially lymphoma. 100 mice were sham exposed and 100 mice were exposed to far-field RF fields (900 MHz, pulse width 0.6 ms, pps 217 Hz) for 1 h/day for 18 months. The SARs for individual mice ranged from 0.01–4.2 W/kg. However since the mice were seen to remain for large periods in closely packed groups of 5, it was determined that mice under these conditions would be exposed to SARs in the range 0.13–1.4 W/kg. Specific pathogen free transgenic mice aged 4–6 weeks were purchased from GenPharm, California and allowed to rest for 10 days prior to entry into the study. The facility was maintained as specific pathogen free (SPF) throughout the study. An SPF facility is free of pathogens likely to affect the test animals. The statistical analyses and review of results are now in progress and the results will be published within the next six months. It is anticipated that follow-up studies may be necessary.

Adey (1988) has suggested that, modulated RF fields may affect membranes by altering the binding characteristics of calcium on surface glycoprotein strands. This RF signal is then transmitted to the cell interior by an unidentified mechanism, presumably via transmembrane proteins, where some change in specific enzyme kinetics could affect processes connected with cell maturation and division. Whilst not acting as a primary carcinogen, it has been argued that electromagnetic fields may act as promoters or co-promoters of carcinogenesis. Thymic lymphocytes (T-cells) are important components of the immune system and respond by directly recognizing antigens. The presence of an antigen triggers enlargement of the cell, mitosis and increased DNA and RNA synthesis. Concanavalin A is thought to mimic this process. Further, cells undergoing mutations or malignant transformation may alter their antigenic properties and evoke a T-cell response. If electromagnetic fields are affecting this process then normal immune response would be impaired. With this rationale Wood and co-workers are currently investigating the effects of pulsed 915 MHz fields on thymic lymphocyte function. In particular they are studying the effect of GSM mobile telephone radiation waveforms on critical components of the immune system, as measured by cellular and membrane calcium levels in thymic lymphocytes. They are also investigating whether RF pulse modulated fields affect the normal responses of these cells to mitogens such as Concanavalin A, co-carcinogens such as phorbol myristate acetate, or antibodies such as anti-CD3 monoclonal antibodies. In addition studies will be conducted to determine whether these RF fields can affect the ability of certain substances to alter cell membrane architecture (e.g. Concanavalin A).

9.3.2   China

Several papers published in China over the past few years have reported biological effects from exposure to chronic low intensity millimetre (mm) wave electromagnetic fields. Effects such as pyknosis of nuclei of megakaryocytes, increased glycogen deposition in the liver and decreases in spermatocytes and spermatogonia in testes, have been reported. Since the mm wave (36 GHz) have a very low depth of penetration, it is possible that the effects observed may be due to an indirect mechanism. Studies by Li and co-workers are continuing to confirm these results and to determine the mechanism involved. In a study on mice exposed to 36 GHz fields, $4\,mW/cm^2$, 30 min/day for 5 days, histological examination of a number of tissues continued to show the above effects, even with the use of a local skin block (Novocaine) applied prior to exposure. Measurement of the rectal temperature indicated no significant elevation. The authors suggest that these results indicate that the mechanism of action to produce the above effects must be non-thermal. Further studies are continuing.

Studies by another group of investigators in China also suggest the existence of non-thermal effects from RF exposure. Jingsui and Huai (1993) studied 450 microwave operators (no frequency of exposure given) who had worked for more than one year in this occupation and for periods of at least 3 months at any one time. These workers were compared with 249 controls. Following observations of a large number of health-related parameters from groups of workers exposed to different ranges of exposure, the authors concluded that adverse health effects appeared when exposures exceeded $1\,mW/cm^2$. The same authors also studied mice exposed to 2.45–3.0 GHz fields (CW 0.5–20 mW/cm^2, or pulsed 0.25–10 mW/cm^2) for 7 days and found a number of differences in health-related parameters. These results also suggested that non-thermal mechanisms were evident. Further studies are continuing to identify these mechanisms.

9.3.3   Japan

One of the most important lines of research currently being undertaken in Japan is a replication of the studies of Kues, Monahan and co-workers (Kues et al., 1985; 1988; Monahan et al., 1988). Kues and co-workers have reported that corneal abnormalities and vascular leakage from the iris were observed in adult cynomolgus monkeys after a 4-hour exposure to 2.45 GHz fields (CW, 20–30 mW/cm^2, local SAR 5.3–7.8 W/kg, or pulsed, 10 s pulses, 100 pps, 1 or 10 mW/cm^2, local SAR 0.26, 2.6 W/kg) for 4 h/day on 3 consecutive days. RF exposures were conducted alone and in combination with ophthalmic drugs (pilocarpine and timolol maleate) applied topically prior to exposure. Corneal damage and iris vascular leakage were observed following exposure to fields as low as $1\,mW/cm^2$. It was suggested that serum proteins from the iris could escape into the anterior chamber and contribute to the production of endothelial lesions.

Kamimura et al. (1994) have been attempting to replicate these studies using the same experimental procedure except that the monkeys were not anaesthetized as they were in the Kues et al. studies. CW power densities exceeding the 30 mW/cm^2 value reported by Kues et al. were used but the same corneal endothelial abnormalities could not be observed. Further there were no abnormalities observed in the vitreous humour, crystalline lens or retina. Further studies are anticipated to extend these results to pulsed fields.

Having previously reported that low dose RF exposure to pregnant mice causes an extension of the gestation period and reduction in the thymus weight of their progeny, Saito and colleagues are continuing their research on mouse embryos (Saito et al., 1994). In their most recent study they report the production of malformations in the foetuses of pregnant rats exposed to 2.45 GHz fields from a 30 W microwave therapy apparatus. The SAR, calculated to be

34.7 W/kg, caused increases in foetal death and a variety of foetal malformations. Further studies are being conducted to determine the mechanisms for the teratogenesis caused by high levels of RF exposure. Obviously exposures at a level of 34.7 W/kg will cause a significant temperature rise.

9.4   CONCLUDING REMARKS

While the amount of research activity in the Asia Pacific Area is low, there is useeful research being conducted. Research in China however is very difficult to evaluate because of the lack of full details on which to make any assessment. It is particularly important that there is replication of results by independent laboratories. This is being carried out and will continue. The results challenging the calcium efflux studies and the reports of enhanced damage to eyes when RF exposure is conducted in combination with ophthalmic drugs is of great interest. New challenges are being presented by the Chinese research that should be investigated further.

REFERENCES

Adey, W.R. (1981) Tissue interactions in nonionizing electromagnetic fields. *Physiol Rev*, **61**, 435–514.

Adey, W.R. (1988) Cell membranes: the electromagnetic environment and cancer promotion. *Neurochem Res*, **13**, 671.

Amemiya, Y. (1994) Research on biological and electromagnetic environments in RF and microwave regions in Japan. *IEICE Trans Communications*, **E77-B**(6), 693–698.

Blackman, C.F., Benane, S.G., Kinney, L.S. *et al.* (1982) Effects of ELF fields on calcium-ion efflux from brain tissue *in vitro*. *Radiation Res.*, **92**, 510–520.

Chiang, H. (1988) *Study of microwave conception and its genetic effects*. Abstract: Bioelectromagnetic Society Meeting, Stamford, Connecticut, June 19–23.

Graham, C., Cohen, H.D., Cook, M.R. *et al.* (1991) *Human cardiac activity in 60 Hz magnetic fields*. Abstract: Bioelectromagnetic Society Meeting, Salt Lake City, Utah, June 23–27.

Jingsui, P. and Huai, C. (1993) *The non-thermal effects caused by microwave radiation*. Abstract: Bioelectromagnetic Society Meeting, Los Angeles, California, June 13–17.

Kamimura, Y., Sato, K., Saiga, T. *et al.* (1994) Effect of 2.45 GHz microwave irradiation on monkey eyes. *IEICE Trans Communications*, **E77-B**(6), 762–765.

Kues, H.A., Hist, L.W., Lusty, G.A. *et al.* (1985) Effects of 2.45 GHz microwaves on primate corneal endothelium. *Bioelectromagnetics*, **6**, 177–188.

Kues, H.A. and Macleod, D.S. (1988) *Histological evaluation of microwave-induced vascular leakage in the iris*. Abstract: Bioelectromagnetic Society Meeting, Stamford, Connecticut, June 19–23.

Li, J.X., Nui, Z-Q., Zhu, P-J. *et al.* (1988a) *Bioeffects of 36.11 GHz mm-wave field on human hepatoma monolayer cultures.* Abstract: Bioelectromagnetic Society Meeting, Stamford, Connecticut, June 19–23.

Li, J.X., Nui, Z-Q., Zhu, P-J. *et al.* 1988b) *Effects of mm-wave irradiation on murine bone marrow cells damaged by gamma-rays.* Abstract: Bioelectromagnetic Society Meeting, Stamford, Connecticut, June 19–23.

Li, J. (1988) *MM-wave bioeffect investigation in China.* Abstract: Bioelectromagnetic Society Meeting, Stamford, Connecticut, June 19–23.

Liu, W-K. and Liu, F. (1991a) *Effects of microwave radiation on sperm morphology in mice.* Abstract: Bioelectromagnetic Society Meeting, Salt Lake City, Utah, June 23–27.

Liu, W-K. and Liu, F. (1991b) *Effects of microwave on sex hormone in rats.* Abstract: Bioelectromagnetic Society Meeting, Salt Lake City, Utah, June 23–27.

Liu, W-K., Tan, X-T., and Sun, T-Y. (1992a) *Effects of microwave radiation on LPO in rats.* Abstract: 1st World Congress for Electricity and Magnetism in Biology and Medicine, Lake Buena Vista, Florida, June 14–19.

Liu, W-K., Tan, X-T., and Sun, T-Y. (1992b) *Influence of non-ionizing radiation on lymphocyte micronucleus rate in the human blood.* Abstract: 1st World Congress for Electricity and Magnetism in Biology and Medicine, Lake Buena Vista, Florida, June 14–19.

Liu, W-K. and Syu, Z-L. (1992) *The observation of -SH in the serum of high frequency workers.* Abstract: 1st World Congress for Electricity and Magnetism in Biology and Medicine, Lake Buena Vista, Florida, June 14–19.

Liu, W-K., Qi, Y. *et al.* (1988) *Effects of microwave radiation on incidence of micronucleus of polychromatic erythrocytes (PCE) in the bone marrow and the shape of sperm in mice.* Abstract: Bioelectromagnetic Society Meeting, Stamford, Connecticut, June 19–23.

van Lohuizen, M., Verbeek, S., Krimpenfort, P. *et al.* (1989) Predisposition to lymphomagenesis in pim-1 transgenic mice: Cooperation with c-myc and N-myc in murine leukaemia virus-induced tumors. *Cell,* **56,** 673–682.

Miura, M. and Okada, J. (1991) Non-thermal vasodilation by radiofrequency burst-type electromagnetic field radiation in the frog. *J Physiol.,* **435,** 257–273.

Monahan, J.C., Kues, H.A., Macleod, D.S. *et al.* (1988) *Lowering of microwave exposure threshold for induction of primate ocular effects by timolol maleate.* Abstract: Bioelectromagnetic Society Meeting, Stamford, Connecticut, June 19–23.

Nie, S. and Yuan, G. (1992) *Effects of microwave irradiation on ACH level and CHAT activity in the mouse brain.* Abstract: The First World Congress for Electricity and Magnetism in Biology and Medicine, Lake Buena Vista, Florida, June 14–19.

Saito, K., Goto, N., Ogasawara, T. *et al.* (1988) Growth patterns in several organs in mice under low-level exposure. *J Growth,* **27**(1), 1–6.

Saito, K., Suzuki, K. and Motoyoshi, S. (1991) Lethal and teratogenic effects of long-term low-intensity radio frequency radiation at 428 MHz on developing chick embryo. *Teratology,* **43,** 609–614.

Saito, K. and Suzuki, K. (1994) Teratogenic effect of microwave irradiation on mouse embryos. *J Robotics Mechatronics,* **6,** 51–54.

Saito, K., Tsuchida, Y., Yamada, K. *et al.* (1993) Effect of exposure to RF of fertilized chicken eggs and pregnant mice on hatchability, organ-weight, and locally delayed hypersensitivity. *J Robotics Mechatronics*, **5**, 244–247.

Schwartz, J.-L., House, D.E. and Mealing, G.A.R. (1990) Exposure of frog hearts to CW or amplitude-modulated VLF fields: Selective efflux of calcium ions at 16 Hz. *Bioelectromagnetics*, **11**, 349–358.

Shao, B.J., Chiang, H., Yao, G.D. *et al.* (1988) *Promoted development of dimethylhydrazine (DMH)-induced colon cancer in mice exposed to 2450 MHz microwave radiation.* Abstract: Bioelectromagnetic Society Meeting, Stamford, Connecticut, June 19–23.

WHO (1993) Electromagnetic Fields 300 MHz – 300 GHz. *Environmental Health Criteria No. 137, World Health Organisation, Geneva.*

Wood, A.W., Lubinas, V., Joyner, K. *et al.* (1993) Calcium efflux from toad heart: A replication study, in *Electricity and Magnetism in Biology and Medicine*, Martin Blank (ed), San Francisco Press, San Francisco, pp. 482–484.

Wu, R.Y., Chiang, H., Shao, B.J. *et al.* (1994) Effects of 2.45 GHz microwave radiation and phorbol ester 12-O-tetradecaniylphorbol-13-acetate on dimethylhydrazine-induced colon cancer in mice. *Bioelectromagnetics*, **15**, 531–538.

Zhao, Z., Zhang, S. *et al.* (1988) *The effects of RFR (<30 MHz) on human beings and a primary study of its protective guide.* Abstract: Bioelectromagnetic Society Meeting, Stamford, Connecticut, June 19–23.

PART IV

Regulation Activities and Standards

10

Regulatory activities in the U.S.A.

Robert F. Cleveland, Jr.

10.1 INTRODUCTION

There is a worldwide explosion in telecommunications and particularly in the use of mobile communications. New technologies are being developed that will facilitate even greater growth in future telecommunications systems. For example, the last decade has witnessed a tremendous increase in the cellular telephone industry, and in the coming years new personal communications systems will become widespread. In the United States the Federal Communications Commission (FCC) is responsible for regulating telecommunications by all users except the U.S. Federal Government itself. The National Telecommunications and Information Administration (NTIA) of the U.S. Department of Commerce regulates use of the radiofrequency (RF) spectrum by the U.S. Government.

These two government agencies allocate frequency bands in the RF spectrum for a variety of civilian and military uses in the United States including broadcasting, mobile telecommunications, satellite communications systems, military and civilian radar and many others. Mobile telecommunications systems that are regulated by the FCC include the cellular radio service, the new personal communications radio service (PCS), and land-mobile radio systems used by businesses and for fire, police and other safety-related communications. Many of these services are included under the category of Commercial Mobile Radio Service or CMRS.

In recent years concern has been expressed over the safety of mobile communications systems, particularly handheld and other devices that are designed to be used in close proximity to users. Various U.S. Government agencies have been involved in investigating this issue to try and determine whether there is a public health risk. In addition to the FCC and the NTIA, the U.S. Food and Drug Administration (FDA), the U.S. Environmental Protection Agency

The views expressed are those of the author and do not necessarily reflect the views of the U.S. Federal Communications Commission.

Mobile Communications Safety
Edited by N. Kuster, Q. Balzano and J.C. Lin
Published in 1997 by Chapman & Hall, London. ISBN 0 412 75000 7.

(EPA), the National Institute for Occupational Safety and Health (NIOSH) and the Occupational Safety and Health Administration (OSHA) of the U.S. Department of Labor all have undertaken various actions to respond to these concerns.

This presentation will attempt to outline the regulatory activities taking place in the United States at the present time (1996) with respect to the issue of potential RF health risks of mobile communications technology. Primary emphasis will be on the activities of the FCC where the author is a scientist in the Office of Engineering and Technology. It is important to keep in mind, that the continuing acquisition of new data and information in this area will undoubtedly have a significant effect on the future direction and the nature of the activities of the FCC and other agencies. Therefore, regulatory activities are subject to change, and by the time this chapter is published some of the information given here may be subject to modification.

10.2   FCC RESPONSIBILITIES AND ACTIVITIES

Because the FCC is responsible for licensing and otherwise regulating most of the mobile communications systems in the United States, it has been directly involved in attempting to ensure that the use of mobile communications technology is safe and does not create a public health risk. The National Environmental Policy Act of 1969 (NEPA) requires all agencies of the U.S. Government to evaluate whether actions they take may have a significant effect on 'the quality of the human environment' (NEPA, 42 United States Code, Section 4321, et seq.). Since 1985, the FCC has designated the potential for human exposure to RF energy from FCC-regulated transmitters as one of several potential environmental consequences requiring evaluation (FCC, 1985a). There are many sources of RF exposure in the environment that are regulated by the FCC, including radio and television broadcast stations, satellite and microwave communications systems, land-mobile and cellular radio systems, amateur radio, radar and industrial RF sources (Cleveland, 1994).

There is no official U.S. Government standard for exposure to RF radiation. Therefore, in its original order adopting rules for RF environmental analysis, the FCC specified that it would use the 1982 guidelines of the American National Standards Institute (ANSI C95.1-1982) as an indicator of whether a transmitting facility or operation might cause a 'significant' environmental effect (ANSI, 1982). It became FCC policy to ensure that all regulated transmitters not expose members of the public and workers to levels of RF energy in excess of the 1982 ANSI protection guides (U.S. Code of Federal Regulations, 47 CFR1.1307,b). Subsequently, the FCC has amended its rules to clearly indicate which transmitters would be of greatest concern. In that regard, routine environmental evaluation has been required of relatively higher-powered transmitting stations, such as commercial radio and television broadcast stations and satellite uplink installations.

Other lower-powered transmitters, such as those used for land-mobile, cellular radio and microwave radio communications have been categorically excluded from undergoing routine environmental evaluation for RF exposure (FCC, 1987). This latter policy was based on the lack of evidence that such transmitters could exceed the 1982 ANSI guidelines due to their lower operating powers, their intermittent operation or their relative inaccessibility to members of the public or to workers.

Due to public interest and concern over the issue of RF exposure and to assist FCC licensees in complying with ANSI guidelines, the FCC has developed various publications and factsheets to assist consumers and telecommunications systems users. The FCC's OET Bulletin 56, 'Questions and Answers about Biological Effects and Potential Hazards of Radiofrequency Radiation,' has proved to be very popular and thousands of copies have been distributed (FCC, 1989). A new edition is expected to be published in 1996. Another popular publication that is more technical in nature is OET Bulletin 65, 'Evaluating Compliance with FCC-specified Guidelines for Human Exposure to Radiofrequency Radiation' (FCC, 1985b). This publication will also be updated in the next one to two years when new guidelines are adopted by the FCC (see discussion below). Factsheets dealing with specific transmitter types are planned for future FCC distribution to the public. The first of these deals with exposure to cellular radio towers and telephones, the subject of many inquiries received by the FCC.

10.3   NEW ANSI/IEEE GUIDELINES

In 1991, the Institute of Electrical and Electronics Engineers (IEEE) approved new RF exposure guidelines, developed by the IEEE's Standards Coordinating Committee 28 (SCC-28) on Non-Ionizing Radiation Hazards, as a replacement for the 1982 ANSI protection guides. In the following year ANSI officially adopted the IEEE standard as a revision of its 1982 guidelines (ANSI/IEEE, 1992). Since then, this standard has increasingly been used either outright or has been the basis for standard-setting activities worldwide.

There are several significant differences between the 1982 and 1992 ANSI guidelines. It is beyond the scope of this paper to explain these differences in detail, but some areas in which significant changes have been made are important with respect to regulatory proposals. For example, the 1992 standard recommends two tiers for exposure rather than one as in the old protection guides. The 1992 guidelines also incorporate modified exposure recommendations for both the lower frequencies below the VHF bands and for the higher microwave frequencies, and new recommendations for induced and contact currents created by RF fields are also included for frequencies between 3 kHz and 100 MHz.

Significantly for mobile communications technology, the 1992 guidelines contain a major revision with respect to evaluation of handheld low-powered devices such as cellular telephones. For low-powered devices, such as cellular telephones, that are used in 'uncontrolled' environments, ANSI/IEEE C95.1-1992 recommends a specific absorption rate (SAR) as averaged over one gram of tissue of 1.6 W/kg. This value is five times less than the 8 W/kg limit recommended by the 1982 ANSI standard, although for 'controlled' environments the low-power device exposure limit remains at 8 W/kg.

The ANSI/IEEE guidelines permit exclusions in controlled environments if the radiated power of a device is 7 W or less at frequencies between 100 kHz and 450 MHz. At frequencies between 450 and 1500 MHz, the radiated power must be limited to $7 \times (450/f)$ W, where f is the frequency in MHz. In uncontrolled environments, the values are one-fifth of those in controlled environments. Consumer devices, such as handheld telephones, would generally be assumed to fall under the uncontrolled category.

In the U. S., operating frequencies for mobile cellular radio transmitters operate in the 824–849 MHz frequency band. Most handheld units now in use operate with maximum power levels of about 600 mW. Vehicle-mounted units and 'bag' phones usually operated with maximum power levels of 3 W. The ANSI/IEEE radiated power exclusion clause permits about 740–765 mW, with a 2.5 cm separation distance maintained between the body and the 'radiating structure' for cellular telephone frequencies. Regardless of whether a device meets the radiated power exclusion criteria or not, compliance can be demonstrated by evaluating exposure in terms of SAR. Table 10.1 shows the limits recommended for low power devices by ANSI/IEEE C95.1-1992.

10.4 FCC PROPOSAL TO ADOPT NEW GUIDELINES

It is incumbent upon the FCC to use guidelines for evaluating environmental RF exposure that are both up to date and scientifically supportable. Therefore, in 1993, the FCC recognized the need to update its environmental rules, and the Commission issued a proposal to adopt the 1992 ANSI/IEEE guidelines, including the new limitations on low-power devices (FCC, 1993).

The FCC's Notice of Proposed Rule Making (NPRM) to adopt new RF guidelines was adopted by the Commission in March, 1993, and released in April, 1993. Originally, four months were allowed for the filing of comments and replies to those comments in the rule-making docket. However, several requests for extensions of time to submit comments and reply comments were filed with the FCC, and four extensions of time were granted. The final deadline for comments and reply comments was April 25, 1994. By that time well

Table 10.1 ANSI/IEEE C95.1-1992 Limits for low power devices.

	Controlled environment	Uncontrolled environment
Average SAR (100 kHz – 6 GHz)	<0.4 W/kg (whole-body) $\leq$0.8 W/kg (partial-body)	<0.08 W/kg (whole-body) $\leq$1.6 W/kg (partial-body)
Radiated power* (100 kHz – 450 MHz)	7.0	1.4
Radiated power* (450–1500 MHz)	$7 \times (450/f^{\dagger})$	$1.4 \times (450/f^{\dagger})$

* Radiated power exclusions do not apply if 'radiating structure' is maintained within 2.5 cm of the body.
† f = frequency in MHz.

over 100 organizations, agencies and individuals had filed comments, and there were over 2500 pages of comments in the docket record. Even more filings have been submitted since the deadline and accepted as 'late filed' or 'ex parte' submissions. The final total of submissions, both comments and reply comments, is around 150.

Comments were filed by many major corporations, by industry trade associations, by other associations, by federal, state and local government agencies, and by individuals. Many of the comments filed contained important data and the results of studies relevant to issues discussed in the NPRM. Table 10.2 shows some of the major organizations filing comments.

Several important issues were discussed in the FCC's NPRM, and comments were requested concerning them. These issues included: (1) interpretation and implementation of the ANSI/IEEE definitions of 'controlled' and 'uncontrolled' environments; (2) evaluation of compliance with limitations on induced and contact currents; (3) whether alternative exposure guidelines should be considered instead of the ANSI/IEEE standard; (4) interpretation and implementation of ANSI/IEEE limits on low-power devices such as handheld cellular telephones; and (5) whether certain lower powered or inaccessible transmitters could be excluded from routine evaluation for compliance.

As expected, a variety of opinions were expressed on these and other important issues. For the most part most respondents filing comments supported at least some aspects of the ANSI/IEEE guidelines. However, some U.S. Government agencies with responsibilities for health and safety, such as the U.S. Environmental Protection Agency (EPA), expressed opposition in their comments to the FCC's adopting the ANSI/IEEE standard without modification.

Both the EPA and the FDA (commenting through its Center for Devices and Radiological Health) were critical of certain features of the ANSI/IEEE standard including its rationale. For example, according to the FDA, the standard, 'lacks a full explanation of its basis'. Furthermore, the FDA continued, 'it is unclear what types of biological effects and exposure conditions are addressed by the standard. For example, very few research studies of long-term, low-level exposures of animals were included in the scientific rationale for the standard, despite the existence of animal studies that suggest an association between chronic low level exposures and acceleration of cancer development.' The FDA noted that the relevance of questions dealing with chronic exposures 'can only increase as the use of portable and handheld devices grows'. The FDA recommended that, 'new research be closely monitored for possible evidence that the levels in the 1992 guideline may need to be reduced' (Gill, 1993).

In its comments to the FCC, the EPA was also critical of aspects of the ANSI/IEEE standard including its basis. Because of its concerns, the EPA urged the FCC to adopt the Maximum Permissible Exposure (MPE) limits recommended in 1986 by the National Council on Radiation Protection and Measurements (NCRP, 1986) instead of the ANSI/IEEE MPE's (Oge, 1993). The NCRP and ANSI/IEEE MPE's are similar in many respects, but the EPA was concerned that insufficient protection was afforded in the microwave region of the spectrum by the ANSI/IEEE guidelines. The EPA also disagreed with the use of 'controlled' and 'uncontrolled' environments in determining which set of MPEs would apply. The NCRP guidelines define exposure populations in terms of 'occupational' and 'public'.

The EPA noted that the ANSI/IEEE 1992 standard contains significant revisions that the EPA considers to be improvements over the 1982 ANSI guidelines. Specifically, the EPA recognized the development of a two-level exposure standard and the extension of the lower frequency range down to 3 kHz as improvements over the previous standard. The EPA also supported FCC consideration of adopting the 1992 ANSI/IEEE limits for induced and contact currents and the criteria for low-power devices in addition to adoption of the NCRP MPE values. With respect to the recommendations for localized SAR, the NCRP recommends one-fifth of 8 W/kg (1.6 W/kg) for public exposure, the same as ANSI/IEEE.

Importantly for the mobile communications industry, there appears to be general support for the ANSI/IEEE recommended limits for handheld, low-powered devices. Most parties commenting in the FCC proceeding did not take issue with the SAR limits recommended for controlled and uncontrolled environments. Although critical of other aspects of the ANSI/IEEE guidelines, the EPA and the FDA did not express opposition to the ANSI/IEEE recommendation of 1.6 W/kg for the localized SAR limit for a low-powered device in an uncontrolled environment.

The FDA did express opposition to the FCC's use of the ANSI/IEEE exclusion clause for low-powered devices that is based on radiated power alone (ANSI/IEEE, 1992, Section 4.2). The FDA based its concern on recent experimental data indicating that some handheld cellular telephones may cause

Table 10.2 Some major organizations filing comments in FCC rule-making proceeding.

Companies	Alcatel SEL, AT&T, Bell South Corp., CBS, Inc., COMSAT Corp., Ericsson Corp., GTE Service Corp., Matsushita Corp., Motorola, Inc., Northern Telecom, Inc., PacTel Corp., Raytheon Co., Southwestern Bell, Sprint Cellular Co. and TRW, Inc.
Associations	American Radio Relay League, Inc., Cellular Telecommunications Industry Assoc., Electromagnetic Energy Assoc., Electronic Industries Assoc., Institute of Electrical & Electronic Engineers, Land Mobile Communications Council, National Assoc. of Broadcasters, National Assoc. of Business & Educational Radio, Personal Communications Industry Assoc., Society of Broadcast Engineers and Telecommunications Industry Assoc.
U. S. Federal Agencies	Department of Defense, Environmental Protection Agency, Federal Aviation Administration, Food and Drug Administration, National Institute for Occupational Safety & Health and Occupational Safety& Health Administration

localized exposures in excess of 1.6 W/kg even though the radiated power limit is met. In a later letter to the FCC, the FDA argued that low-power, handheld devices should be certified by their manufacturer as not exceeding the local SAR limit, as determined under 'realistic worst-case conditions' (Jacobson, 1994).

In addition to the question of whether radiated power can be used to establish compliance, there are other related issues with respect to evaluation of handheld devices that need to be addressed. These issues include the following:

1. If radiated power is to be used as a basis for evaluating devices, can the exclusions be extended to frequencies greater that the 1.5 GHz upper limit now in the ANSI/IEEE standard? For example, can transmitters operating in the new Personal Communications Service in the U. S. (1850–1990 MHz) be subject to radiated power exclusions? A letter from the IEEE to the FCC indicates that this may be acceptable (Adair, 1993).

2. Some confusion has been expressed over use of the terms 'radiated power' and 'radiating structure' used in the ANSI/IEEE low-power guidelines. Apparently, the IEEE SCC-28 Committee may issue future interpretations of

these and other terms. In the meantime, it has been suggested that the IEEE Standard definition of radiated power be used in this context.*

3. Is it possible to develop radiated power exclusion criteria when the separation distance is less than the 2.5 cm distance specified in the ANSI/IEEE standard? As more data on SAR due to handheld devices is acquired, it may be possible to establish a lower threshold for radiated power at which compliance is assured.

4. What methods are acceptable for determining compliance? Should there be standardized procedures when using implantable probes for measuring localized SAR in head models? Are computer-based techniques, such as finite difference time domain (FDTD) analysis, accurate and do they agree with measured values?

5. Are there factors other than SAR, such as modulation, that are important in determining if exposures are safe? Most future handheld devices will use digital modulation schemes, such as TDMA or CDMA.

Over time there will undoubtedly be answers to most of these questions, particularly as more research is carried out with these systems. In the short term there is a need for a threshold to use in evaluating handheld devices such as cellular telephones, even if it proves to be an interim threshold. It appears that the 1.6 W/kg limit will serve as that threshold for the present.

Concerning certification of compliance for handheld devices with SAR limits, several parties commenting to the FCC urged that uniform measurement and evaluation standards be established. For example, Ericsson Corporation recommended that the FCC 'designate an appropriate ANSI-accredited standards generating body to promulgate standardized measurement and calibration procedures for facilities, phantom (human) models, and antenna models ...'. It is worth noting that in the U. S. the Electromagnetic Energy Association (EEA) and Wireless Technology Research, L.L.C. (WTR) are initiating activities aimed at some sort of standardization of procedures (EEA, 1994; FDA, 1995). The EEA is proposing to become Secretariat of an 'ANSI-Accredited Committee for Product Performance Relative to the Safe Use of Electromagnetic Energy'. WTR plans to sponsor risk management research with a focus on certification and design of wireless devices to ensure compliance with safety standards.

With respect to mobile communications transmitters that are not handheld, it appears that most of these would comply with ANSI/IEEE specified limits. For example, data submitted to the FCC by several organizations indicates that vehicular-mounted antennas would generally comply if mounted at the center of the vehicle's roof. Also, most base-station installations should comply with indicated limits for 'uncontrolled' environments. There does seem to be a

---

* The IEEE Standard Dictionary of Electrical and Electronics Terms (5th Ed.) defines radiated power output as: 'The average power output available at the antenna terminals, less the losses of the antenna, for any combination of signals transmitted when averaged over the longest repetitive modulation cycle.'

possibility, however, that in 'controlled' situations higher powered land-mobile transmitters, such as those used in paging operations, could result in areas near antennas where access would have to be restricted. The FCC and the EPA conducted a joint study of a few such installations in 1994 and found this to be the case at some sites visited (Cleveland *et al.*, 1995).

FCC staff have reviewed the comments received in response to the NPRM, and a decision on most of the issues raised is expected in mid-1996. The new U.S Telecommunications Act of 1996 requires the FCC to adopt updated RF guidelines by early August of 1996 (Telecommunications Act of 1996, Pub. L. No. 104–104, 110 Stat. 56, 1996). This action should have been taken by the time of publication of this book.

10.5   INTERIM FCC DECISIONS

Since issuance of its NPRM the FCC has approved the development of a new Personal Communications Service (PCS) to be operated in U.S. in the frequency band of 1850 to 1990 MHz. This new service will be highly competitive with existing cellular radio services in the U.S., and projections have been made that it will greatly expand wireless mobile communications in the coming years. Millions of consumers are expected to purchase handheld PCS units.

When considering approval of PCS the FCC realized that it needed to provide PCS manufacturers and service providers with guidance on RF exposure in the near term. Therefore, to avoid delaying introduction of PCS, the FCC decided to adopt the ANSI/IEEE guidelines on an interim basis for PCS transmitters (FCC, 1994a). In adopting this policy for PCS the FCC noted that the final decision on guidelines would be made in the pending rule-making proceeding and that any guidelines subsequently adopted would supersede the PCS decision. However, because of the similarities between the various limits that have been proposed, and due to the widespread acceptance of the 1.6 W/kg local SAR value, it was thought to be unlikely that future guidelines would be significantly at variance with the ANSI/IEEE recommendations for PCS frequencies.

In the FCC's adoption of PCS an interim decision was also made with regard to the use of the ANSI/IEEE radiated power exclusion clause for low-power devices. If the ANSI/IEEE equation for radiated power exclusion in uncontrolled environments is extrapolated out to the PCS frequencies an indicated level for acceptable radiated power would be about 315 to 340 milliwatts (mW). The FCC felt that some sort of exclusion value should be acceptable, since there must be some lower limit on the radiated power necessary to exceed the 1.6 W/kg value. A threshold was needed to avoid a situation where, for example, expensive SAR evaluation would be required of devices that might use only a few mW of power.

However, because of the FDA's expressed concern over use of the ANSI/IEEE power exclusions the FCC believed that it would be premature to adopt these exclusions without modification and extend them to PCS frequencies. Therefore, the FCC decided to adopt, also on an interim basis, a more conservative power exclusion value of 100 mW for PCS devices pending the acquisition of additional exposure data and a final decision in the rule-making proceeding. As is required by the ANSI/IEEE standard, this exclusion only applies when the 'radiating structure' is maintained at least 2.5 cm from the body. If the exclusion criteria are not met then evaluation of SAR is necessary.

Interim decisions to use ANSI/IEEE limits have also been made in the FCC's proceeding so establishing the new Mobile Satellite Service (FCC, 1994b). Consumer devices to be used in the MSS service will be required to comply with ANSI/IEEE 1992 specifications for 'uncontrolled' environments pending adoption of official guidelines. As with PCS, the final guidelines adopted will take precedence, but the FCC recognized the need for immediate guidance for this new service.

10.6   ACTIVITIES OF OTHER U. S. FEDERAL AGENCIES

10.6.1   The FDA

The Radiation Control for Health and Safety Act of 1968 authorized the U. S. Food and Drug Administration (FDA) to develop performance standards for the emission of radiation from electronic products. This applies for both ionizing and non-ionizing forms of radiation. With regard to RF and microwave emissions the Center for Devices and Radiological Health (CDRH) of the FDA has established a performance standard for microwave ovens that limits the amount of microwave radiation an oven can leak (FDA, 1981). RF performance standards for other devices have not been established.

With regard to the issue of handheld cellular telephones, in 1993, the FDA released a 'talk paper' entitled 'Update on Cellular Phones' (FDA, 1993). In this paper the FDA discussed the issue of potential health hazards due to RF emissions from handheld cellular telephones. The FDA noted that the telephones of concern are those that operate in close proximity to the user's head and not telephones operated with vehicle-mounted antennas or other antennas that are not near a person's body.

According to the FDA paper, there is insufficient evidence to determine whether or not there may be a hazard due to exposure from handheld telephones. The FDA stated that it is working closely with other federal government agencies and with industry to assure that further research is undertaken to provide the answers to these questions of public health.

Under U. S. law, the FDA does not review the safety of cellular telephones prior to marketing, as it does with new drugs or medical devices. However, the

FDA noted that it could impose restrictions on cellular telephones 'if health problems were to arise after marketing'. Such restrictions could take the form of a performance standard on cellular telephone manufacturers that might require that the telephones emit RF energy below a certain level. The talk paper emphasized that existing scientific data do not justify the FDA's taking such action. However, it was stated that the agency is 'exploring' with manufacturers ways to minimize exposure, such as changes in antenna design and better instructions for users.

The FDA has also conducted consultations and meetings with representatives of other federal agencies and with industry representatives concerning potential health effects of cellular telephones. For example, joint workshops have been held in conjunction with the industry-sponsored Scientific Advisory Group on Wireless Technology (now renamed Wireless Technology Research, L.L.C., 'WTR') to discuss areas of mutual concern and progress in the WTRs program for investigating public health issues related to wireless communications. Other federal agencies have also participated in these workshops and an inter-agency group has been established to monitor progress in this area. Cooperation has also been encouraged by the U.S. General Accounting Office (GAO). In a report issued in 1994, the GAO recommended that the FDA, FCC and the WTR work together 'to maximize the usefulness, independence, and objectivity of the [WTR's] planned research initiative' (GAO, 1994).

10.6.2   The EPA

In 1986, the U.S. Environmental Protection Agency (EPA) published a proposal soliciting comment on various alternative approaches to limit exposure of the general public to RF radiation (EPA, 1986). However, a decision was eventually made to indefinitely delay EPA activities related to developing exposure guidelines (Guimond, 1988).

In 1993, the EPA held a two-day workshop on the potential biological effects and hazards of RF radiation (EPA, 1993). Among the goals of this conference was the need to address the question of whether the EPA should take action(s) to control human exposure to RF energy. In 1994, as a result of recommendations generated by this conference and also because of a 1992 recommendation of the EPA's Science Advisory Board (Loehr et al., 1992), the EPA's Office of Radiation and Indoor Air decided to proceed with the development of voluntary guidelines for exposure of the general public to RF radiation. This latest EPA effort was intended to elaborate further on EPA's comments, filed with the FCC, that were critical of certain aspects of the ANSI/IEEE C95.1-1992 protection guidelines. As discussed previously, in its comments to the FCC, the EPA had recommended that, with respect to field intensity levels, the FCC use the RF protection MPE values of the NCRP instead of the ANSI/IEEE MPEs. The new guidelines had been expected to be similar to the NCRP MPE values for exposure of the general public. Guidance on acceptable levels of exposure due to handheld devices was also expected to be part of the EPA recommendations.

In the short term, the EPA had planned to issue independent guidelines for public exposure based on known health effects. The EPA's program was to have consisted of two phases. The first would constitute the development of the 'interim' exposure guidelines based on known effects, and the second would be a longer-term effort to consider modulated RF signals and 'non-thermal' effects. This latter effort was being conducted in cooperation with the NCRP.

An inter-agency working group was formed to provide input to the EPA. The working group consists of representatives of six U. S. federal agencies: the EPA, FCC, FDA, NIOSH, NTIA and OSHA. The EPA guidelines would have been voluntary and would not have constituted a mandatory standard. In light of the lack of any official standard from the U. S. Government there was widespread speculation that EPA guidelines would become a *de facto* standard in the U. S. for the general public. However, late in 1995, the EPA changed its policy and will not be developing guidelines in the near future.

10.6.3   Other Federal Agencies

There are other agencies of the U. S. Government that have an interest in the RF hazards issue. NTIA in the U. S. Department of Commerce was mentioned earlier. As part of NTIAs spectrum of management functions it is concerned that RF sources meet appropriate safety guidelines, and the NTIA is part of the EPA's inter-agency RF working group.

Also, a part of the working group are NIOSH and OSHA. Both of these agencies are concerned with issues related to occupational safety and health and RF exposures in the workplace. NIOSH, an agency of the Center for Disease Control and part of the U. S. Department of Health and Human Services, primarily conducts research and investigations into workplace hazards. Several years ago NIOSH was developing occupational exposure recommendations for RF radiation but those recommendations have never been issued. NIOSH does conduct research and investigations into RF hazards, and NIOSH staff have published numerous papers and reports dealing with RF effects and dosimetry. However, mobile-communications facilities have not been the subject of many of these studies.

OSHA, part of the U. S. Department of Labor, does not have official RF safety guidelines. However, OSHA staff do sometimes cite transmitting facilities, such as broadcast stations, for failure to comply with other OSHA regulations related to access to areas where high RF fields exist. In that regard, OSHA personnel usually use the ANSI/IEEE 1992 guidelines as criteria for safe exposure levels (Curtis, 1995).

Several other federal agencies have an interest in RF safety due to their routine use of RF transmitters. For example, the U.S. Departments of the Army, Air Force and Navy all operate thousands of transmitters of all types including radar, satellite uplinks and mobile-communications systems. These agencies, under the Department of Defense, have programs in place to protect personnel from exposure in excess of established guidelines such as ANSI/IEEE C95.1-1992.

10.7   CONCLUSION

To briefly summarize, the primary regulatory activity currently underway in the U.S. with respect to mobile telecommunications systems is being undertaken by the FCC to adopt new RF exposure guidelines that will help ensure that handheld devices and other FCC-regulated transmitters do not constitute a potential health hazard. Other agencies such as the FDA and the EPA are not presently proposing regulations but have undertaken various efforts in the past to, respectively, investigate the potential for health hazards from handheld telephones and, in the case of the EPA, to develop exposure guidelines for the public. Decisions and final actions related to the FCC proceeding are expected soon.

Note: During the time since this article was originally written, the FCC has adopted, on August 1, 1996, new guidelines for evaluating RF exposure. The FCC's guidelines were based both on NCRP and ANSI/IEEE recommendations for power density, field strength and specific absorption rate. The FCC declined to adopt the ANSI/IEEE exclusion clause based on radiated power alone and also declined to adopt limits on induced and contact currents at this time. A summary of the FCC's action and the complete text of the Report and Order are available at the following address on the World Wide Web: http://www.fcc.gov/oet/.

Questions concerning the FCC's actions in this area can also be sent via e-mail to: rfsafety@fcc.gov. The citation in the U.S Federal Register for a summary of the Order is: 61 Federal Register 41006 (August 7, 1996).

REFERENCES

Adair, E.R., Co-Chairman, IEEE SCC-28 (1993) Letter to Thomas P. Stanley, FCC, October 11, 1993.

ANSI (1982) American National Standard Safety Levels with Respect to Human Exposure to Radio Frequency Electromagnetic Fields, 300 kHz to 100 GHz. ANSI C95.1-1982.

ANSI/IEEE (1992) Safety Levels with Respect to Human Exposure to Radio Frequency Electromagnetic Fields, 3 kHz to 300 GHz. IEEE C95.1-1991, adopted by the American National Standards Institute as ANSI/IEEE C95.1-1992. Copies can be obtained in the United States from the IEEE, telephone [1] 800 678 4333.

Cleveland, R.F., Jr. (1994) Radiofrequency Radiation in the Environment: Sources, Exposure Standards and Related Issues, in *Biological Effects of Electric and Magnetic Fields*, Vol. 1 (Sources and Mechanisms), (eds D.O. Carpenter and S. Ayrapetyan), Academic Press, Inc., San Diego, CA.

Cleveland, R.F., Jr., Sylvar, D.M., Ulcek, J.L. *et al.* (1995) *Measurement of Radiofrequency Fields and Potential Exposure from Land-mobile Paging and Cellular Radio Base Station Antennas.* Presented at 17th Annual Meeting, Bioelectromagnetics Society, Boston, Massacusetts, U. S. A.

Curtis, R.A., OSHA Health Response Team (1995) *Elements of a Comprehensive RF Protection Program: Role of RF Measurements.* Presentation at National Association of Broadcasters Broadcast Engineering Conference, Las Vegas, Nevada, April 12, 1995.

EEA (1994) Information from briefing given by the Electromagnetic Energy Association for the FCC and the FDA, December 12, 1994.

EPA (1986) *Federal Radiation Protection Guidance – Proposed Alternatives for Controlling Public Exposure to Radiofrequency Radiation.* Notice of Proposed Recommendations, 51 Federal Register, No. 146, pp. 27 318–27 339, July 30, 1986.

EPA (1993) Radiofrequency Radiation Conference, sponsored by EPA, Office of Air and Radiation and Office of Research and Development. April 26–27, 1993, Bethesda, Maryland, U. S. A.

FCC (1985a) Report and Order, Gen. Docket 79–144, 100 FCC 2d 543, and Memorandum Opinion and Order, 50 Federal Register 38653.

FCC (1985b) Evaluating Compliance with FCC-specified Guidelines for Human Exposure to Radiofrequency Radiation. *OET Bulletin*, **65**.

FCC (1987) Second Report and Order, Gen. Docket 79–144, 2 FCC Record 2064 and 2 FCC Record 2526.

FCC (1989) Questions and Answers about Biological Effects and Potential Hazards of Radiofrequency Radiation. *OET Bulletin*, **56**, Third Edition.

FCC (1993) *Guidelines for Evaluating the Environmental Effects of Radiofrequency Radiation.* Notice of Proposed Rule Making, ET Docket 93–62, 8 FCC Record 2849, 58 Federal Register 19393.

FCC (1994a) Memorandum Opinion and Order, Gen. Docket 90–314. Amendment of the Commission's Rules to Establish New Personal Communications Services at para. 245–249, 9 FCC Record 4957. See also, 47 Code of Federal Regulations (CFR) Section 24.52.

FCC (1994b) Report and Order, ET Docket 92–28. Amendment of Section 2.106 of the Commission's Rules to Allocate the 1610–1626.5 MHz and 2483.5–2500 MHz Bands for Use by the Mobile-Satellite Service, Including Non-geostationary Satellites at para. 32–35, 9 FCC Record 536.

FDA (1981) Performance Standards for Microwave and Radio Frequency Emitting Products, 21 CFR 1030.10 (as amended).

FDA (1993) Update on Cellular Phones. FDA Talk Paper, February 4, 1993. U. S. Food and Drug Administration, U. S. Department of Health and Human Services,

Public Health Service, Rockville, Maryland 20857, U. S. A.

FDA (1995) Workshop sponsored by FDA and Wireless Technology Research, L.L.C., March 17, 1995.

GAO (1994) Status of Research on the Safety of Cellular Telephones, November 1994.

Gill, L.J., Office of Science and Technology, CDRH, FDA (1993) Comments to the FCC in ET Docket 93–62, November 10, 1993.

Guimond, R., EPA, (1988) Letter to Robert Cleveland, FCC, September 28, 1988.

Jacobson, E., CDRH, FDA (1994) Letter to Richard Smith, FCC, December 12, 1994.

Loehr, R.C. *et al.*, EPA Science Advisory Board (1992) Letter to William K. Reilly, Administrator, EPA, January 29, 1992.

NCRP (1986) Biological Effects and Exposure Criteria for Radiofrequency Electromagnetic Fields. *NCRP Report, 86, Bethesda, Maryland 20814, U. S. A.*

Oge, M.T., Office of Radiation and Indoor Air, EPA (1993) Comments to the FCC in ET Docket 93–62, November 9, 1993.

11

Regulatory environment in the EU

Mark Bogers

11.1 INTRODUCTION

This chapter describes the regulatory environment regarding safety within the European Union (EU). After the assession of three States of EFTA (Austria, Finland and Sweden), the EU consists now of 15 European Member States.

The rapid development of the cellular market in the EU, and in particular the GSM service, has raised concerns about the non-ionizing radiation levels to which the public and workers are increasingly exposed. These concerns deal with:

- the large scale deployment of infrastructural equipment, and the consequent high density of GSM base stations in metropolitan areas;

- handheld equipment, use of which results in near-field exposure of the brain;

- the potential effect of electromagnetic radiation on medical implants (cardiac pacemakers and hearing aids).

In the absence of regulatory regimes and well-documented scientific data, the installation of GSM base stations has been challenged in some Member States, slowing down the deployment of the GSM service.

Concerns regarding the health effects of handheld equipment were reinforced when reports on the use of GSM handheld equipment showed thermal effects (i.e. increase of temperature) in the brain and the eyes due to the near-field exposure of the skull. These effects are now well documented and it is generally felt, that 2 W GSM equipment do not invoke hazardous thermal effects. In addition there were reports on other biological effects, commonly referred to as non-thermal effects. There is however no evidence that these biological effects are hazardous.

Mobile Communications Safety
Edited by N. Kuster, Q. Balzano and J.C. Lin
Published in 1997 by Chapman & Hall, London. ISBN 0 412 75000 7.

11.2 STATUS QUO

11.2.1 Regulatory responsibilities

The Treaties of Rome and Maastricht lay down the regulatory competences of the European institutions. With regard to the safety of mobile communications, the Articles of the Treaty of relevance can be divided into two groups:

- Articles aiming at achieving the free movement of goods;
- Articles dealing with workers' protection and health issues.

Articles dealing with the free movement of goods

Articles 30 to 36 forbid Member States to create undue barriers to trade.

Conflicting safety regulations for mobile equipment could in principle create a barrier to trade and would thus contravene these articles. The European Commission, the executive arm of the European Union, may propose Directives to harmonize national legislation, to be adopted by the Council of Ministers and the European Parliament in accordance with Article 100a. This article, introduced after the revision of the Treaty of Rome in 1985, is the legal basis for regulation of the European Commission of safety levels for mobile equipment.

It should be emphasized that Member States cannot demand stricter safety levels than those set by the European authorities under Article 100a Directives. Such demands would breach Article 30.

Article 30

> Quantitative restrictions on imports and all measures having equivalent effect shall, without prejudice to the following provisions, be prohibited between Member States.

Article 100a

1. By way of derogation from Article 100 and are where otherwise provided in this Treaty, the following provisions shall apply for the achievement of the objectives set out in Article 8a. The Council shall, acting by a qualified majority on a proposal from the Commission in cooperation with the European Parliament and after consulting the Economic and Social Committee, adopt the measures for the approximation of the provisions laid down by law, regulation or administrative action in Member States which have as their object the establishment and functioning of the internal market.
2. Paragraph 1 shall not apply to fiscal provision, to those relating to the free movement of persons nor to those relating to the rights and interests of employed persons.
3. The Commission, in its proposals envisaged in paragraph 1 concerning health, safety, environmental protection and consumer protection, will take as a base a high level of protection.

4. If, after the adoption of a harmonization measure by the Council acting by a qualified majority, a Member States deems it necessary to apply national provisions on grounds of major needs referred to in Article 36, or relating to protection of the environment or the working environment, it shall notify the Commission of these provisions. The Commission shall confirm the provisions involved after having verified that they are not a means of arbitrary discrimination or a disguised restriction on trade between Member States. By way of derogation from the procedure laid down in Article 169 and 170, the Commission or any Member State may bring the matter directly before the Court of Justice if it considers that another Member State is making improper use of the powers provided for in this Article.

5. The harmonization measures referred to above shall, in appropriate cases, include a safeguard clause authorizing the Member States to take or one or more of the non-economic reasons referred to in Article 36, provisional measures subject to a Community control procedure.

Articles dealing with health issues

Although competence for workers' protection is with the Member States, the European Commission has the right to propose Directives setting minimum levels of protection, to be adopted by the Council of Ministers and the European Parliament in accordance with Article 118a.

In contrast with measures issued under Article 100a, Member States have the right to adopt stricter safety regulations than those set under such Directives. This reflects the differing views within the EU on workers' protection (also on ecology).

Article 118a

1. Member States shall pay particular attention to encouraging improvements, especially in the working environment, as regards the health and safety of workers, and shall set as their objective the harmonization of conditions in this area, while maintaining the improvement made.

2. In order to help achieve the objective laid sown in the first paragraph, the Council, acting by a qualified majority on a proposal from the Commission, in cooperating with the European Parliament and after consulting the Economic and Social Committee, shall adopt, by means of directives, minimum requirements for gradual implementation, having regard to the conditions and technical rules obtaining in each of the Member States. Such directives shall avoid imposing administrative, financial and legal constraints in a way which would hold back the creation and development of small and medium-sized undertakings.

3. The provisions adopted pursuant to this Article shall not prevent any Member State from maintaining or introducing more stringent measures for the protection of working conditions compatible with this Treaty.

Table 11.1 Summarization of the situation in the Member States and the EFTA as regards regulations (legally binding documents) and standards (non-binding recommendations on safety levels).

EU	Law/ Directive	Regulation	Standard	Other document	Recommendation
CEC	EWG 93 42 EWG 90 385 CEC Draft				
Austria			ON ÖVE MW		
Belgium	RGPT			Belgacom Santé	
Denmark				DMW	IRPA
Finland	FIN A	FIN D FIN O FIN C		FIN SG 9.2 FIN SG 9.3	
France					IRPA
Germany	GBIG	BPT1 BPT2	VDE VDE MW VDE CP VDE Draft VDE M Draft	BFE BFS	
Greece					IRPA
Ireland					IRPA
Italy	IT 1–5		IT Draft		IRPA
Luxemburg					VDE Draft
Netherlands		NL		NEL 3	ACGIH
Portugal					
Spain					
Sweden		AFS AFS MW		SWE	
United Kingdom			NRPB BSI MW		

EFTA					
Iceland					
Liechtenstein	LIL				
Norway	NOR 1			NOR 2	

11.2.2   The current legislative situation

The current legislative situation within the EU (and in the EFTA countries) is rather fragmented. A study performed by CENELEC* – 'Biological effects on the human body (including implants) of electromagnetic radiation in the frequency range of 80 MHz – 6 GHz' – for the European Commission analyzed 131 documents (laws, regulations, standards and recommendations) worldwide. It reported that safety laws and regulations specifically dealing with the effects of electromagnetic radiation emitted by mobile communications equipment are in place in six of the Member states.

It further found that most of these laws and regulations did not specify limits but gave general requirements. An interesting finding was the fact that most laws and regulations only dealt with exposure levels and did not set safety levels for equipment. One has to recognize however, that within the GSM community handheld equipment with a peak transmission power greater than or equal to 2 W (average power greater than or equal than 0.25 W) are considered safe and that no minimum distance between the antenna and the head needs to be maintained.

Although specific legislation setting safety levels for such equipment is almost non-existent, it has been recognized by the European Commission that existing Directives dealing with safety issues can, in conjunction with harmonized European standards, properly address such issues. Regarding safety levels for mobile communications equipment, the following Directives, based upon Article 100a, apply:

1. The Low Voltage Directive (73/23/EEC, 19 February 1973, as modified by Council Directive 93/68/EEC of 22 July 1993 on the harmonization of the laws of the Member States relating to electrical equipment designed for use within certain voltage limits).

2. The Terminal Type Approval Directive (91/263/EEC, notably Article 4a and 4b).

In order to set immunity levels for implants, the following Directives apply:

3. The EMC Directive (89/336/EEC, notably Article 4b).

4. The Medical Implants Directive (90/385/EEC).

---

* CENELEC (Comite Electrotechnique), CEN (Comite Europeenne de Normalisation) and ETSI (the European Telecommunications Standards Institute) are the three recognised European Standards Organizations. CENELEC is competent in the area of electrotechnical equipment.

Table 11.2 Emission limits and minimum distances for low power transmitters in some of the Member States.

	Frequency range	Power	Min. Distance Work	Public
ON (Austria)	$f < 1\,\text{GHz}$	7 W	None	
		7–25 W	$r = 6 \times P^{0.5}\,\text{cm}^*$	
AFS (Sweden)	$f < 1\,\text{GHz}$	7 W	None	
NL (Netherlands)	$f < 1\,\text{GHz}$	7 W	None	
IRPA (WHO)	No restriction	7 W	None	
IRPA T (WHO)	450 MHz	0.5 W	None	
Draft	analogous	1 W	2 cm	4 cm
		5 W	10 cm	20 cm
		20 W	20 cm	40 cm
&	900 MHz	0.5 W	None	
	analogous	1 W	2.5 cm	5 cm
		5 W	12.5 cm	25 cm
		20 W	25 cm	50 cm
BFS (Germany)	900 MHz	2 W	None	
	GSM	4 W	1.5 cm	3 cm
	digital	8 W	2.5 cm	5 cm
		20 W	4 cm	8 cm
	1800 MHz	1 W	None	
	(DCS 1800)	2 W	1.5 cm	3 cm
	digital	8 W	3.5 cm	7 cm
		20 W	6 cm	12 cm
BFE (Germany)	No restriction	10 W	None	
BUWAL 1	900 MHz[†]	2–3 W	None	
(Switzerland)	934 MHz	2–3 W	None	

* r = minimum distance
  P = radiated power
[†] Natel C

11.3 CURRENT AND FUTURE ACTIONS

The European Commission has launched several actions to harmonize the legal situation within the Union. Both on the product side and the human exposure side, standards and measures are under development.

11.3.1   Product standards

Although in the context of this book it is not useful to elaborate the legal concepts of the 'New Approach', in detail, it is important to note that for industrial products, standards play an important role in the assessment of whether or not products may be placed on the market. Compliance with harmonized European standards, mandated under 'New Approach' Directives gives presumption of conformity with the 'essential requirements' that products have to meet.

Within this context, the European Commission has mandated the European Standards Organizations under Directives 73/23/EEC and 91/263/EEC,

- to draft harmonized standards covering the thermal effects of mobile communications equipment (mandate M/032);

- to draft a work programme identifying standards covering the non-thermal effects of mobile communications equipment (mandate M/033).

Work under these mandates is progressing. It is expected, that the standard developed under M/032 will not, in contrast with currently existing product standards or recommendations, define radiated power (i.e. emission) levels for handheld equipment. The main element of the standard will be a method for measuring exposure levels in a 'phantom' head. Such a procedure would take better account of the fact that the exposure of the head is not only related to the radiated power but also to the design of the product itself (notably the antenna). Although mandate M/033 called for a work programme on standards for non-thermal effects it is likely that CENELEC will conclude that, in the absence of scientific evidence that such effects are hazardous, no such safety standards are required.

Regarding the immunity of medical implants, Directives 90/385/EEC requires products to be sufficiently immune to electromagnetic waves. In defining product safety standards, immunity standards for medical implants must be taken into account.

'New Approach' The new approach to technical harmonization and standards – Council Resolution 85/C/136/01.

Mandate M/032 European standard specifying safety limits for thermal aspects of human exposure to EMR emitted by mobile communication equipment.

Mandate M/033 Preparation of a work programme for standardization and related activities in the field of safety requirements on non-thermal aspects for mobile communication equipment exposing humans to EMR.

11.3.2   Worker protection

In order to set minimum safety levels within the Union to protect workers from the effects of physical agents, a draft Directive has been proposed by the European Commission under Article 118a.

This Directive covers not only the effects of electromagnetic radiation but also other physical phenomena (e.g. noise levels). It follows the view that exposure levels are to be set by the public authorities rather than relying on standards. Unlike the measures in the previous sections, therefore, exposure levels are written into the Directive. The draft Directive distinguishes between three areas of exposure:

1. inherently safe, unlimited duration of exposure;
2. limited duration of exposure;
3. inherently unsafe exposure.

11.4   RELATION BETWEEN EXPOSURE LEVELS AND PRODUCT STANDARDS

Safety levels for products should be based on, and should develop in accordance with, the state of the technology. There is therefore no direct link between safety levels for products and exposure levels set, for instance, under the draft 'physical agents' Directive. If products are not inherently safe (i.e. don't exceed legally enforced exposure levels under all usage conditions), measures limiting their use or enforcing special conditions of use are required. This may be best illustrated by taking an extreme example: The safety of cars, which are notoriously more dangerous then mobile phones. A car must adhere to safety standards which have evolved over the last century (a car of 1905 would now be considered inherently unsafe). Unlike mobile phones, there are and never will be inherently safe cars. The use of a car has therefore been regulated so as to protect the user to such an extent that driving has become one of the most regulated activities of humankind. Traffic rules and driving hour limitations are, however, to a great extent independent of safety requirements for cars.

By the same token authorities may set a limit duration for use or enforce a certain distance between humans and the antenna for handheld equipment, which is legally placed on the market.

11.5   CONCLUDING COMMENTS

Taking into account the development in the mobile communications market, resulting in an increased exposure of humans to electromagnetic waves, it is necessary that there be in place a proper and harmonized regulatory system within the EU, consisting of the two elements outlined in the previous sections. With the development of equipment safety standards and a possible adoption of the 'physical agents' directive such a system would become reality.

APPENDIX 11.A LEGISLATION AND GUIDELINES

EU	Law/Directive
CEC	EWG 93 42 – June 1993: Richtlinie 93/42/EWG über Medizinprodukte, Amtsblatt der Europäischen Gemeinschaften, Nr. L169/1. EWG 90 385 – June 1990: Richtlinie 90/385/EWG zur Angleichung der Rechtsvorschriften der Mitgliedstaaten über aktive implantierbare medizinische Geräte, Amtsblatt der Europäischen Gemeinschaften, Nr. L189/17. CEC Draft – Commission of the European Communities/Draft (Febr. 1993) Vorschlag für eine Richtlinie des Rates über Mindestvorschriften zum Schutz von Sicherheit und Gesundheit der Arbeitnehmer vor der Gefährdung durch physikalische Einwirkungen. CEC, Amtsblatt der Europäischen Gemeinschaften, Nr. C 77.
Belgium	RGPT – Belgium Law: Protection des travailleurs (R.G.P.T., Titre II, Art. 103), Decision du medecin du travail sur état de santé des travailleurs (R.G.P.T., Titre II, Art. 123), Travailleurs soumis aux examens médicaux (R.G.P.T., Titre II, Art. 124), Belgium.
Finland	FIN A – March 1991: Radiation act (592/91). Helsinki, Finland.
Germany	GBIG – Bundesimmissionsschutzgesetz, § 7 und § 23. Germany.
Italy	IT 1 – Regional Law of Abruzzo (June 1991) Normativa regionale in materia di prevenzione dell'inquinamento da onde elettromagnetiche. Legge Regionale, N. 20. Bollettino Ufficiale della Regione Abruzzo, Anno XXII, N. 19, p 528–531. Direzione Redazione e Amministraz. Presso la Presidenza della Giunta Regionale, Via Cristoforo Colombo, 212, 00147 Roma, Italia. IT 2 – Regional Law of Piemonte (Oct. 1986) Criteria tecnici per la tutela sanitaria ed ambientale relativa agli impianti di teleradiocomunicatione. Giunta Regionale del Piemonte. Commissariato del Governo nella Regione Piemonte, Commissione di Controllo, Torino, Italy. IT 3 – Regional Law of Lazio (July 1993) Piano regionale degli insediamenti radiotelevisivi. Legge Regionale 11, N. 56. Bollettino Ufficiale della Regione Lazio, Anno XX, N. 27, p 1–44. Direzione Redazione e Amministraz. Presso la Presidenza della Giunta Regionale, Via Cristoforo Colombo, 212, 00147 Roma, Italia. IT 4 – Regional Law of Veneto (July 1993) Tutela igienico sanitaria della popolazione dalla esposizione a radiazioni non ionizzanti generate da impianti per teleradiocomunicazioni. Legge Regionale 9, N. 29. Bollettino Ufficiale della Regione Lazio, N. 58, p 6730–6737. Direzione Redazione e Amministraz. Presso la Presidenza della Giunta Regionale, Via Cristoforo Colombo, 212, 00147 Roma, Italia. IT 5 – Regional Law of Toscana (July 1989) Raccomandazioni sui Limiti di Esposizione ai Campi Elettromagnetici non Ionizante, Giunta Regionale, Commissione Regionale per la Prevenzione dei Rischi da espozione a campi elettromagnetici non ionizzante, Toscana, Italia.

EFTA	Law/Directive
Liechtenstein	LIL – Liechtensteinisches Landesgesetzblatt Nr. 25 (July 1970) Verordnung III zum Gesetz über die Arbeit in Industrie, Gewerbe und Handel (Arbeitsgesetz), Gesundheitsvorsorge und Unfallverhütung in industriellen Betrieben, Art. 31, Art. 58, Art. 78, Fürstliche Regierung, Liechtenstein.
Norway	NOR 1 – The Norwegian act of worker protection and working environment. Chapter II, requirements concerning the working environment, § 8 letter d. Oslo, Norway.

EU	Regulation
Finland	FIN D – Ministry of Social Affairs and Health (Dec. 1991) Supervision of non-ionizing radiation decree (1513/91) Helsinki, Finland. FIN O – Ministry of Social Affairs and Health (Dec. 1991) Order on limits of exposure to non-ionizing radiation (1474/91). Helsinki, Finland. FIN C – Council of State (June 1985) Decision on high-frequency equipment and their inspection Helsinki, Finland.
Germany	BPT1 – Bundesministerium für Post und Telekommunikation (1992) Amtsblattverfügung Nr. 95, Gewährleistung des Schutzes von Personen in elektromagnetischen Feldern, die von festen Funksendestellen ausgesendet werden. Bonn, Germany. BPT2 – Bundesministerium für Post und Telekommunikation: Amtsblattverfügung Nr. 77/1994: Änderungen und Ergänzungen zur Amtsblattverfügung Nr. 95/1992, Bonn, Germany.
Netherlands	NL – 1993: Arbo jaarboek 1993. Labour safety regulations. Staatstoezicht Volksgezondheid en Cultuur, Zoetermeer, Netherlands.
Sweden	AFS – National Institute of Occupational Safety and Health (June 1987) Högfrekventa elektromagnetiska fält. (Human exposure to electromagnetic fields in the frequency range 3 MHz to 300 GHz). Arbetarskyddsstyrelsens författningssamling, AFS 1987:2, Liber Distribution, S-162 89 Stockholm, Sweden. AFS MW – National Institute of Occupational Safety and Health (Oct. 1979) Mikrovagsugnar (Microwave ovens). Arbetarskyddsstyrelsens författningssamling, AFS 1979:6, Liber Distribution, S-162 89 Stockholm, Sweden.

EU	Standard
Austria	ON – ÖNORM S1120 (July 1992) Microwave and Radiofrequency electromagnetic fields – Permissible limits of exposure for the protection of persons in the frequency range 30 kHz to 3000 GHz, measurements. Österreichisches Normungsinstitut, Heinestr. 38, A-1021 Wien, Austria.
	ÖVE MW – ÖVE-HG 335, Teil 2 [2500] (1985) Sicherheitsanforderungen für Elektrogeräte für den Hausgebrauch und ähnliche Zwecke. Mikrowellenkochgerä te. Österreichischer Verband für Elektrotechnik, Eschenbachgasse 9, A-1010 Wien, Austria.
Germany	VDE – DIN 57 848 VDE 0848 Part 2 (July 1984) Hazards by electromagnetic fields. Protection of persons in the frequency range from 10 kHz to 3000 GHz. VDE-Verlag, Bismarckstr. 33, 10 625 Berlin, Germany.
	VDE MW – DIN VDE 0700 Part 25 (July 1985) Appliances for heating food by means of microwave energy. VDE-Verlag, Bismarckstr. 33, 10 625 Berlin, Germany.
	VDE CP – DIN-VDE 0750 Part 9 (August 1992) Safety of implantable cardiac pacemacers; German Version EN 50061:1988. VDE-Verlag, Bismarckstr. 33, 10 625 Berlin, Germany.
	VDE Draft – DIN-VDE 0848 Part 2 [Draft] (Oct. 1991) Safety in electromagnetic fields; Protection of persons in the frequency range from 30 kHz to 300 GHz. VDE-Verlag, Bismarckstr. 33, 10 625 Berlin, Germany.
	VDE M Draft – DIN-VDE 0848 Part 1 [Draft] (Oct. 1991) Safety in electrical, magnetic and electromagnetic fields; Methods for measurement and calculation. VDE-Verlag, Bismarckstr. 33, 10 625 Berlin, Germany.
Italy	IT Draft – Italian Standard (1982) Protezione dei lavoratori e della populazione dall'esposizione a campi elettromagnetici e a radiofrequenze a microonde. Ministero della Sanità, Italy.
United Kingdom	BSI MW – British Standards Institute BS 3456 Part 102 (1988) Specification for safety of commercial electrical appliances using microwave energy for heating footstuffs. BSI, London, UK.
	NRPB – British National Radiological Protection Board NRPB-Volume 4 NO 5 (1993) Documents of the NRPB, Board Statement on Restrictions on Human Exposure to Static and Time Varying Electromagnetic Fields and Radiation. NRPB, Chilton, Didcot, Oxon OX11 ORQ, UK.

EU	Other Document
Belgium	Belgacom – Belgacom (July 1993) Copie Service Central de Sécurité-Hygiène. Protection du personnel contre les rayonnements électromagnetiques non ionisants. Belgacom, Départment de la Transmission, 1210 Bruxelles, Rue des Palais 42, Belgium. Sante – Santé et Travail; Dr. D. Slaets (August 1993) GSM and microwaves – biological effects of microwaves. Statement of Santé et Travail.
Denmark	DMW – Demko: Specification for safety of household- and similar electrical appliances, dealing with microwaves. Denmark.
Finland	FIN SG 9 – Finnish Centre for Radiation and Nuclear Safety (Dec. 1991) Radiation safety of pulsed radars. ST-guide. STUK, P.O.Box 268, SF-00101 Helsinki, Finland. FIN SG 9.3 – Finnish Centre for Radiation and Nuclear Safety (April 1992) Radiation safety on mastworks at FM/TV stations. ST-guide. STUK, P.O.Box 268, SF-00101 Helsinki, Finland.
Germany	BFE – Berufsgenossenschaft der Feinmechanik und Elektrotechnik (Oct. 1982) Sicherheitsregeln für Arbeitsplätze mit Gefährdung durch elektromagnetische Felder. Merkblatt für die Unfallverhütung. Berufsgenossenschaft der Feinmechanik und Elektrotechnik, Gustav-Heinemann-Ufer 130, D-5000 Köln 51, Germany. BFS – Bundesamt für Strahlenschutz (Dec. 1991) Schutz vor elektromagnetischer Strahlung beim Mobilfunk. Empfehlung der Strahlenschutzkomission. Bundesamt für Strahlenschutz, Geschäftsstelle der Strahlenschutzkomission. Germany.
Netherlands	NEL3 – Publication, 90-01: Richtlijnen voor radiofrequente straling bij zendinrichtingen, Netherlands.
Sweden	SWE – National Institute of Radiation Pretection (1978) Guideline on exposure of the general population to EM fields. National Institute of Radiation Pretection, Box 60204, 104 01 Stockholm, Sweden.
EFTA	
Norway	NOR 2 – National Institute of Radiation Hygiene (Feb. 1982) Adiministrative normer for radiofrekvent straling for yrkeseksponerte? National Institute of Radiation Hygiene, Osterndalen 25, 1345 Osteras, Norway.
Worldwide	Recommendation
WHO	IRPA (WHO) – International Non-Ionizing Radiation Committee/ International Radiation Protection Association (1988) Guidelines on limits of exposure to radiofrequency electromagnetic fields in the frequency range from 100 kHz to 300 GHz. Health Physics, Vol. 54, No. 1, p. 115–123.
WHO	IRPA T (WHO), Draft – International Commission for Non-Ionizing Radiation Protection/Draft (April 1992) Protection against electromagnetic radiation from mobile telephones. Statement of the International Commission for Non-Ionizing Radiation Protection.

12

Regulatory activities in the Asia-Pacific area

Masao Taki and Michael H. Repacholi

12.1 INTRODUCTION

Wireless communications are rapidly penetrating into the Asia-Pacific area as well as other areas in the world. In most countries in Asia the positive aspects of wireless communications have far outweighed any negative impacts such as concern about the health consequences of exposure to electromagnetic fields radiated by wireless communication systems. As such there has been little pressure on governments to intentionally control human exposure to electromagnetic waves.

Among the countries in Asia-Pacific area, Japan, Australia and New Zealand are the countries where regulatory activities to limit human exposure to electromagnetic fields have been taken. In this chapter, we describe the regulatory activities ongoing in these three countries, as well as a brief overview of the recent deployment of wireless communication systems in the Asia-Pacific area.

12.2 WIRELESS COMMUNICATIONS IN THE ASIA-PACIFIC AREA

The rapid increase in the number of subscribers of cellular telephones in the Asia-Pacific area has been remarkable. The growth of subscribers in the ten countries having the largest numbers of subscribers of cellular telephones at the end of 1995 are shown in Fig. 12.1. Japan, China and Australia have the second, the sixth and the seventh largest numbers respectively. Subscriber growths have also been very large in China and South Korea. This figure shows that the Asia-Pacific area is now a very important region in the world with regard to the use of cellular telephones.

Mobile Communications Safety
Edited by N. Kuster, Q. Balzano and J.C. Lin
Published in 1997 by Chapman & Hall, London. ISBN 0 412 75000 7.

In some countries in this area the demand for the development of private communications drives the growth. Some other Asia-Pacific nations are still developing the infrastructure for their communication networks. Wireless technologies are expected to provide a rapid means of establishing basic telephone services for their enormous populations, and hence the explosive growth in these communication systems.

In some countries devices with higher output power are sometimes preferred because larger areas can be covered with a smaller number of base stations. Thus devices with output powers of 3–8 W are sometimes used as well as devices with the same specification as the United States or Europe.

The cellular telephone systems established in this region mostly follow the specification of analog systems in the United States or Europe such as AMPS, TACS and NMT. Recently the digital systems of GSM and NADC have been introduced. The indifference to the possible safety problem of electromagnetic exposure in most countries in this area could partly be attributed to the fact that the technology of cellular telephones was not developed within the countries themselves but imported from the United States or Europe and its benefits far outweigh the safety concerns of the public.

Japan, with the second largest number of subscribers in the world, has unique specifications based on its own standards. NTT (Hi and Lo cap) system is an analog system of Japanese standard. PDC is the Japanese digital system similar to NADC or IS-54 TDMA system (Padgett *et al.*, 1995). The JTACS and NTACS systems, based on European TACS, are also used in a limited portion of the analog cellular systems in Japan.

12.3   REGULATORY ACTIVITY IN JAPAN

12.3.1   Role of government agencies

Various government agencies are involved with the human safety with respect to exposure to electromagnetic fields in Japan. The Ministry of Posts and Telecommunications (MPT) is responsible for the use of electromagnetic waves below 3 THz, using its responsibility under the Radio Law. The MPT issued a protection guideline for human exposure to electromagnetic waves in 1990 (TTC/MPT, 1990; Amemiya, 1994). The details of the activities of the MPT and of the guideline will be described in the following subsection.

The Agency of Natural Resources and Energy (ANRE) in the Ministry of International Trade and Industry (MITI) is responsible for the safety of electrical appliances under the Electrical Appliance and Material Control Law. Electrical appliances defined in this law must comply with the mandatory standards in the Ministerial Ordinance of Standards for Electrical Appliance, enacted in 1962. This includes the regulation of radiation from microwave ovens. The maximum

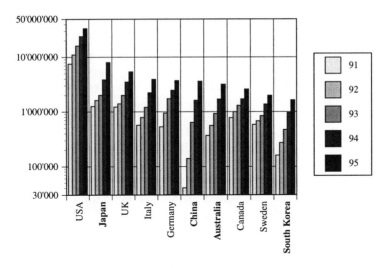

Fig. 12.1 Subscribers of cellular telephones from the end of 1991 to 1995.

permissible value of leakage radiation from microwave ovens is $1\,mW/cm^2$ at 5 cm distance during operation and $5\,mW/cm^2$ after an open and shut test of 100 000 times. There are other requirements on the radiation from electrical appliances in this standard, which are not concerned with human health, but regulates unintentional radiation to avoid electromagnetic interference.

The ANRE is also responsible for the safety of electric power facilities. Regulation of electric field strength at the edge of the 'right of way (ROW)' below $3\,kV/m$ was enacted in 1976 by the Ministerial Ordinance of Standards for Electrical Equipments (Matsumoto *et al.*, 1994). However no guideline of power frequency magnetic fields has been produced by the ANRE.

The Environment Agency (EA) was established in 1971 to have jurisdiction over the protection of the natural environment from the impact by physical or chemical agents. The concerns of the EA have been oriented to the protection of natural environment and public health from pollution and public nuisance. Electromagnetic fields is one of the environmental issues within the scope of its jurisdiction, but no regulatory activity has been taken with regard to the control of this energy for a long time. The EA came to be concerned about the health effect of environmental electromagnetic fields, especially of electric power lines, and established an investigative committee on the biological effects of electromagnetic fields in 1990. This resulted in an interim report being issued in 1992 (Japan Environment Assoc., 1992). The deliberations were suspended but resumed in 1994 with the release of the epidemiological studies on ELF from the Scandinavian countries. The activity of the EA on this problem has been limited and they have only organized investigative committees.

The Ministry of Health and Welfare (MHW) is responsible for the safety of medical appliances. Human safety of therapeutic and diagnostic applications of electromagnetic energy is within the scope of its responsibility. The electromagnetic interference by wireless communication devices with medical devices including cardiac pacemakers is an important problem related to its responsibility. This problem is very complex due to its interministerial nature.

12.3.2   Regulatory activity by the MPT

Japan had long been largely unconcerned about the health problem of electromagnetic field exposures. The general public had not expressed much concern about reported health effects from environmental electromagnetic fields. Occupational exposures were implicitly controlled within the framework of general occupational safety. Anecdotal health effects of electromagnetic field exposure were sometimes reported but greater concerns were oriented to the evident problems such as water or air pollution.

In 1988 the situation changed. An interpellation was presented in the Diet (Japanese parliament) that the MPT (whose jurisdiction covers any application of radio waves) should also be controlling excessive human exposures to electromagnetic waves. With this interpellation as an opportunity, the Minister of Posts and Telecommunications requested that the Telecommunication Technology Council (TTC) report on protection guideline for human exposure to electromagnetic waves. The report was submitted in 1990 and contained RF protection guidelines (TTC/MPT Guideline) and recommended procedures for measurement. The major part of this guideline was adopted as RCR (Research and Development Center for Radio Systems) standard for radio frequency exposure protection (RCR STD-38) in 1993. This is a voluntary standard for manufacturers and operators associated with RCR. RCR is a private standard-setting organization closely cooperating with the MPT. This guideline was also adopted by the Japanese Society of Hyperthermic Oncology for protection of personnel from occupational exposure during hyperthermic treatment in 1993 (QAC/JSHO, 1993).

12.3.3   TTC/MPT guideline

The TTC/MPT guideline has similarities to both ANSI/IEEE C95.1-1992 standard and INIRC/IRPA guideline (IRPA, 1988). The guideline is constituted of the 'fundamental guide' and the 'administrative guide'. The fundamental guide provides the basis for the guideline in terms of the quantities closely related to biological phenomena such as SAR and induced current. The SAR limits in the fundamental guide are 0.4 W/kg averaged over any 6 minutes with regard to the whole-body averaged SAR and 8 W/kg with regard to the maximum local SAR within 1 g tissue except extremities and skin, where the SAR limit is 25 W/kg for any 1 g tissue. The limit values in the fundamental guide are comparable with those in other major guidelines. The administrative guide is a practical guideline which provides means to control the electromagnetic environment. It is therefore presented in terms of directly measurable quantities such as electric and magnetic field strengths.

The administrative guide has a two-tier structure consisting of 'condition P' and 'condition G'. Condition P corresponds to the controlled environment and condition G to the uncontrolled environment in the ANSI/IEEE standard, respectively. On the other hand the fundamental guide makes no difference between these two categories. The difference in the exposure limits between the condition P and G in the administrative guide is not derived from the difference in physical tolerance but from the difference in the uncertainty of exposure conditions and in the reliability of the measurements and control of the electromagnetic fields.

Basically there are no substantial differences in the exposure limit values in the administrative guide of the TTC/MPT guideline from the ANSI/IEEE C95.1-1992 standard and the INIRC/IRPA guideline. The main difference exists, however, in the exclusion clause for low power devices among these three guidelines. This is important for wireless communication systems. The TTC/MPT guideline excludes, in its auxiliary guide in the administrative guide, low power devices with RF nominal output power 7 W or less operating at frequencies lower than or equal to 3 GHz for both condition P and G.

The nominal output power of low power radiation devices is well-defined in the specification of the devices, and the exposure conditions during its ordinary use are usually well specified. So the exclusion clause makes no difference in the safety factors between condition P and G in contrast with the exposure limits for electric and magnetic field strengths in the administrative guide.

The exclusion clause is based on the maximum local SAR criterion in the fundamental guide. To ensure the consistency of this clause with the fundamental guide, calculated SARs in a spherical head model irradiated by electromagnetic fields from a $\frac{1}{2}$ wavelength dipole antenna were examined. It should be noted that the distance between the head and the antenna was assumed 7 cm as a typical distance.

The INIRC/IRPA guideline also excludes those with 7 W or less without limitation of frequency for both occupational and general public, although it is noted that the International Commission on Non-Ionizing Radiation Protection (ICNIRP) has rectified this situation in its statement (ICNIRP, 1996). The ANSI/IEEE standard, being more recent, has now addressed this issue. The exclusion clause has two-tier structure with a larger safety factor for the uncontrolled environment. At 1.5 GHz, for example, the maximum radiated power of the low power devices to be excluded is 420 mW that is only 6% of the 7 W exclusionary clause level of the TTC/MPT guideline.

12.3.4   Current state and future actions

In 1993 a digital cellular system operating at 800 MHz (PDC-800) started service in Japan, followed by 1.5 GHz system (PDC-1500) in 1994. Telephones were only for rent in the cellular systems, but this was deregulated in 1994. These events stimulated the explosive growth in the cellular telephone industry in Japan. The Personal Handyphone System (PHS) (Padgett *et al.*, 1995), which is a low power personal communication system like CT2 and DECT, started in July 1995. This has further accelerate the penetration of personal wireless communications. Numbers of subscribers of PHS was 2.42 millions and that of cellular telephones was 11.75 millions at the end of May 1996.

Under these circumstances the construction of new base stations for wireless communication systems has become a burden for the operators because the residents near the site are becoming concerned about possible health effect of chronic exposure to electromagnetic waves. In some cases construction of antennas for base station have been withdrawn because of opposition by nearby residents.

The Product Liability Law was enacted in 1994 in Japan. This will enhance the interest of general public in the safety of industrial products including wireless communication devices. It should be noted that the majority of Japanese people welcome the progress in private communication systems and have little fear of health effects.

It is five years since the TTC/MPT guideline was issued. The ANSI standard in the United States has been revised during this period. The dosimetry of exposure, especially for portable radios, has made progress. The TTC/MPT guideline should be reviewed now whether it is consistent with the latest knowledge about health effect of electromagnetic waves.

In order to investigate the current state of human protection from electromagnetic wave exposure, an investigative committee was established by the MPT in September 1995. The scope of deliberation covered various aspects of the protection guideline. It investigated whether the TTC/MPT guideline was necessary to be revised. The necessity of two-tier structure and validity of the exclusion of low power devices were discussed. It has been pointed out that the typical distance of 7 cm assumed in the rationale for the exclusion clause is often much larger than the distance in the ordinary use of recent wireless devices.

As a result of deliberation the committee recommended that the auxiliary guide for low power devices should be rewritten to be definite about the restriction, especially for the general public. It also recommended coordination with the international guidelines such as that of ICNIRP. In addition it recommended promotion of researches on biological effects of electromagnetic waves to accumulate a scientific data base in our own country.

In addition to the direct electromagnetic interaction with tissue, attention has been growing on the indirect health effects through interference with medical devices and implants, especially with cardiac pacemakers. Although the importance of this problem has been well recognized by various government organizations involved in this problem, no regulatory activity has been taken. Voluntary activities by manufacturers and medical personnel to prevent hazardous interference has been encouraged. The use of wireless communication devices is prohibited in some hospitals to avoid electromagnetic interference with medical devices and implants.

Recently, the Electromagnetic Compatibility (EMC) Conference in Japan has started deliberation on this matter. The EMC Conference is an organization established in 1987 to deal with problems of electromagnetic compatibility. It is chaired by the Director of the Telecommunications Bureau of the MPT and the government organizations involved in EMC problems, i.e. the MPT, MITI, MHW, EA, the Ministry of Labor, the Ministry of Transport and the National Police Agency, participate in this conference as well as industrial associations and scientists from universities.

An interim guideline has been issued in March 1996 which recommends control of the use of cellular telephones in hospitals. It also recommends a distance of at least 22 cm between a cellular telephone device and a cardiac pacemaker when a patient implanted with a cardiac pacemaker uses a cellular telephone. This guideline is voluntary and interim one at present. Further deliberation continues.

12.4   REGULATORY ACTIVITY IN AUSTRALIA AND NEW ZEALAND

In Australia and New Zealand the responsibility for developing standards for the exposure to electromagnetic fields has been taken by the voluntary standards setting agencies: Standards Association of Australia and Standards New Zealand. Australia first developed a standard for limiting exposure to RF fields in 1985. This standard was reaffirmed in Australia in 1990 and adopted by New Zealand in the same year. At present a revision of the 1990 standard is being prepared and has almost been completed by the Joint Australia/New Zealand (A/NZ) Standards Committee TE/7 on Human Exposure to Electromagnetic Fields. Once completed it will supersede the previous Australian standard AS 2772.1-1990 and New Zealand standard NZS 6609.1:1990 Radiofrequency radiation Part 1: Maximum exposure levels – 100 kHz to 300 GHz and their Amendment 1 – 1994.

The A/NZ standard is based on the IRPA Guidelines (IRPA, 1988) and subsequent draft amendments. The standard provides limits of exposure to radiofrequency fields in the frequency range from 3 kHz to 300 GHz.

The purpose of the A/NZ Standard is to provide guidance on human exposure to radiofrequency (RF) fields and to set limits intended to avoid any adverse effects on health. It applies to the exposure of workers due to their employment and the incidental exposure of the general public, but it does not apply to patients undergoing medical diagnosis or treatment. This Standard does not address the problem of electromagnetic interference (EMI) with electromedical and other equipment.

The standard has been developed following a review of the relevant scientific literature and is in accordance with the recommendations of the World Health Organization (WHO), the International Commission on Non-Ionizing Radiation Protection (ICNIRP), the International Radiation Protection Association (IRPA) and other major national standards. The limits of exposure to RF fields in this standard for both the general public and workers are the same as the international guidelines on exposure limits to RF fields published by the IRPA, ICNIRP and all major RF standards. Alignment with international standards is also in accord with Australia's and New Zealand's obligations under the World Trade Organization's Technical Barriers to Trade Agreement.

While the committee responsible for this standard considered both thermal and non-thermal effects of RF exposure, it found, as has been found by all major international and national review committees developing standards in all Western countries, that when established peer-reviewed scientific literature is used, exposure limits can only be based on thermal effects at frequencies above about 10 MHz. All reviews of the scientific literature show that, while non-thermal exposure may cause transient perturbations in some tissue and isolated cells, no adverse health impact has been found from exposure at these levels below the limits of the standard after almost 40 years of research. Below about 10 MHz currents induced in the body by RF fields become more important than tissue heating as the basis for setting exposure safety levels.

In setting limits, the lowest RF exposure level that caused adverse biological effect that could be confirmed by independent laboratory studies was used as the threshold. For exposures in the frequency range above about 10 MHz this threshold was found to be an absorption of RF power in the body equivalent to 4 W/kg. An example of the biological effects detected at this level is a reduced endurance to perform tasks in experimental animals when their core temperature was raised by the RF exposure by at least 1 °C. If the rectal temperature was raised less than 1 °C, no detectable effect was found on performance.

To derive the exposure limits from this threshold RF level, a safety factor of 10 was incorporated so that workers would not be exposed to more than 1/10th of the threshold level (i.e. 0.4 W/kg). For the general public an additional safety factor of 5 was incorporated into their exposure limits, since the public cannot be expected to take any precautions to avoid exposure. Thus the exposure limits for the general public are set at 1/50th of the threshold level (i.e. 0.08 W/kg).

There is no evidence of any harmful effects in people exposed to the threshold value of 4 W/kg. While workers cannot be exposed to levels more than 1/10th of this threshold and the general public to more than 1/50th, research continues to provide new information about the effects of RF exposure. The purpose of the

Table 12.1 Maximum exposure levels – aware users

Operating frequency MHz			Mean output power (nominal) W
0.100	–	450	7
450	–	1500	$7 \times 450/f$
1500	–	2500	2.1

Table 12.2 Maximum exposure levels – general users

Operating frequency MHz			Mean output power (nominal) W
0.100	–	450	1.4
450	–	1500	$1.4 \times 450/f$
1500	–	2500	0.42

NOTE: Nominal power refers to the specific power prior to the allowed tolerance. In the case of cellular mobile telephones, the allowed tolerance is up to 2 dB (Austel Technical Standards TS005 and TS018). For allowed tolerances up to 3 dB, the 'deemed to comply' provisions will not result in local SAR values exceeding the basic SAR limit of 1.6 W/kg.

safety factors is to make allowance for the limitations of the scientific data base and for any new results which may show harmful effects below the threshold exposure level. However there is some reassurance from the fact that the current set of exposure limits have remained constant for over 12 years. The exposure limits in the standard are considered to provide large safety factors, however good practice suggests unnecessary exposure should be avoided at levels close to the limits.

An amendment to the Australian/New Zealand Standard was made in 1994 to remove the 7 W exclusion clause (SA/SNZ, 1994) The 7 W exclusion clause was replaced by a 'deemed to comply' provision for aware users (occupational exposure) as shown in Table 12.1. These provisions are based on limiting the spatial peak SAR averaged over 1 g of tissue to a value not exceeding 8 W/kg. There is a separate 'deemed to comply' provision for the general users (public) as shown in Table 12.2. These provisions are based on limiting the spatial peak SAR averaged over 1 g of tissue to a value not exceeding 1.6 W/kg.

The Australian/New Zealand standard is normally reviewed every five years, but if any research results suggest that there should be changes to this standard, they will be considered promptly.

12.5   CONCLUDING COMMENTS

The current state of wireless communications in the Asia-Pacific area has been briefly reviewed and the regulatory activities in Japan, Australia and New Zealand have been described. The only countries cooperating on standards development are Australia and New Zealand. Unfortunately, there are no other cooperative activities in this area to develop common wireless communication systems or common regulation on human protection.

Most countries in Asia are not seriously concerned about the possible health risk of exposure to electromagnetic waves. As no definitive evidence of adverse health effects by current wireless communication systems has been presented, this lack of concern will continue. However, in some countries, particularly Australia and New Zealand, and to some extent Japan, residents near base station sites for mobile telephone systems are concerned about the unclear health hazard of long-term low-level exposure. These community fears may spread over the countries where there are no serious concerns about safety of wireless communications at present. The countries where wireless communication technology has been developed should not export the ungrounded fear of health effect together with the industrial products and technology. For this reason it is necessary to accumulate plain, enlightening evidences of the safety of electromagnetic exposures by wireless communication systems.

REFERENCES

Amemiya, Y. (1994) Researches on biological and electromagnetic environment in RF and microwave regions in Japan. *IEICE Trans.*, **E77-B**, 693–698.

ICNIRP (1996) International Commission on Non-Ionizing Radiation Protection. Health issues related to the use of handheld radiotelephones and base transmitters: A statement from ICNIRP. *Health Physics, 70*, 587–593.

IRPA (1988) International Radiation Protection Association. Guidelines on limits of exposure to radiofrequency electromagnetic fields in the frequency range from 100 MHz to 300 GHz, *Health Physics, 54*, 115–123.

Matsumoto, G. and Shimizu, K. (1994) Biological effects of ELF electric fields – Historical review on bioengineering studies in Japan. *IEICE Trans.*, **E77-B**, 684–692.

Padgett, J.E., Günther, C.G. and Hattori, T. (1995) Overview of wireless personal communications. *IEEE Communications Magazine*, January, 28–41.

TTC/MPT (1990) Protection guidelines for human exposure to radiofrequency electromagnetic waves. *A report of Telecommunications Technology Council for the Ministry of Posts and Telecommunications, Deliberation No.38.*

QAC/JSHO (1993) Quality Assurance Committee of Japanese Society of Hyperthermic Oncology. Guide for the protection of occupationally exposed personnel in hyperthermia treatment from the potential hazards to health. *Int. J. Hyperthermia,* 8, 613–624.

SA/SNZ (1994) Radiofrequency Radiation Part 1: Maximum exposure levels – 100 kHz to 300 GHz. Standards Australia/Standards New Zealand, AS 2772.1/NZS 6609.1/Amdt 1/1994-05-16. (Available from Standards New Zealand, Standards House, 155 The Terrace, Private Mail Bag 2439, Wellington, New Zealand.)

PART V

Final Considerations

13

Criteria for the assessment of the EMF literature

Michael H. Repacholi and Masao Taki

13.1 INTRODUCTION

In a field where a large number of biological effects have been reported and not replicated, it is extremely important that studies reporting effects that could impact on human health, meet certain criteria before they are be added to the database of established effects. This paper provides some of the essential criteria necessary for the development of such a scientific database which can be used to derive health risk assessments.

When conducting a review of scientific research one has to consider the types of experiments being conducted, and their purpose. *In vitro* experiments provide different information to studies conducted on whole animals or indeed epidemiological investigations of human populations. Further, one cannot accept research results and authors' conclusions as valid without assessing how they compare with the results of other researchers. The process for addressing these issues is given below.

13.2 TYPES OF BIOLOGICAL RESEARCH

Biological research is divided into three major categories:

(i) *In vitro* studies conducted on isolated components of biological systems such as solutions of molecules (e.g. DNA), cultures of cells, or pieces of tissue. These studies are important for determining possible mechanisms by which RF fields interact with biological systems and for identifying appropriate end-points and exposure conditions to be tested in whole animals. Determining mechanisms of interaction is important to give an understanding of how RF fields act at the molecular or cellular level, and

Mobile Communications Safety
Edited by N. Kuster, Q. Balzano and J.C. Lin
Published in 1997 by Chapman & Hall, London. ISBN 0 412 75000 7.

thus allow an extrapolation to the whole animal level. Studying simple systems allows interactions to be detected that may be masked in the complexity of interactions that occur normally at the whole animal level. It is because of this that biological effects found to occur at the molecular or cellular level cannot be assumed to occur at the whole animal level. Thus biological end-points found *in vitro* must still be tested *in vivo*.

(ii) *In vivo* studies are conducted on complete biological systems such as laboratory animals. The great advantage of these studies is that they are conducted under carefully controlled laboratory conditions where all environmental and exposure parameters are kept constant. The only difference between exposed and unexposed animals should be the actual exposure to RF fields they receive. Since experiments cannot normally be conducted on humans, animal studies are very useful for making health risk assessments related to human exposure. However, when evaluating animal studies, it is important to remember that the results of these studies are only applicable to humans if the effects observed occur in a number of different animal models. This is necessary because one particular animal model may be extremely sensitive to a particular end-point and have characteristics that are not observed in humans.

(iii) Human studies can be conducted on volunteers in the laboratory or on different populations of people in the living and working environment. Laboratory studies are conducted with the approval of the volunteer and usually a human experimentation ethics committee, and have the advantage of allowing exposures under strictly controlled conditions (as with animal studies). However the end-points that can be studied are limited. End-points such as cancer and mortality can be researched on cancer patients but obviously cannot be studied on laboratory volunteers.

Studies on populations are called epidemiological studies and have the advantage of being non-intrusive. They compare the differences in the incidence of, or mortality from, some predetermined disease or diseases in the populations. Generally one group is exposed to RF fields and is compared with a group not exposed or at least having a much lower exposure to RF fields. The major difficulty is to obtain two identical groups in sufficient numbers where the only difference is their exposure. This can become a significant problem when studying rare diseases such as cancer (Taub, 1995). However, these studies can indicate differences in the incidence of disease, especially when the presumed causal factor has a large effect as identified by large risk ratios. When the risk ratios are small, there can be some difficulty in attributing this difference to the RF exposure and not some other factor in the living or working environment that is not detected as a difference between the two groups (e.g. chemical exposure in the workplace).

13.3   CRITERIA FOR ASSESSMENT OF RESEARCH RESULTS

When reviewing the scientific literature, certain criteria must be met if claims of a positive or negative effect are to be accepted into the database as established. This is extremely important when conducting health risk assessments for the development of standards (Repacholi *et al.*, 1991; WHO, 1993). These criteria include:

1. Experimental techniques, methods and conclusions should be as completely objective as possible, using biological systems appropriate to the end-points studied. To safeguard against bias, researchers should use double-blind techniques. Appropriate controls must be used for valid comparison of results. The sensitivity of the experiment must be such that there is a reasonable probability that an effect could be detected if it exists.

2. All data analyses should be fully and completely objective, no relevant data should be deleted from consideration and uniform analytical methods used. Data from experiments within the same protocol should be internally consistent.

3. The published descriptions of the methods should be given in sufficient detail that a critical reader would be convinced that all reasonable precautions have been taken to meet requirements 1 and 2.

4. Results should demonstrate an effect of the relevant variable at a high level of statistical significance using appropriate tests. The effects of interest should ordinarily be shown by a majority of test organisms and the responses found should be consistent.

5. Results should be quantifiable and susceptible to confirmation by independent researchers. Preferably the experiments should be repeated and the results confirmed independently; or the claimed effects should be consistent with results of similar experiments, where the biological systems are comparable.

6. Results should be viewed with respect to previously accepted scientific principles before ascribing them new ones.

While it will not be possible for all the above criteria to be applied to all experiments, these criteria provide a guide when determining what effects are established and can be used in a health risk assessment, and those that merely raise a hypothesis that needs to be tested, or those results which should be considered as preliminary and needing confirmation. Information from the various types of laboratory and human studies, including the limitations in the amount of information they can provide, is also taken into account when conducting health risk assessments.

REFERENCES

Repacholi, M.H. and Stolwijk, J.A.J. (1991) Criteria for evaluating scientific literature and developing exposure limits. *Radiation Protection in Australia*, **9**(3), 79–84.

Taub, G. (1995) Epidemiology faces its limits. *Science*, **269**, 164–169.

WHO (1993) Electromagnetic Fields 300 Hz – 300 GHz. *Environmental Health Criteria No. 137, World Health Organisation, Geneva.*

Acronyms

AAMI	Association for the Advancement of Medical Instrumentation
AC	Alternating current
ADPCM	Adaptive differential pulse code modulation
ALL	Acute lymphoblastic leukemia
AM	Amplitude modulation
AMPS	Advanced Mobile Phone Service
ANRE	Agency of Natural Resources and Energy
ANSI	American National Standards Institute
BBB	Blood-brain barrier
BP	3,4-benzpyrene
CENELEC	Comité Européen de Normalisation Electrotechnique
CDMA	Code division multiple access
CDPD	Cellullar Digital Packet Data (U.S.)
CDRH	Center for Devices and Radiological Health
cGMP	Cyclic-guanosine monophosphate
ChAT	Choline acetyltransferase
COST	Coopération Européenne dans le domaine de la recherche Scientifique et Technique (European cooperation in the field of scientific and technical research)
CMRS	Commercial Mobile Radio Service
CNS	Central nervous system
EA	Environment Agency
EBEA	European Bioelectromagnetics Association
ECG	Electrocardiogram
EEA	Electromagnetic Energy Association
EEG	Electroencephalography
ELF	Extremely low frequency
EMF	Electromagnetic fields
EMC	Electromagnetic compatibility
EMI	Electomagnetic interference
ENEA	Agency for New Technologies, Energy and Environment
ENU	N-Ethyl-N-Nitrosourea
EPA	Environmental Protection Agency
ERP	Effective radiated power
ETACS	Extended Total Access Telecommunication System

ETDMA	Enhanced TDMA (with DSI – digital speech interpolation)
ETSI	European Telecommunications Standards Institute
FACS	Fluorescence-activated cell sorter
FCC	Federal Communications Commission
FE	Finite-element
FDTD	Finite-difference time-domain
FDA	Food and Drug Administration
FDD	Frequency division duplex
FM	Frequency modulation
GABA	Gamma-aminobutyric acid
GAO	General Accounting Office
GMP	Guanosine mono-phosphate
GSM	Groupe Spéciale Mobile (originally) currently Global System for Mobile Communication (ETSI, Europe)
GTEM	Gigahertz transverse electromagnetic cell
GTP	Guanosine triphosphate
HPD	Haematoprophyrin derivative
IARC	International Agency for Research on Cancer
ICD	Implantable cardiac defibrillators
IEC	International Electrotechnical Commission
IEEE	Institute of Electrical and Electronics Engineers
ICINRP	International Commission on Non-Ionizing Radiation Protection
INIRC	International Non-Ionizing Radiation Commitee
IRIDIUM	Low Earth Orbit Satalite Cellular System (Motorola)
IRPA	International Radiation Protection Association
ISO	International Organisation for Standardization
JSHO	Japanese Society of Hyperthermal Oncology
JTACS	Japanese Total Access Telecommunication System
LPO	Lipid peroxidase
MCCC	Mobile Communications Coordination Commitee
MoM	Method of moment
MHW	Ministry of Health and Welfare
MITI	Ministry of International Trade and Industry
MPE	Maximum permissible exposure
MPT	Ministry of Posts and Telecommunications
MTE	Mobile telecommunications equipment
MRS	Magnetic resonance spectroscopy
NADC	North American Digital Cellular
NAMPS	Narrowband Advanced Mobile Phone Service
NCRP	National Council on Radiation Protection and Measurements
NEC	Numerical Electromagnetic Code
NEPA	National Environment Policy Act 1969
NIOSH	National Institute for Occupational Safety and Health
NMT	Nordic Mobile Telephone (Europe)

NO	Nitric oxide
NRPB	National Radiological Protection Board (GB)
NTACS	Narrowband Total Access Telecommunication System
NTIA	National Telecommunications and Information Administration
NTT	Nippon Telephone and Telegram
OATS	Open area test site
ODC	Ornithine decarboxylase
OSHA	Occupational Safety and Health Administration
OR	Odds ratio
PACS	Personal Access Communications Services
PCS	Personal Communications Radio Service
PDC	Personal Digital Cellular (Japan)
PHP	Personal Handy Phone (Japan)
PHS	Personal Handyphone System
PKC	Protein kinase C
PSCI	Posterior subcapsular iridescence
PTH	Parathyroid hormone
QAC	Quality Assurance Committee
QPSK	Quaternary phase shift keying
RCR	Research and Development Center for Radio Systems
RESNA	Rehabilitation Society of North America
RF	Radio frequency
RFI	Radio frequency interference
RNA	Ribonucleic acid (rRNA, mRNA)
RR	Risk ratio
SA/SNZ	Standards Australia/Standards New Zealand
SAR	Specific absorption rate
SBET	Society of Biomedical Equipment Technicians
SMR	Standard mortality rate
SMR	Specialized mobile radio
SPF	Specific pathogen free
TACS	Total Access Telecommunication System
TDD	Time division duplex
TEM Cell	Transverse electromagnetic cell
TDMA	Time division multiple access
TIA	Telecommunications Industry Association (U.S.)
TPA	Tetradecanoyl phorbol acetate (phorbol esters)
TTC	Telecommunication Technology Council
TWA	Time weighted average
VDE	Verband Deutscher Elektrotechniker (German Assosiation of Electrical Engineers)
VEP	Visual evoked potentia
UHF	Ultra high frequency
U.S.	United States

VHF	Very high frequency
WHO	World Health Organisation
WTR	Wireless Technology Research

Index